Adverse Cutaneous Drug Eruptions

Chemical Immunology and Allergy

Vol. 97

Adverse Cutaneous Drug Eruptions

Volume Editor

Lars E. French Zurich

43 figures, 30 in color, and 34 tables, 2012

KARGER

Basel · Freiburg · Paris · London · New York · New Delhi · Bangkok · Beijing · Tokyo · Kuala Lumpur · Singapore · Sydney

Chemical Immunology and Allergy
Formerly published as 'Progress in Allergy' (Founded 1939),
continued 1990–2002 as 'Chemical Immunology'
Edited by Paul Kallós 1939–1988, Byron H. Waksman 1962–2002

Prof. Dr. med. Lars E. French
Department of Dermatology
Zurich University Hospital
Gloriastr 31
CH–8091 Zurich (Switzerland)
E-Mail lars.french@usz.ch

Bibliographic Indices. This publication is listed in bibliographic services, including Current Contents® and PubMed/MEDLINE.

www.karger.com
Printed in Germany on acid-free and non-aging paper (ISO 9706) by Kraft Druck GmbH, Ettlingen
ISSN 1660–2242
e-ISSN 1662–2898
ISBN 978–3–8055–9970–2
e-ISBN 978–3–8055–9971–9

Contents

Preface

As a result of improved treatment outcomes, longer patient survival, extended treatment courses, and polymedication of an ageing population, patients are exposed to drugs more frequently and for longer time periods, increasing the risk of sensitization to medications. As a consequence, the frequency of adverse drug reactions is regularly increasing.

The skin is one of the most frequently involved organs in adverse drug reactions. Cutaneous adverse reactions to drugs are observed in 0.1–1% of patients during premarketing clinical trials, and postmarketing analyses suggest that their incidence can be as high as 1–8% for certain types of drugs (NSAIDS, antibiotics, antiepileptics), and among hospitalized patients the incidence of these reactions ranges from 1 to 3%.

The majority of adverse cutaneous drug eruptions are benign in nature, comprised largely by the maculopapular type of drug eruption and urticaria. Nonetheless, studies suggest that roughly a third of drug eruptions require hospital management and are considered as severe, although fortunately only 2% of cutaneous drug eruptions are really life-threatening.

As a consequence, it is estimated that between 5 and 9% of all hospital costs are related to adverse drug eruptions, and – cutaneous adverse drug eruptions representing 20–30% of all drug eruptions – the burden of these on the health care system is considerable.

Although the pathomechanism of the benign and severe forms of cutaneous drug eruptions remains incompletely understood, great progress in this field of medicine has been made in the past few years. Improvements range from the clinical classification that is essential for a better understanding to the identification of genetic susceptibilities to certain drugs, and consequently the development of the first preventive genetic screening measures for selected patient groups and drug classes.

In this book, a selected group of experts have provided an up-to-date, condensed and clinically relevant overview of the field of cutaneous drug eruptions ranging from the epidemiological basics and novel knowledge of genetic predisposition to the available therapeutic measures including rapid drug desensitization.

We hope to provide physicians, be it generalists or specialists, and non-physicians (nurses and scientists) with a useful tool for a better diagnosis, understanding and management of cutaneous drug eruptions in daily practice.

Lars E. French, Zurich

French LE (ed): Adverse Cutaneous Drug Eruptions.
Chem Immunol Allergy. Basel, Karger, 2012, vol 97, pp 1–17

Epidemiology of Cutaneous Adverse Drug Reactions

Maja Mockenhaupt

Dokumentationszentrum schwerer Hautreaktionen, Department of Dermatology,
University Freiburg – Medical Center, Freiburg, Germany

Abstract

Epidemiologic investigations of cutaneous adverse drug reactions (cADR) are important to evaluate their impact in dermatology and health care in general as well as their burden for affected patients. Few epidemiologic studies have been performed on frequent non-life-threatening cADR including reactions of both delayed and immediate hypersensitivity, such as maculopapular exanthema, fixed drug eruption and urticaria. Concerning rare but life-threatening severe cutaneous adverse reactions, e.g. toxic epidermal necrolysis (TEN), Stevens-Johnson syndrome (SJS), acute generalized exanthematous pustulosis and drug reaction with eosinophilia and systemic symptoms, several epidemiologic studies have been performed to date, some of which are still ongoing. Such studies enabled the calculation of reliable incidence rates and demographic data, but also allowed to perform risk estimation for drugs. The spectrum of drugs causing cADR differs substantially when separating the various clinical conditions. Whereas antibiotics are by far the most frequent inducers of milder cADR like maculopapular exanthema, they have a much lower risk to induce SJS/TEN, for which high-risk drugs are anti-infective sulfonamides, allopurinol, certain anti-epileptic drugs, nevirapine and nonsteroidal anti-inflammatory drugs (NSAIDS) of the oxicam type. In contrast, acute generalized exanthematous pustulosis is predominantly caused by the antibiotics pristinamycin and aminopenicillins, followed by quinolones, (hydroxy-)chloroquine and sulfonamides. Drug reaction with eosinophilia and systemic symptoms can be induced by a number of drugs known to cause SJS/TEN, such as certain antiepileptics and allopurinol, but also other medications (e.g. minocyclin).

Essentials in a Nutshell

- Epidemiologic studies on cutaneous adverse drug reactions (cADR) are important to evaluate their impact in dermatology and health care in general as well as their burden for affected patients
- For milder, non-life-threatening adverse drug reactions (ADR), only rough estimates of the incidence exist, whereas for severe cADR reliable incidence rates have been calculated

- Risk estimates for drugs causing cADR have been provided by case-control studies on rare severe reactions such as Stevens-Johnson syndrome (SJS)/toxic epidermal necrolysis (TEN) and acute generalized exanthematous pustulosis (AGEP), but not for milder cADR
- Antibiotics are the most frequent inducers of milder cADR like maculopapular exanthema (MPE), but they have a much lower risk to induce SJS/TEN, for which the high-risk drugs are anti-infective sulfonamides, allopurinol, certain anti-epileptic drugs, nevirapine and oxicam nonsteroidal anti-inflammatory drugs (NSAIDs)

Introduction

Based on the definition of the World Health Organization (WHO), an ADR is 'a response to a medicine which is noxious and unintended, and which occurs at doses normally used in man' [1]. The majority of ADR (up to 80%) are dose dependent and predictable, whereas the remaining 20% occur independent of the doses taken and are not predictable. The latter may be immunologically mediated reactions, which are often referred to as drug allergy and which either involve IgE or T cells. In contrast, nonimmunologically mediated reactions are also called 'idiosyncratic' [2]. Since a large proportion of ADR affects the skin, epidemiologic studies have been performed in relation to cutaneous manifestations. However, these studies often comprise various cutaneous ADR of different mechanism and clinical appearance. Except for anaphylaxis of different etiology, systematic large-scale epidemiologic studies have only been performed for severe cutaneous adverse reactions (SCAR) allowing to obtain reliable data on incidence and demography. In contrast, few studies on the epidemiology of milder cutaneous ADR have been undertaken and published.

Clinical Pattern of Cutaneous Adverse Drug Reactions

The majority of adverse drug reactions affecting the skin are non-serious and not life-threatening eruptions. However, many patients with such a reaction are admitted to the hospital since in the beginning a serious and life-threatening condition is suspected or cannot be excluded.

Non-Life-Threatening Cutaneous Adverse Drug Reactions

Milder cutaneous ADR include MPE, fixed drug eruption (FDE), morbilliform eruption, urticaria, purpura, vasculitis and many other clinical manifestations. All of these reactions, except perhaps FDE, are not exclusively caused by medications but can also be induced by various kinds if infections [3]. In some of them, infections even seem to be the more likely etiology, e.g. in urticaria or vasculitis, whereas others almost obligatorily occur when both certain infections and specific medications are present, e.g. EBV infection and aminopenicillins leading to MPE. The clinical pattern of these frequently occurring, less severe conditions are known by many physicians, but to confirm the clinical diagnosis the evaluation by a dermatologist and the result of a skin biopsy is needed. Whether drugs caused a specific reaction or not is sometimes difficult to determine, and a detailed medication history has to be obtained. Further allergologic workup may follow 2–4 months after the skin eruption has resolved.

Life-Threatening Cutaneous ADR

These conditions are also called SCAR. They include SJS and TEN, but also AGEP and drug reaction with eosinophilia and systemic symptoms (DRESS) [4]. The precondition for these studies and the analysis of data was a clinical consensus definition of skin reactions in the spectrum of SJS/TEN. In addition, well-defined diagnostic scores were elaborated for AGEP and DRESS.

Stevens-Johnson Syndrome/Toxic Epidermal Necrolysis

These reactions are characterized by erythematous skin and extensive detachment of epidermis and erosions of mucous membranes [4]. Nowadays, SJS and TEN are considered as a single disease entity of different severity but with common causes and mechanisms. The differentiation is made based on the extent of skin detachment. That is limited to less than 10% of the body surface area (BSA) in SJS, widespread with more than 30% of the BSA in TEN, and in-between defined as SJS/TEN overlap [4, 5]. The histopathology shows subepidermal blistering and necrotic keratinocytes either in wide dissemination or full-thickness necrosis of the epidermis, which is due to extensive apoptosis. Based on the almost identical histopathology of SJS/TEN and erythema (exsudativum) multiforme, SJS/TEN is often thought to be part of a broader EM spectrum [4]. For decades, EM with mucosal involvement (EM majus, EMM) was considered as SJS leading to false assessment of the etiology, which in EMM predominantly comprises infections and not medications [5]. However, a consensus definition allows differentiating SJS from EMM based on the clinical presentation [6, 7].

Acute Generalized Exanthematous Pustulosis

AGEP is characterized by the sudden occurrence of dozens of sterile, nonfollicular pinhead-sized pustules on edematous erythema predominantly in the main body folds. The reaction is frequently accompanied by fever and leukocytosis, especially neutrophilia. The pustules appear within only a few hours and resolve within a few days leaving a typical postpustular desquamation. Complications are rare and may occur in patients with an overall poor medical condition [8].

The histopathology reveals subcorneal and/or intraepidermal pustules, a sometimes pronounced edema in the papillary dermis and perivascular infiltrates consisting of neutrophils and some eosinophils [8]. The presence of pustules frequently leads to a misdiagnosis of an infectious condition and explains how an ADR may be overlooked.

Drug Reaction with Eosinophilia and Systemic Symptoms

For many years, the term drug hypersensitivity syndrome summarized numerous severe drug reactions [9]. More recently, a specific entity of drug hypersensitivity syndrome was separated from other ADR and re-named in Europe as DRESS, and in Japan as drug-induced hypersensitivity syndrome (DIHS) [10, 11]. DRESS/DIHS is characterized by a highly variable skin eruption, multi-organ involvement, lymphocyte activation (lymph node enlargement, lymphocytosis, atypical lymphocytes), eosinophilia, frequent virus reactivation [10, 11].

The main features such as skin eruption, fever, and organ involvement can also be attributed to a wide range of infections and to concomitant and underlying diseases. Therefore, each symptom has to be thoroughly investigated for its relation to the reaction. Not all symptoms or signs are always recognized in time, and asymptomatic features like eosinophilia and atypical lymphocytes may be overlooked. Furthermore, visible skin lesions and elevated specific laboratory values may occur at different times throughout the course of DRESS/DIHS [10, 11].

Epidemiologic Studies on Cutaneous Adverse Drug Reactions

Studies monitoring cutaneous ADR, e.g. the Boston Collaborative Drug Surveillance Programme, revealed important information on type of reaction and potentially inducing drugs, but were not designed to study the incidence and prevalence of the reactions, which could only be roughly estimated. More recently, two prospective studies have been undertaken to investigate the epidemiology of cutaneous ADR in a hospital setting. The first study from France analyzed cutaneous ADR due to systemic drugs in a specific hospital over a period of 6 months. All patients were examined and clinically diagnosed by a dermatologist, whereas medication intake was reviewed by a pharmacologist. Based on 48 inpatients with a diagnosis of cADR, the prevalence was calculated as 3.6 per 1,000 hospitalized patients [12]. The second study from Mexico was a prospective cohort study over 10 months and revealed a prevalence of 7 per 1,000 hospitalized patients with cADR (35/4,765 inpatients) [13]. A mandatory electronic reporting system for immunologically mediated drug reactions in South Korea identified 2,682 cases of ADR, both cutaneous and noncutaneous, among 55,432 admissions in a period of 7 months.

After review by allergologists, 532 were classified as 'significant drug hypersensitivity reactions', 100 of these were new events, of which 70% had cutaneous manifestations. The overall incidence of ADR was estimated as 1.8 per 1,000 hospital admissions [14].

Epidemiologic Studies on Severe Cutaneous Adverse Reaction

Several epidemiologic studies on SCAR were performed in Europe in the last 25 years. First, two hospital-based retrospective studies over a period of 5 years were undertaken in France and Germany in the 1980s [15, 16]. Second, a prospective population-based registry on severe skin reactions was initiated in Germany in 1990 with the aim to ascertain all hospitalized cases of SJS/TEN [17], and in parallel, an international case-control study on SCAR – the so-called SCAR study – was conducted in France, Germany, Italy, and Portugal between 1989 and 1995 [18, 19]. Later, from 1997 to 2001, the European ongoing case-control surveillance of SCAR – also referred to as EuroSCAR – was undertaken in Austria, France, Germany, Israel, Italy, and the Netherlands [20]. In addition to SJS/TEN, AGEP was investigated [21]. The European registry on SCAR to drugs and collection of biological samples – also called RegiSCAR – was established, which initially collected cases of SJS/TEN, AGEP and DRESS in the same six countries as the EuroSCAR study, but later expanded to Taiwan, UK, South Africa and Spain [22].

These epidemiologic studies first established clinical networks for active case ascertainment.

In the German Registry, a population-based approach was chosen with a network of approximately 1,700 hospitals including all departments of dermatology and pediatrics, all burn units, and all departments of internal medicine with intensive care facilities. Potential cases are reported by phone, fax or e-mail to the registry center. A physician checks the inclusion criteria and, in case they are met, arranges a visit in the reporting/treating hospital.

In order to achieve a high coverage rate, all departments receive quarterly letters addressed to a nominated contact person. Prepaid postcards asking whether cases of SCAR occurred in the past 3–4 months that have not yet been reported are added to these letters and should be returned. A high percentage of postcards are returned to the registry center, but departments that do not respond over a certain period of time receive a reminder phone call. Due to such active and systematic ascertainment, the registry is considered to be exhaustive for detection of SJS and TEN cases in Germany [17].

For the SCAR and EuroSCAR studies, cases from the German Registry were included, whereas specific networks were established in the other participating countries. These were not operating nationwide, but followed the same rules for case ascertainment. However, only prospectively ascertained and directly interviewed community cases of SJS/TEN (i.e. patients who developed the reaction in the community and were admitted because of SCAR) were included [18–21]. For the case-control analysis, 3 control patients were matched for age, gender, region and date of interview to each case patient. Controls were patients hospitalized for acute conditions including infections (e.g. pneumonia), trauma (e.g. fractures), and abdominal emergencies (e.g. appendicitis, ruptured ovarian cyst, strangulated hernia), which were not related to an underlying chronic disease. Not only cases but also controls were validated by checking for appropriateness of diagnosis and eligibility and inappropriate controls were excluded [18].

In the current RegiSCAR study, also cases occurring in the hospital (so-called in-hospital cases) are included. Besides SJS/TEN, AGEP and DRESS are included in the study. The networks of the German Registry and the EuroSCAR study are used for the RegiSCAR project. Within RegiSCAR, a cohort of patients is followed for long-term sequelae and quality of life after SCAR. Furthermore, blood samples are taken and stored centrally for pathophysiologic investigations [22].

All patients with SCAR included in these studies were/are interviewed by a trained health care professional investigator (physician, pharmacist, study nurse) using a standardized questionnaire. The interview includes questions regarding the current illness, demographic data, recent and past medical history, recent infections as well as detailed information on medication use. All collected cases are reviewed by a dermatologic expert committee with no information on exposures using clinical data, photographs and histopathology for clinical case validation. Cases are classified as definite, probable or possible severe skin reactions or are excluded based on the consensus definition [6, 7].

Incidence and Demographic Data

Stevens-Johnson Syndrome/Toxic Epidermal Necrolysis

Although data in the retrospective studies were not primarily collected for epidemiologic purposes, an incidence rate of 1.2 per one million inhabitants per year for TEN in France, and of 0.93 per one million per year in Germany could be estimated [15, 16]. Incidences between 1.4 and 6 per million person-years were reported for SJS and TEN in other countries. However, the huge variation among incidence rates may be caused by smaller reference populations, different diagnostic criteria and further methodological issues (e.g. the use of automated databases with variable coding to identify cases) [23].

Over the past 20 years, the prospective population-based registry in Germany has calculated an incidence of 1–2 cases of SJS/TEN per one million population per year (varying between 1.53 and 1.89) [17, 24].

SJS/TEN occur in different age groups. In the German Registry, the average age of patients with validated SJS/TEN was 53.4 years (1–94 years) for over 2,200 patients.

36% of SJS patients are ≤40 years of age, while 75% of the patients with SJS/TEN overlap and 72% of the patients with TEN are >40 years of age. In contrast, 83% of the patients with EMM are ≤40 years of age. More specifically, children and adolescents of ≤17 years account for 45% of EMM patients, whereas the percentage of this age group is only 13% in SJS. Less than 8% of EMM and SJS cases cannot clearly be distinguished, but these cases seem to follow the demographic characteristics of EMM. Men are more often affected with EMM (66%) and women with SJS/TEN (57–63%) [4].

Among patients with SJS/TEN in Europe, about 5% have been shown to be infected with HIV, with a lower percentage in recent years. Although the distribution of age and gender differs from that of non-HIV-infected patients, mortality rate and outcome are comparable [4, 25].

Mortality is high, with 9% in SJS, 29% in SJS/TEN overlap, 48% in TEN, and altogether almost 25% [4]. Compared to previous years, the mortality rate seems even higher, probably reflecting the increased age of patients (in an older general population) and with it the underlying diseases. Because it is often difficult to determine the actual cause of death in SJS/TEN patients, death within 6 weeks after the onset of the reaction is considered to be directly related to the severe adverse reaction. Risk factors for death in the acute stage of the disease are large amount of skin detachment, old age and underlying diseases (e.g. renal and/or hepatic insufficiency, acute malignant disorders). However, the cohort study within RegiSCAR has revealed a higher death rate one year after the acute stage of the disease [26].

Acute Generalized Exanthematous Pustulosis

The EuroSCAR study collected the largest validated cohort of patients with AGEP. Due to the fact that the case-control study did not work on a population-based scale, reliable incidence data for AGEP are not available. However, it seems that AGEP is more frequent in some European countries than in others, which could be explained by the availability of specific drugs with a high risk to induce AGEP.

Of the 150 potential AGEP cases collected within EuroSCAR, 97 were finally validated as probable and definite. The majority of cases (78/97) derived from France. The mean age was 56 years (range 4–91 years), and 80% of the patients were women. A death rate of almost 4% was calculated [21].

Drug Reaction with Eosinophilia and Systemic Symptoms

The fact that a wide variety of adverse reactions had been reported under the denomination of hypersensitivity syndrome (HSS) for decades, and that no epidemiologic studies were performed on the disease, may explain why no reliable incidence data are available for what is nowadays called DRESS or DIHS. The existing data suggest that the incidence of HSS related to anticonvulsants may vary between 1 in 1,000 and 1 in 10,000 exposed patients [9].

Of the 201 potential DRESS cases collected within RegiSCAR, 117 were finally validated as probable and definite. Interestingly, 66 patients were female with a median age of 41.5 years, whereas 51 were male with a significantly higher median age of 57 years. The death rate was lower than the previously reported 10% with 2 deaths in 117 patients [27].

Etiology of Cutaneous Adverse Drug Reactions

Numerous case reports and case series report on a huge variety of drugs considered to be responsible for different types of cutaneous adverse reactions. In addition, one drug or drug group may induce clinically different reactions, whereas a specific adverse reaction may be caused by many different drugs. Some drugs seem to have a high risk for cutaneous adverse reactions, especially if a viral infection is present in parallel, as stated above for aminopenicillins and EBV. In the few epidemiologic studies mentioned before, beta-lactam antibiotics accounted for 21% of the cutaneous ADR in the French study [12], while antibiotics were thought to be responsible for 32% of the reactions in the Korean study, followed by 26% due to contrast media [14]. In Singapore, antimicrobial and anti-epileptic agents were the most common causative drugs (75%), including penicillins (25%), cephalosporines (16%), co-trimoxazole (9%), phenytoin (8%), and carbamazepine (6%), whereas allopurinol (5.7%) was less frequently determined as an etiologic factor. However, these percentages refer to different types of cADR of both delayed and immediate type hypersensitivity (63% MPE, 18% urticaria) [28]. In a 20-year survey of cutaneous adverse reactions in Switzerland (Comprehensive Hospital Drug Monitoring), penicillins were identified as the culprit drug in 8%, co-trimoxazole in 2.8% of the cases. In that study, more than 90% of the reactions were diagnosed as MPE, the remaining as urticaria (5.5%), vasculitis (1.4%) and FDE (0.5%) [29].

Etiology and Medication Risk of Severe Cutaneous Adverse Reaction

Stevens-Johnson Syndrome/Toxic Epidermal Necrolysis

Case-control studies are considered as the gold standard of risk estimation for drugs. In the EuroSCAR study, risk estimates are based on 379 community cases of SJS/TEN (i.e. patients who developed the adverse reaction outside the hospital and who were admitted because of symptoms of SCAR) and 1,505 controls, all with a determined index day and adequate information on drug exposures. The analysis strategy looked specifically at medications with prior alerts, recently marketed drugs, but also drugs with a known risk for SJS/TEN and those with the problem of confounding. Confounding arises when, for example, a drug is used for an indication that may have

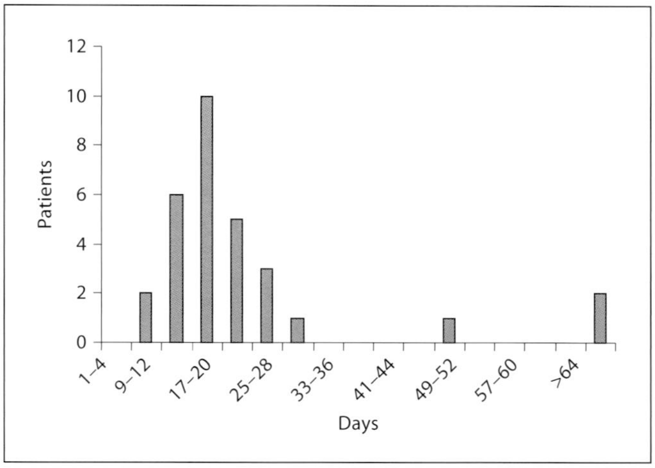

Fig. 1. Time latency between beginning of drug use and onset of SJS/TEN. Example of a highly suspected/strongly associated drug (carbamazepine).

caused the reaction by itself, such as a certain infection. It can also be a problem when a drug is administered in order to treat symptoms that may already reflect the onset of the adverse reaction (e.g. fever, malaise), which is frequently observed for analgesics and antipyretics [18–20].

Among the newly marketed drugs lamotrigine and nevirapine were strongly associated with SJS/TEN. The manufacturers of both drugs had proposed to avoid adverse reactions by slow titration of the dosis (lead-in periods), which obviously could not prevent the occurrence of SCAR like SJS/TEN [20].

For a number of previously suspected drugs such as anti-infective sulfonamides (especially co-trimoxazole), allopurinol, carbamazepine, phenytoin, phenobarbital, and NSAIDs of the oxicam type, a high risk could be confirmed [19, 20].

Most of the highly suspected/strongly associated drugs were prescribed and taken for a longer period of time. Almost all SJS/TEN patients exposed to these drugs (85–100%) had started treatment <8 weeks before onset of the reaction (table 1). The median time latency between beginning of drug use and onset of the reaction was less than 4 weeks (15 days for carbamazepine, 24 days for phenytoin, 17 days for phenobarbital, 20 days for allopurinol) (fig. 1). The majority of patients exposed to allopurinol (56/66) were recent users in contrast to only one of 27 controls. The univariate relative risk for recent use was 261 (36–infinite) versus a multivariate relative risk of 0.9 (0.3–2.4) for long-term use. No significant risk persisted after 8 weeks of use, neither for allopurinol nor for other strongly associated drugs. The typical pattern for these drugs is characterized by recent start of use and infrequent comedication with another highly suspected/strongly associated drug (table 1) [20].

Some other drugs previously suspected of increasing the risk for SJS/TEN were shown to be associated with a significant but lower risk. Among these suspected/associated drugs are various antibiotics, among which penicillins have the lowest relative risk estimates, and acetic acid NSAIDs such as diclofenac (table 2). Valproic acid was

Table 1. Estimation of relative risks (RR) for drugs with a high risk for SJS/TEN [20]

Drug/duration of use	Case patients (n = 379)	Control patients (n = 1,505)	Univariate RR (95% CI)	Multivariate RR (95% CI)	Cases with use of other highly suspected drugs started within 8 weeks
Recently marketed drugs					
Nevirapine	21 (5.5%)	0	>22	n.d.	0
≤8 weeks	20	0	>22		0
>8 weeks	1	0	>0.1		0
Lamotrigine	14 (3.7%)	0	>14	n.d.	1 (7%)
≤8 weeks	14	0	>14		1 (7%)
>8 weeks	0	0	n.d.		0
Long-term marketed drugs					
Cotrimoxazole	24 (6.3%)	1 (0.1%)	102 (14–754)	n.d.	4 (17%)
≤8 weeks	19	0	>20		0
>8 weeks	5	1	21 (2.3–172)		4 (80%)
Other anti-infective sulfonamides[1]	13 (3.4%)	1 (0.1%)	53 (7.0–410)	n.d.	0
≤8 weeks	13	1	53 (7.0–410)		0
>8 weeks	0	0	n.d.		0
Allopurinol	66 (17.4%)	28 (1.9%)	11 (7.0–18)	18 (11–32)	7 (11%)
≤8 weeks	56	1	261 (36 to ∞)	n.d.	2 (4%)
>8 weeks	10	27	1.4 (0.7–3.0)	0.9 (0.3–2.4)	5 (50%)
Cabamazepine	31 (8.2%)	4 (0.3%)	33 (12–95)	72 (23–225)	1 (3%)
≤8 weeks	29	0	>32	n.d.	0
>8 weeks	2	4	2.0 (0.4–121)	n.d.	1
Phenytoin	19 (5.0%)	3 (0.2%)	26 (7.8–90)	17 (4.1–68)	3 (16%)
≤8 weeks	17	0	>17	n.d.	2 (12%)
>8 weeks	2	3	2.7 (0.4–16)	n.d.	1
Phenobarbital	20 (5.3%)	5 (0.3%)	17 (6.2–45)	16 (5.0–50)	3 (15%)
≤8 weeks	17	1	71 (9.4–532)	n.d.	2 (12%)
>8 weeks	3	4	3 (0.7–13)	2.4 (0.2–23)	1 (33%)
Oxicam-NSAIDs[2]	11 (2.9%)	7 (0.5%)	6.4 (2.5–17)	16 (4.9–52)	1 (9%)
≤8 weeks	11	3	15 (4.1–54)	50 (12–211)	1 (9%)
>8 weeks	0	4	0 (0–6.2)	n.d.	0

n.d. = Not done because of <3 cases or controls.

[1] Includes sulfasalazine (5 cases,1 control), sulfadiazine (5, 0), sulfadoxine (2, 0), sulfafurazole (2, 0).

[2] Includes meloxicam (2 cases, 2 controls), piroxicam (6, 4), tenoxicam (3, 1).

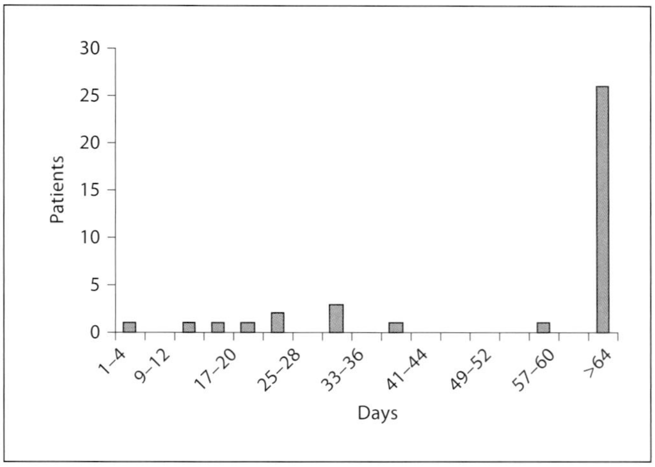

Fig. 2. Time latency between beginning of drug use and onset of SJS/TEN. Example of a non-associated drug (furosemide for more than 2 months).

demonstrated to have no increased risk for SJS/TEN [uvRR = 9.4 (3.9–23), mvRR = 2.0 (0.6–7.4); time latency of more than 30 weeks], as had been assumed earlier [19, 20].

A variety of other drugs and drug groups commonly used, such as beta-blockers, ACE inhibitors, calcium channel blockers, sulfonamide-related diuretics and sulfonylurea antidiabetics, insulin, and propionic acid NSAIDs (e.g. ibuprofen) were not associated with a detectable risk to induce SJS/TEN (fig. 2, table 3) [20].

Outside case-control studies, risk estimation can be done by linking data on drug use in certain populations – e.g. SJS/TEN patients – to prescription data for certain medications. Thus, the population-based data of the German Registry were compared to nationwide prescription data, and drug-based incidences were calculated for various NSAIDs. The analysis revealed overall low risks for most NSAIDs except for those of the oxicam type [30].

Due to the fact that the risk for SJS/TEN is highest in new users of drugs, numbers of new users could be estimated from numbers of dispensed prescriptions in Germany, average prescribed doses and duration of use in the IMS Disease Analyzer – Mediplus Database, and assumptions which relate new use to growth in national dispensings. This approach was based on data of all hospitalized patients with SJS/TEN ascertained by the German Registry, who had used various antiepileptic drugs. The analysis revealed that more than 90% of SJS/TEN cases occurred in the first 63 days of drug use. Increase in dispensings was 5% for carbamazepine, 65% for lamotrigine, 6% for phenobarbital, –16% for phenytoin, 26% for valproic acid in a period of 4 years. The risk estimates were calculated after assumptions about frequency of incident use had been made, and varied between 1 and 10 per 10,000 new users for different antiepileptic drugs except for valproic acid [31].

Another approach for risk estimation in large cohorts of SJS/TEN cases is the use of a standardized algorithm for causality assessment. In 2010, an algorithm for causality assessment in SJS/TEN called algorithm for assessment of drug causality in Stevens-

Table 2. Estimation of RR for drugs with a significant but lower risk for SJS/TEN [20]

Drug/duration of use	Case patients (n = 379)	Control patients (n = 1,505)	Univariate RR (95% CI)	Multivariate RR (95% CI)	Cases with use of highly suspected drugs started within 8 weeks
Acetic acid NSAIDs[1]	27 (7.1%)	21 (1.4%)	5.4 (3.0–10)	5.6 (2.6–12)	7 (26%)
≤8 weeks	24	11	9.2 (4.5–19)	13 (5.2–31)	7 (29%)
>8 weeks	3	10	1.2 (0.3–4.4)	0.7 (0.1–3.3)	0
Macrolides[2]	18 (4.8%)	10 (0.7%)	7.5 (3.4–16)	6.8 (2.6–18)	8 (44%)
Quinolones[3]	13 (3.4%)	5 (0.3%)	10.7 (3.8–30)	6.9 (1.8–27)	6 (46%)
Cephalosporins[4]	19 (5.0%)	7 (0.5%)	11.3 (4.7–27)	7.3 (2.4–22)	12 (63%)
Tetracyclines[5]	7 (1.9%)	5 (0.3%)	5.6 (1.8–18)	6.3 (1.6–25)	1 (14%)
Aminopenicilins[6]	18 (4.8%)	18 (1.2%)	4.1 (2.1–8.0)	2.4 (1.0–5.9)	10 (56%)

[1] Includes diclofenac (21 cases, 17 controls), indomethacin (1, 2), lonazolac (2, 0), etodolac (1, 1), aceclofenac (1, 0), sulindac (1, 0), ketorolac (0, 1).
[2] Includes azithromycin (3 cases, 1 control), clarithromycin (4, 5), erythromycin (3, 0), midecamycin (0, 1), pristinamycin (1, 0), roxithromycin (4, 2), spiramycin (3, 1).
[3] Includes ciprofloxacin (6 cases, 2 controls), grepafloxacin (1, 0), levofloxacin (1, 0), norfloxacin (4, 2), ofloxacin (1, 1).
[4] Includes cefaclor (0 cases, 2 controls), cefalexin (3, 0), cefapirin (1, 0), cefatrizine (2, 0), cefixime (3, 2), cefonicide (1, 2), cefotiam (2, 0), cefpodoxime (0, 2), ceftibutem (0, 1), ceftriaxone (3, 0), cefuroxime (5, 0).
[5] Includes doxycycline (3 cases, 5 controls), metacycline (1, 0), minocycline (3, 0).
[6] Includes amoxicillin (17 cases, 18 controls), bacampicillin (1, 0).

Table 3. Estimation of RR for drugs most likely not associated with SJS/TEN [20]

Drug/duration of use	Case patients (n = 379)	Control patients (n = 1,505)	Univariate RR (95% CI)	Multivariate RR (95% CI)	Cases with use of highly suspected drugs started within 8 weeks
Beta-blockers	37 (9.8%)	122 (8.1%)	1.2 (0.8–1.8)	0.9 (0.5–1.5)	19 (51%)
ACE inhibitors	44 (11.6%)	120 (8.0%)	1.5 (1.1–2.2)	0.9 (0.5–1.5)	23 (52%)
Calcium channel blockers	45 (11.9%)	104 (6.9%)	1.8 (1.3–2.6)	1.4 (0.8–2.4)	24 (54%)
Thiazide diuretics	26 (6.9%)	80 (5.3%)	1.3 (0.8–2.1)	0.7 (0.4–1.4)	17 (65%)
Furosemide	41 (10.8%)	49 (3.3%)	3.6 (2.3–5.5)	1.8 (0.9–3.4)	24 (59%)
Propionic acid NSAIDs	16 (4.2%)	35 (2.3%)	1.9 (1.0–3.4)	1.5 (0.6–3.4)	8 (50%)
Sulfonylurea anti-diabetics	11 (2.9%)	35 (2.3%)	1.3 (0.6–2.5)	0.8 (0.3–2.4)	5 (45%)
Insulin	10 (2.6%)	22 (1.5%)	1.8 (0.9–3.9)	1.0 (0.3–3.3)	6 (60%)

Johnson syndrome and toxic epidermal necrolysis (ALDEN) was published. It provides structured help for the identification of drug(s) responsible for SJS/TEN in individual cases [32]. It includes the findings of epidemiologic studies, which were able to provide risk estimates for drugs inducing SJS/TEN, and is based on the following criteria: time latency between beginning of drug use and index day (i.e. onset of the adverse reaction), drug present in the body before index day (taking into account the drug's half-life as well as the patient's liver and kidney function), information on prechallenge/rechallenge and dechallenge (if available), type of drug/notoriety (based on drug lists that require a regular update) and alternative causes. Numerical score values lead to a causality assessment for each individual drug a patient has taken or was administered, ranging from very unlikely, unlikely, possible, probable to very probable [32].

Drugs could be identified as causes of SJS/TEN in approximately 75% of the cases, i.e. in at least 25% of the cases no culprit drug can be determined, although cases of SJS/TEN without any drug use are rare. Some patients are only exposed to long-term medication, which cannot be accused to have caused the adverse reaction. Viral infections and mycoplasma pneumoniae infection have also been reported as etiologic factors and a possible interaction of infection and medication as well as the interaction of different drugs remains to be clarified. Frequently, it is difficult to decide whether certain symptoms, e.g. oronasal soreness and conjunctival injection, are signs of an acute infection or the onset of the severe skin reaction itself, which may lead to difficulties in determining the index day and false causality assessment.

Because there are no reliable in vitro or in vivo tests to determine the link between a specific drug and SJS/TEN in an individual case, the detection of the culprit drug mainly relies on the time interval between beginning of drug use and onset of the adverse reaction. For safety reasons, oral provocation tests with the suspected drug cannot be recommended, although the reaction may not occur again, as studies performed in Finland in the 1970s could show [33]. Patch tests with the potentially culprit drug are safe but often false negative [24].

Acute Generalized Exanthematous Pustulosis

Although case series frequently list the medications thought to have caused the reaction, risk estimation based on the case-control approach was first performed by the EuroSCAR study. Of the 97 patients with AGEP, 13 were exposed to macrolide antibiotics in the week before the index day, 10 of which were associated with pristinamycin, a macrolide only marketed in France. The adverse reaction occurred after only one day of use in 9 cases, and after 2 days in one case. A high odds ratio was also calculated for aminopenicillins, for which the exposure time was less than 15 days in all cases and often very short. The results were similar for quinolones. Seven cases versus 2 controls were exposed to chloroquine or hydroxychloroquine, 7 cases versus 10 controls to diltiazem. The fact that none of these cases was exposed to

Table 4. Estimation of RR (as OR) for drugs with a high risk to induce AGEP [21]

Drug or drug group	Case patients (n = 97)	Control patients (n = 1,009)	OR (95% CI)[a]	Cases with use of other highly suspected drugs started within 8 weeks[b]
Pristinamycin	10 (10)	0	∞ (26 to ∞)	1 (10%)
Aminopenicillins	18 (19)	17 (2)	23 (10–54)	3 (17%)
Quinolones	9 (9)	5 (0.5)	33 (8.5–127)	3 (33%)
(Hydroxy-) chloroquine	7 (7)	2 (0.2)	39 (8.0–191)	0
Sulfonamides	4 (4)	0	∞ (7.1 to ∞)	0
Terbinafine	4 (4)	0	∞ (7.1 to ∞)	1 (25%)
Diltiazem	7 (7)	10 (1)	15 (5.0–48)	0

[a] Multivariate OR if at least 3 cases and 3 controls exposed, otherwise univariate.
[b] Recent use of other highly suspected drugs (i.e. any other drug listed in the table).

another drug with a high risk for AGEP suggests that these antimalarials and diltiazem carry a high risk for AGEP, which was not demonstrated for other ACE inhibitors (table 4). The time latency between beginning of drug use and onset of AGEP varied between a median of one day for antibiotics and sulfonamides (41 cases) and a median of 11 days for other drugs including chloroquine/hydroxychloroquine and diltiazem [21].

Drug Reaction with Eosinophilia and Systemic Symptoms

To date, information on drugs inducing DRESS/DIHS is based on case reports and case series. Often, the reaction itself was named after the drug that was considered to be the culprit, e.g. allopurinol HSS, dapsone syndrome, anticonvulsant syndrome, etc. Within the RegiSCAR study, drug exposure was analyzed in 117 validated cases of DRESS. A median of 5 (interquartile range 2–8) drugs were taken in the month before onset of the reaction. In 77% of the cases one, and in 3% two equally (very) probable culprit drugs could be identified, whereas in 4% causality remained undetermined and in 7% unlikely. Antiepileptic drugs including carbamazepine, phenytoin and lamotrigine were thought to be responsible in 36% of the cases, followed by allopurinol in 18%, and sulfonamides in 12%, while other reported drugs were less frequent. The median time latency between beginning of drug use and onset of DRESS was 28 (±17) days for all drugs with a probable or very probable causality assessment [27].

Furthermore, viral reactivation and antiviral T cell response seem to play an important role in the development of DRESS/DIHS, especially in recurrent cases and persisting reactions [11, 34]. Nevertheless, it is not clear whether the reactivation of HHV6 and other members of the human herpes virus family are involved in the etiology of the disease or should be interpreted as a complication [10].

Genetic Epidemiology on Cutaneous Adverse Drug Reactions

A genetic susceptibility for cutaneous ADR has long been suspected. However, not until recently were studies able to determine a risk for specific types of reactions related to certain drugs in patients with a particular pattern of HLA alleles, which may be different in various ethnic groups. Thus, HLA-A*3101 was detected in European patients with carbamazepine-induced hypersensitivity reactions, especially MPE, but not severe reactions like SJS/TEN [35]. A very strong association between carbamazepine-induced SJS/TEN and HLA-B*1502 was observed in Han Chinese patients, which could not be confirmed for Europeans. However, HLA-B*5801 was found in Han Chinese with SJS/TEN and DRESS due to allopurinol (100%) as well as in Europeans with SJS/TEN (55%). These findings are very important because they clearly demonstrate that, first, the genetic predisposition to develop SCAR is highly associated with specific drugs, and, second, ethnicity matters much more than previously thought [36].

References

1 World Health Organization: International drug monitoring: the role of national centres. World Health Organ Tech Rep Ser 1972;498:1–25.

2 Johansson SG, Bieber T, Dahl R, Friedmann PS, Lanier BQ, Lockey RF, Motala C, Ortega Martell JA, Platts-Mills TA, Ring J, Thien F, Van Cauwenberge P, Williams HC: Revised nomenclature for allergy for global use: report of the nomenclature review committee of the World Allergy Organization. October 2003. J Allergy Clin Immunol 2004;113: 832–836.

3 Bork K: Cutaneous Adverse Drug Reactions; in Burgdorf WHC, Plewig G, Wolff HH, Landthaler M (eds): Braun-Falco's Dermatology, ed 3. Heidelberg, Springer, 2009, chapter 33, pp 456–472.

4 Mockenhaupt M: Severe cutaneous adverse reactions; in Burgdorf WHC, Plewig G, Wolff HH, Landthaler M (eds): Braun-Falco's Dermatology, ed 3. Heidelberg, Springer, 2009, chapter 34, pp 473–484.

5 Auquier-Dunant A, Mockenhaupt M, Naldi L, Correia O, Schröder W, Roujeau JC for the SCAR Study Group: Correlations between clinical patterns and causes of erythema multiforme majus, Stevens-Johnson syndrome, and toxic epidermal necrolysis. Arch Dermatol 2002;138:1019–1024.

6 Bastuji-Garin S, Rzany B, Stern RS, Shear NH, Naldi L, Roujeau JC: Clinical classification of cases of toxic epidermal necrolysis, Stevens-Johnson syndrome, and erythema multiforme. Arch Dermatol 1993;129:92–96.

7 Schröder W, Mockenhaupt M, Schlingmann J, Schneck B, Hering O, Schöpf E: Clinical Re-classification of severe skin reactions and evaluation of their etiology in a population-based registry; in Victor N, Blettner M, Edler L, Haux R, Knaup-Gregori P, Pritsch M, Wahrendorf J, Windeler J, Ziegler S (eds): Medical informatics, biostatistics and epidemiology for efficient health care and medical research: contributions from the 44th annual conference of the GMDS. Heidelberg, Urban & Vogel, 1999, pp 107–110.

8 Sidoroff A, Halevy S, Bouwes Bavinck JN, Vaillant L, Roujeau JC: Acute generalized exanthematous pustulosis (AGEP) – a clinical reaction pattern. J Cutan Pathol 2001;28:113–119.
9 Sullivan JR, Shear NH: The drug hypersensitivity syndrome: what is the pathogenesis? Arch Dermatol 2001;137:357–362.
10 Kardaun SH, Sidoroff A, Valeyrie-Allanore L, Halevy S, Davidovici BB, Mockenhaupt M, Roujeau JC: Variability in the clinical pattern of cutaneous side-effects of drugs with systemic symptoms: does a DRESS syndrome really exist? Br J Dermatol 2007; 156:609–611.
11 Shiohara T, Iijima M, Ikezawa Z, Hashimoto K: The diagnosis of a DRESS syndrome has been sufficiently established on the basis of typical clinical features and viral reactivations. Br J Dermatol 2007; 156:1083–1084.
12 Fiszenson-Albala F, Auzerie V, Mahe E, Farinotti R, Durand-Stocco C, Crickx B, Descamps V: A 6-month prospective survey of cutaneous drug reactions in a hospital setting. Br J Dermatol 2003; 149:1018–1022.
13 Hernandez-Salazar A, Rosales SP, Rangel-Frausto S, Criolio E, Arche-Dubon C, Orozco-Topete R: Epidemiology of adverse cutaneous drug reactions. A prospective study in hospitalized patients. Arch Med Res 2006;37:899–902.
14 Park CS, Kim TB, Kim SL, Kim JY, Yang KA, Bae YJ, Cho YS, Moon HB: The use of an electronic medical record system for mandatory reporting of drug hypersensitivity reactions has been shown to improve the management of patients in the university hospital in Korea. Pharmacoepidemiol Drug Saf 2008;17:919–925.
15 Roujeau JC, Guillaume JC, Fabre JP, Penso D, Fléchet ML, Girre JP: Toxic epidermal necrolysis (Lyell's syndrome): incidence and drug etiology in France, 1981–1985. Arch Dermatol 1990;126: 37–42.
16 Schöpf E, Stühmer A, Rzany B, Victor N, Zentgraf R, Kapp JF: Toxic epidermal necrolysis and Stevens-Johnson syndrome. An epidemiologic study from West-Germany. Arch Dermatol 1991;127:839–842.
17 Rzany B, Mockenhaupt M, Baur S, Schröder W, Stocker U, Mueller J, Holländer N, Bruppacher R, Schöpf E: Epidemiology of erythema exsudativum multiforme majus (EEMM), Stevens-Johnson syndrome (SJS) and toxic epidermal necrolysis (TEN) in Germany (1990–1992). Structure and results of a population-based registry. J Clin Epidemiol 1996;49: 769–773.
18 Kelly JP, Auquier A, Rzany B, Naldi L, Bastuji-Garin S, Correia O, Shapiro S, Kaufman D: An international collaborative case-control study of severe cutaneous adverse reactions (SCAR). Design and methods. J Clin Epidemiol 1995;48:1099–1108.
19 Roujeau JC, Kelly JP, Naldi L, Rzany B, Stern RS, Anderson T, Auquier A, Bastuji-Garin S, Correia O, Locati F, Mockenhaupt M, Paoletti C, Shapiro S, Shear N, Schöpf E, Kaufman DW: Medication use and the risk of Stevens-Johnson syndrome or toxic epidermal necrolysis. N Eng J Med 1995;333: 1600–1607.
20 Mockenhaupt M, Viboud C, Dunant A, Naldi L, Halevy S, Bouwes Bavinck JN, Sidoroff A, Schneck J, Roujeau JC, Flahault A: Stevens-Johnson syndrome and toxic epidermal necrolysis: assessment of medication risks with emphasis on recently marketed drugs. The EuroSCAR-study. J Invest Dermatol 2008;128:35–44.
21 Sidoroff A, Dunant A, Viboud C, Halevy S, Bouwes Bavinck JN, Naldi L, Mockenhaupt M, Fagot JP, Roujeau JC: Risk factors for acute generalized exanthematous pustulosis (AGEP) – results of a multinational case-control study (EuroSCAR). Br J Dermatol 2007;157:989–896.
22 Orpha News Europe: the newsletter of the rare disease task force. www.orphanet.net/actor/EuropaNews/2006/060124.html.
23 Strom BL, Carson JL, Halpern AC, Schinnar R, Snyder ES, Shaw M, Tilson HH, Joseph M, Dai WS, Chen D, Stern RS, Bergmann U, Stolley PD: A population-based study of Stevens-Johnson syndrome: incidence and antecedent drug exposures. Arch Dermatol 1991;127:831–838.
24 Mockenhaupt M, Norgauer J: Cutaneous adverse drug reactions: Stevens-Johnson syndrome and toxic epidermal necrolysis. Allergy Clin Immunol Int 2002;14:143–150.
25 Fagot JP, Mockenhaupt M, Bouwes Bavinck JN, Naldi L, Viboud C, Roujeau JC: Nevirapine and the risk of Stevens-Johnson syndrome or toxic epidermal necrolysis: preliminary results of a case-control study. AIDS 2001;15:1–6.
26 Mockenhaupt M, Sekula P, Roujeau JC, Sidoroff A, Kardaun S, Liss Y, Bounoua M, the RegiSCAR-study group: Mortality and long-lasting sequelae in patients with severe cutaneous adverse reactions. Pharmacoepidem Dr S 2008;17:115–116.
27 Kardaun SH, Sekula P, Mockenhaupt M, Chu CY, Creamer D, Sidoroff A, Naldi L, Roujeau JC: Drug reaction with eosinophilia and systemic symptoms (DRESS): Results from the RegiSCAR-study. Eur Ann Allergy Clin Immunol 2010;42:45.

28 Thong BV, Leong KP, Tang CY, Chung HH: Drug allergy in a general hospital: results of a novel prospective inpatient reporting system. Ann Allergy Asthma Immunol 2003;90:342–347.
29 Hunziker T, Künzi UP, Braunschweig S, Zehnder D, Hoigne R: Comprehensive hospital drug monitoring (CHDM): adverse skin reactions, a 20 year survey. Allergy 1997;52:388–393.
30 Mockenhaupt M, Kelly JP, Kaufman D, Stern RS: The risk of Stevens-Johnson syndrome and toxic epidermal necrolysis associated with nonsteroidal antiinflammatory drugs: a multinational perspective. J Rheumatol 2003;30:2234–2240.
31 Mockenhaupt M, Messenheimer J, Schlingmann J, Tennis P: Risk of Stevens-Johnson syndrome and toxic epidermal necrolysis in new users of anti-epileptics. Neurology 2005;64:1134–1138.
32 Sassolas B, Haddad C, Mockenhaupt M, Dunant A, Liss Y, Bork K, Haustein UF, Vieluf D, Roujeau JC, LeLouet H for the RegiSCAR-group: ALDEN an algorithm for assessment of drug causality in Stevens-Johnson-syndrome and toxic epidermal necrolysis. Comparison with case-control analysis. Clin Pharmacol Ther 2010;88:60–68.
33 Kauppinen K: Cutaneous reactions to drugs. With special reference to severe bullous mucocutaneous eruptions and sulphonamides. A clinical study. Acta Derm Venereol Suppl 1972;68:1–89.
34 Picard D, Janela B, Descamps V, D'Ibcan M, Jacquot S, Rogez S, Mardivirin L, Moins-Teisserenc H, Toubert A, Benichou J, Joly P, Musette P: Drug reaction with eosinophilia and systemic symptoms (DRESS): a multiorgan antiviral T cell response. Sci Transl Med 2010;2:46–62.
35 McCormack M, Alfirevic A, Bourgeois S, Farrell JJ, et al: HLA-A*3101 and carbamazepine-induced hypersensitivity reactions in Europeans. N Engl J Med 2011;364:1134–1143.
36 Phillips EJ, Chung WH, Mockenhaupt M, Roujeau JC, Mallal SA: Drug hypersensitivity: pharmacogenetics and clinical syndromes. J Allergy Clin Immunol 2011;127(3 suppl):60–66.

Prof. med. Maja Mockenhaupt
Dokumentationszentrum schwerer Hautreaktionen (dZh)
Department of Dermatology, University Freiburg – Medical Center
Hauptstrasse 7
DE–79104 Freiburg (Germany)
Tel. +49 761 270 67230, E-Mail dzh@uniklinik-freiburg.de

French LE (ed): Adverse Cutaneous Drug Eruptions.
Chem Immunol Allergy. Basel, Karger, 2012, vol 97, pp 18–31

Genetics and the Potential for Predictive Tests in Adverse Drug Reactions

Munir Pirmohamed

The Wolfson Centre for Personalised Medicine, Department of Molecular and Clinical Pharmacology, University of Liverpool, Liverpool, UK

Abstract

Drug hypersensitivity reactions are an immune-mediated reaction to otherwise innocuous antigens derived from drugs. These reactions can affect many different organs, with the skin being the commonest. Skin involvement can range in severity with hypersensitivity syndrome (or DRESS) and the blistering reactions (Stevens-Johnson syndrome, toxic epidermal necrolysis), also termed serious cutaneous adverse drug reactions, being the most severe and most feared. There is increasing evidence for the role of the immune system in the pathogenesis of these reactions, with drug-specific T cells having been identified in many patients. Until recently, very little was known about the predisposition to these reactions. However, the availability of more accurate molecular typing methods, and the ability to analyse the whole genome in an unbiased fashion, has led to some remarkable findings of the role of the HLA genes as genomic biomarkers of predisposition. The 'revolution' started with abacavir where the predisposition to hypersensitivity was linked to HLA-B*57:01, which was confirmed in a clinical trial, and where its implementation has shown to reduce the incidence of hypersensitivity in a cost-effective manner. Since then, associations have also been shown for allopurinol (HLA-B*58:01)- and carbamazepine (HLA-B*1502 and HLA-A*3101)-induced serious cutaneous adverse drug reactions. The latter is interesting since the association with HLA-B*1502 is present in certain South-Eastern Asian populations, and the predisposition is phenotype specific (only for SJS/TEN). The utility of this biomarker has been shown in a prospective cohort study performed in Taiwan. By contrast, the association with HLA-A*3101 is seen in more diverse ethnic groups, and predisposes to mild as well more severe cutaneous reactions associated with carbamazepine. It is important to note that strong HLA associations have also been shown with a number of drugs that cause liver injury including flucloxacillin, lumiracoxib, lapatinib and ximelagatran, indicating that the immune system is also important in the pathogenesis of other forms of drug-induced organ toxicity. The crucial question as to whether these HLA alleles are truly causative or acting as surrogate markers of predisposition, however, is still unclear, and will require further investigations in larger patient cohorts, through the use of bioinformatic techniques, fine mapping using next generation sequencing technologies and functional studies.

Essentials in a Nutshell

- Genetic factors predisposing to certain types of cutaneous drug eruptions induced by selected drugs have been identified particularly in the HLA genes
- The most important of these include:
  - HLA-B*5701 and abacavir hypersensitivity (AHS), where pre-prescription genotyping has been shown to reduce the incidence of AHS
  - HLA B*5801 and allopurinol-induced hypersensitivity syndrome and SJS/TEN
  - HLA-B*1502 or A*3101 and carbamazepine (CBZ)-induced SJS/TEN depending on the ethnic background
- Predictive genetic testing for HLA-B*1502 in Taiwanese population has been shown to reduce the incidence of carbamezepine-induced SJS-TEN
- Identification of further genetic biomarkers for cutaneous drug eruptions is likely to help predict, and reduce the incidence of such adverse reactions

Introduction

Adverse drug reactions (ADRs) are common, accounting for 6.5% of all hospital admissions [1], and occurring in 15% of in-patients [2]. The burden on any health-care system is large in terms of number of beds occupied by patients with ADRs and the direct costs [3]. Indirect societal costs are also likely to be substantial but have not been accurately quantified. ADRs can take many forms, affect any bodily system and range from mild (fortunately the commonest type of reaction) to life-threatening. Lazarou et al. [4] estimated that ADRs were between the 4th and 6th commonest cause of death in the US in 1994, a figure borne out by data from the UK from our large prospective epidemiological study [1].

ADRs can be divided into two basic types: type A and type B [5] (table 1). ADRs affecting the skin, cutaneous drug eruptions, fall into the category of type B or bizarre adverse reactions – these reactions were defined as not being predictable from the known pharmacology of the drug. However, as our knowledge increases, some of these reactions will become predictable through genetic tests (and other types of tests). Thus, this simple classification, as with all classifications, has its limitations, but nevertheless is useful as a framework for both clinical and research purposes. It is also still in keeping with the fact that the factors predisposing individuals to most type B reactions with individual drugs are unknown. It is also important to state that type A (dose dependent, predictable from the known pharmacology of the drug) also show some genetic predisposition, for example, warfarin-related dose requirements and predisposition to bleeding risk [6].

Cutaneous drug eruptions form part of the spectrum of reactions that are allergic in origin, sometimes also called drug hypersensitivity reactions. The exact incidence

Table 1. Features of type A and type B ADRs

Characteristic	Type A	Type B
Dose dependency	usually shows a good relationship	no simple relationship
Predictable from known pharmacology	yes	not usually
Host factors	genetic factors may be important	dependent on (usually uncharacterised) host factors
Frequency	common	uncommon
Severity	variable, but usually mild	variable, proportionately more severe
Clinical burden	high morbidity and low mortality	high morbidity and mortality
Animal models	usually reproducible in animals	no known animal models

is unclear, but estimates suggest that they represent anything from 5 to 15% of all ADRs depending on the setting of the study and its design [7]. Severe hypersensitivity can require or prolong hospitalisation, and is usually not detected in clinical trials during drug development, but identified through post-marketing surveillance, when a large number of individuals are exposed to a particular drug. The importance of this relates to the fact that in order to conduct genetic studies of cutaneous drug eruptions, it is usually necessary to identify and recruit patients, and collect samples in the post-marketing phase when the drug is being used clinically. It is very unlikely, at least in the near future, that we will be in a position that allows us to predict the occurrence of, and predisposing factors for, cutaneous drug eruptions before the drug is licensed.

Investigation into the Genetics of Cutaneous Drug Eruption

In order to investigate the genetic basis of a cutaneous ADR, several issues need to be considered. These aspects are important if we are ever to realise the prospects of predicting and preventing cutaneous ADRs. These are outlined below.

First, there are many reasons to study the genetic basis of a cutaneous ADR, ranging from personal interest to the fact that the ADR may represent a public health problem because of its frequency and/or severity. The most important issue to consider is whether it will be possible to identify adequate numbers of patients with that ADR, and appropriate controls. Most investigators to date have focused on specific drugs and their ability to cause ADRs which may lead to identification of drug-specific genetic predisposing factors. An alternative may be to focus on a specific phenotype, for example toxic epidermal necrolysis on the basis that some common factors may predispose to the phenotypic manifestation irrespective of the underlying drug aetiology. Conventional power calculations may not be possible because the effect size of a genetic predisposing factor may be unknown. For the identification of genetic loci predisposing to common diseases, such as type II diabetes mellitus, investigators have had to resort to studying more than 40,000 patients [8]. Clearly, this would not be possible with cutaneous ADRs, particularly those which are severe, because of the rarity of these reactions [9], the transient nature of the reactions, the fact that most are never reported to regulatory agencies [10], and even when recorded in case-notes, the description is usually poor with bland terms such as 'rash' being used without any narrative of the morphology, distribution, duration, and associated manifestations. Furthermore, even when a small number of cases are required, it is very rare for one centre to have an adequate sample size, and hence, multi-centre international collaboration is often necessary. To this end, we have recently formed the InternaTional Consortium on Drug Hypersensitivity [11], supported by the international Serious Adverse Events Consortium [http://www.saeconsortium.org/], whose mission is to identify and recruit patients of different ethnicities to identify genetic predisposing factors for drug hypersensitivity reactions.

Second, cutaneous drug eruptions can present with many different clinical manifestations, even when the same drug is implicated, in different patients. It is likely that the pathogenesis of these different reactions will vary, and therefore a mixture of phenotypes may reduce the likelihood of identifying genetic predisposing factors. Furthermore, although different phenotypes may share the same genetic predisposing factor, the effect size may be phenotype dependent. Thus, phenotype standardisation is extremely important in order to facilitate recruitment of patients in a standardised fashion both within and between centres. Pragmatic criteria for the characterisation of patients with serious cutaneous ADRs have been published recently [12], with the term drug-induced skin injury being introduced to be consistent with terms drug-induced liver and kidney injury used for other organs.

Third, several different methods can be used for identifying genetic predisposing factors. Family linkage studies, which were successful in identifying the loci for Mendelian diseases such as cystic fibrosis, are not of use in identifying genetic predisposing factors for ADRs, since it would be difficult to find families where individuals who had the same disease, had been prescribed the same drug and had (or had not) developed the same ADR were available. Most studies to date have focused on candidate gene approaches, based on the knowledge of the pharmacokinetic and pharmacodynamic properties of the drug. Although the identification of a predisposing factor by this method provides evidence of biological plausibility, the major disadvantage for idiosyncratic reactions, including those affecting the skin, is that we do not fully understand the mechanisms leading to these reactions. Rapid progress in genotyping technologies over the past few years has led to increasing utilisation of genome-wide association study (GWAS) approaches. Over 992 studies had been published by August 2011 – a catalogue of the studies is available at http://www.genome.

gov/gwastudies [13]. The GWAS approach allows an unbiased assessment of genetic predisposing loci, which may allow the identification of novel susceptibility factors. The GWAS approach is often regarded as hypothesis generating and data driven, with replication of the findings being crucial. GWAS technologies can allow the simultaneous interrogation of up to 5 million SNPs. Of the 992 studies published to date, only a small subset relate to the genetics of drug response. Similar to all pharmacogenetic studies, the success of any GWAS will depend on several factors including the effect size and allele frequency of genetic variants responsible for the relevant phenotype, the sample size, the population under study and study design [14]. It is also important to remember that GWAS approaches lead to the identification of common variants, occurring with an allele frequency of at least 2% in the population. As mentioned above, a large sample size is particularly difficult to achieve for drug-induced cutaneous eruptions (and indeed other idiosyncratic reactions) given their low incidence and the difficulties sometimes encountered in defining an accurate phenotype. Although there is a clear advantage of using GWAS to study hypersensitivity, it is also important to remember that very few novel loci outside the MHC have been discovered to date [15]. Clearly, the HLA genes are the usual candidates for drug hypersensitivity (see below), and as such careful study here is likely to lead to significant findings, as for example was demonstrated for AHS and HLA-B*5701 [16–18]. Finally, it is now also possible to use sequencing technologies to identify genetic predisposing factors. The availability and rapidly decreasing cost of sequencing provides for the opportunity to sequence specific loci of interest, all exons in the genome (exome sequencing – 1% of the human genome) and whole genomes. The advantage of next generation sequencing is that it provides an assessment of both common and rare variants: the latter are not detected using GWAS approaches, and have been postulated to have larger effect sizes than the common variants [19]. However, sequencing approaches have not been used to assess the genetic contribution to cutaneous ADRs to date.

Fourth, many genetic association studies have suffered from the fact that an initial identification of genetic susceptibility has not been replicated by other investigators leading to many false positive findings in the literature. Because of the high likelihood of false positive findings in GWAS, it is crucial that any positive findings are replicated in different cohorts of patients. When such patient groups are not available, functional analysis of the associated variants is necessary to provide some biological plausibility to the findings.

Finally, although we can now conduct unbiased whole genome studies, it is still necessary to have some idea of the function of the variant that is found to be associated with the phenotype. This adds to the biological plausibility but may also allow the identification of novel mechanisms of the ADR, and future possibilities for intervention. The occurrence of an adverse cutaneous drug reaction can be rationalised into 4 stages: (a) the conversion of a non-toxic non-reactive drug into a reactive metabolite capable of binding to protein (a process called bioactivation); (b) the imbalance between bioactivation and detoxification processes (also called bioinactivation) that leads to persistence of the toxic metabolite; (c) the ability of the body's immune system to respond to the novel antigen(s) that is (are) formed from the toxic metabolite, and (d) the resulting processes that lead to tissue injury. Most genetic studies conducted to identify predisposing factors for cutaneous ADRs can be divided into those that have focused on the metabolism and disposition of the drugs (stages a and b) and the immune response to the drug (metabolite) which leads to tissue injury (stages c and d). Indeed, the early studies largely focused on drug metabolism genes but did not yield any impressive findings [20, 21]. Clinically, cutaneous ADRs are thought to have an immune basis: for example, recurrence on rechallenge often occurs much sooner than on the primary exposure, and there may be accompanying symptoms such as fever, lymphadenopathy, and eosinophilia [22]. Furthermore, laboratory evidence showing the presence of drug-specific T cells has also added to the evidence that these reactions are immune mediated [23–26]. For this reason, the major histocompatibility complex region on the short arm of chromosome 6, where the HLA alleles reside, has been the focus of many studies, and has recently led to some exciting findings (discussed below). The HLA alleles are the most polymorphic genes in the human genome, with the HLA-B locus shown to have the highest number of alleles [15]. The HLA alleles show such a high degree of variation in order to protect us from infectious agents by mounting an immune response which can lead to the destruction of the microorganism by the body's immune system. However, the same variation that protects against infectious diseases can also predispose certain individuals to autoimmune diseases and drug hypersensitivity reactions including those affecting the skin.

Genetic Predisposing Factors for Cutaneous Adverse Drug Reactions

There have been many studies investigating genetic factors predisposing to cutaneous ADRs, most of which have been negative, have not been replicated and/or have not resulted in findings that could have clinical implications. The most significant findings to date have been with HLA alleles (table 2), a selection of which are described below.

*Abacavir Hypersensitivity and HLA-B*5701*

Abacavir is a nucleoside reverse transcriptase inhibitor used as an anti-HIV agent in combination with other antiretrovirals. Approximately 5–7% of patients develop AHS [27]. The reaction is CD8+ T cell mediated as evidenced by skin biopsies taken from patients with positive patch tests to abacavir [28]. The association between the HLA class I allele HLA-B*5701 and AHS was first reported by Mallal et al. [18] in an Australian population, quickly replicated by a study from North America [16] and subsequently by a study from the UK [17]. Progress since then has been rapid:

Table 2. Reported HLA associations with drugs and other chemicals

Drug	Class of drug	HLA allele	Population and references	Phenotype
Allopurinol	uricosuric	B*5801	Han Chinese [57], Thai [58], Japanese [52], Malay [46]	HSS, SJS/TEN
CBZ	antiepileptic	B*1502	Han Chinese [41–43], Thai [44–45], Malay [46], Indian [47]	SJS/TEN
		A*3101	Caucasian [56], Japanese [68]	MPE, HSS, SJS/TEN
Phenytoin	antiepileptic	B*1502	Han Chinese [43], Thai [44]	SJS/TEN
Oxicam	NSAID	A2, B12	Caucasians [69]	SJS/TEN
Sulphamethoxazole	antibiotic	A29, B12, DR7	Caucasians [70]	SJS/TEN
Abacavir	antiretroviral	B*5701	Caucasians [16, 18, 36, 71], African-Americans [35, 72]	HSS
Aminopenicillins	antibiotic	A2, Drw52	Caucasians [73]	HSS
Nevirapine	antiretroviral	DRB1*01	Caucasian-Australian[74]	various including MPE, HSS and SJS/TEN
		DRB1*01	Caucasian-French [75]	
		Cw8,B14	Caucasian-Italian [76]	
		Cw8	Japanese [77]	
		B*3505	Thai [78]	
		Cw4	Thai [79]	
Aspirin	NSAIDS	DRB1*1302, DQB1*0609	Korean, Caucasian [80, 81]	aspirin hypersensitivity
Iodine contrast media		DR	Caucasians-Spanish [82]	MPE
Gold	treatment of rheumatoid arthritis	DR5	Caucasians-Spanish [83]	MPE
Lamotrigine	antiepileptic	B*5801, A*6801	Caucasians [84]	HSS, SJS/TEN
Co-trimoxazole	antibiotic	A30 B13 Cw6	Caucasians-Turkish [85]	FDE
Feprazone	analgesic	B22	Undefined [86]	FDE

Adapted from Alfirevic and Pirmohamed [15]. HSS = Hypersensitivity syndrome; MPE = maculopapular exanthema; FDE = fixed drug eruption.

- Pre-treatment testing for AHS has been demonstrated to be cost effective, first in the UK [17], and subsequently in other countries [29–31].
- The use of HLA-B*5701 in clinical settings has been shown to reduce the frequency of hypersensitivity in Australia [32], UK [33] and France [34], showing that the genetic testing can have a powerful influence in reducing the burden associated with serious ADRs.
- B*5701 is a useful genetic marker for prediction of hypersensitivity in several ethnic groups including those with black African ancestry [35].
- The clinical utility of pre-treatment B*5701 testing has been shown in a prospective randomised controlled clinical trial (PREDICT-1) [36].
- Simple tests to detect HLA-B*5701 are available, and include the use of the HCP5 SNP rs2395029 which is in almost complete (although not total) linkage disequilibrium with HLA-B*5701 [37], real-time PCR techniques [38], and flow cytometry techniques [39].
- In vitro studies have demonstrated that abacavir-treated antigen-presenting cells positive for HLA-B*5701, but not the related alleles B*5702 or B*5801, can stimulate abacavir specific CD8+ T cell responses [40]. The latter provides evidence of the functional relevance of B*5701 in the mechanism of AHS.
- The drug label for abacavir has been altered by the FDA and by the European Medicines Agency which recommends or mandates testing for HLA-B*5701 prior to the prescription of abacavir.

The prevention of AHS through the use of a genetic test represents the paradigm for translation of pharmacogenetics into the clinic. A high negative predictive value but a relatively low positive predictive value (48%) characterises the test [36]. Therefore, nearly 50% of HLA-B*5701-positive individuals will not develop hypersensitivity in response to abacavir, and thus, other genetic or non-genetic factors may play a role in AHS.

Carbamazepine-Induced Hypersensitivity Reactions

CBZ is widely used in the treatment of epilepsy, trigeminal neuralgia and bipolar disorder. It causes cutaneous ADRs which can manifest in many different ways, the three commonest, from mildest to the most severe, being (a) maculopapular exanthema, which typically do not require any specific treatment apart from drug withdrawal, (b) hypersensitivity syndrome where the skin eruption is accompanied by systemic manifestations and extra-cutaneous involvement, most commonly the liver, and (c) Stevens-Johnson syndrome and toxic epidermal necrolysis (SJS/TEN), which are associated with 10–30% mortality.

CBZ-induced SJS/TEN has shown a strong (OR >1,000) association with HLA-B*1502 in the Han Chinese population [41–43]. The association has also been replicated in several other Asian populations including Thai [44, 45], Malay [46] and

Indian [47], but not in Caucasians [48–50] and Japanese [51–52]. Interestingly, the frequency of SJS/TEN is higher in most Asian populations than in Caucasians, as is the frequency of the B*1502 allele (http://www.allelefrequencies.net) which provides circumstantial evidence for its potential functional relevance. Following these findings, the drug label for CBZ was changed by several regulatory agencies, including the EMA and FDA. Apart from being ethnicity specific, the association with HLA-B*1502 is phenotype specific in that it is only valid for SJS/TEN, but has not been shown to be important for maculopapular exanthema and hypersensitivity syndrome [42].

Patients who develop hypersensitivity to one aromatic antiepileptic drug (AED) may also show cross-reactivity to structurally related AEDs [53]. Several case reports have shown that the HLA-B*1502 allele may be important in patients with phenytoin and oxcarbazepine-induced SJS [43, 44, 54]. These findings however need to be validated in a larger number of ethnically diverse populations.

Recently, in a prospective cohort study in Taiwan, Chen et al. [55] genotyped 4,877 patients due to start on CBZ for HLA-B*1502. They avoided the use of CBZ in 7.7% of patients who were positive for HLA-B*1502, while those who were negative for this allele were given CBZ as per usual practice. After a follow-up of 3 months for all patients, no patients developed SJS, when at least 10 cases would have been expected. This prospective study showed the utility of pre-prescription genotyping in preventing CBZ-induced SJS in the Chinese population despite the rarity of the reaction.

A genome-wide association study undertaken by ourselves has recently shown a strong association with CBZ hypersensitivity and HLA-A*3101 in Caucasian patients [56]. This was originally shown in patients with hypersensitivity syndrome, and then replicated in another cohort of patients with CBZ-induced maculopapular exanthema. Sequence-based typing for the HLA alleles confirmed the association with HLA-A*3101, while further validation was also obtained by direct assessment of this allele in another group of Caucasian patients with a variety of phenotypes including SJS. Thus, unlike the association with HLA-B*1502 in Chinese patients which was specific for SJS/TEN, the association with HLA-A*3101 seems to be important for all forms of cutaneous eruptions mentioned above. The pathogenesis of this association needs further study; in particular with the distinct and strong associations with two HLA class I alleles, it will be interesting to determine whether both are causal alleles or whether they are in linkage disequilibrium with another causal variant in the MHC.

Allopurinol-Induced Serious Cutaneous Adverse Drug Reactions

Allopurinol is used for the treatment of gout. It causes hypersensitivity reactions, which like CBZ, can manifest in different ways, ranging from mild reactions to serious cutaneous adverse reactions (SCAR) such as hypersensitivity syndrome and SJS/TEN.

In 2005, Hung et al. [57] showed that HLA-B*5801 was strongly associated with allopurinol-induced SCAR, with 100% of 51 cases, compared with only 15% of 135 tolerant patients (odds ratio 580, 95% CI 34–9,781) being positive for the allele. The association has subsequently been replicated in Caucasians [49], Japanese [52], Thai [58] and South Korean [59] patients, indicating that the same allele can predispose patients of different ethnicities to a serious immunological reaction with the same drug. There are however some caveats: first, no prospective studies have been undertaken to show the utility of pre-prescription genotyping; second, it is not clear whether the milder exanthematous eruptions are associated with HLA-B*5801 [60], and third, we do not know whether HLA-B*5801 is the causal allele. Despite these reservations, the association between HLA-B*5801 and allopurinol-induced SCAR represents another remarkable example of how a distinct HLA allele can predispose to a serious cutaneous ADR.

Predisposition to Drug-Induced Blistering Disease

The examples of genetic associations described in the preceding sections are drug specific. However, if one considers that there may be some common final pathway(s) that lead to the same phenotypic manifestations, for example the blistering reactions, it may be theoretically possible to identify genetic predisposing factors that are not restricted to one drug. In order to investigate this, a recent study undertook a genome-wide approach by typing for 1 million SNPs in 96 cases of either SJS or TEN caused by a number of drugs [61]. Various loci including an SNP in the SLC transporter SLC22A23 were identified but failed to reach genome-wide significance (lowest p value detected was 10^{-6}). The odds ratios were typically in the region of 2 indicating that they were unlikely to show any clinical utility. The study shows that there may be some genetic predisposing factors for diseases such as SJS/TEN which are not drug specific, but these are certainly not going to be as clinically significant as those which have been identified with individual drugs such as CBZ and allopurinol. Nevertheless, further studies with greater statistical power are warranted in this area as the genetic loci identified may shed light on the mechanisms involved, and potentially provide novel targets for therapeutic intervention.

Conclusions and Future Perspectives

Predisposition to idiosyncratic ADRs such as those affecting the skin has always been hypothesised as being due to genetic factors. However, it is only now that we are beginning to uncover such genetic factors, some of which have made the difficult transition to clinical practice. To date, the most impressive findings have arisen from analysis of the HLA alleles in clinically well-characterised patient groups with different types of cutaneous reactions. It is also important to note that while this book focuses on cutaneous ADRs, the HLA system has also been shown to be important with respect to predisposing to liver injury with a number of drugs including flucloxacillin [62], co-amoxiclav [63], lapatinib [64], lumiracoxib [65] and ximelagatran [66].

The ultimate aim of undertaking research in this area is to implement any genetic predisposing factors into clinical practice to effect patient benefit. The best example where this has been achieved is AHS, where the period from the discovery of HLA-B*5701 as a predisposing factor to the use of the genetic test in clinical practice was 4 years in some countries, and 6–8 years in most countries. However, AHS pharmacogenetics probably represents the exception rather than the norm. We know that there are many translational gaps in medical research with most discoveries not even resulting in any clinical benefit, and even when they do, the time span between discovery and implementation is on average 17 years [67]. Careful planning, the availability of multidisciplinary teams, and the ability to recruit well-phenotyped patients from multiple, often international, centres is going to be key in demonstrating clinical validity and clinical utility of genetic biomarkers, and allow for successful implementation into clinical practice.

Acknowledgements

M.P. wishes to thank the Department of Health (NHS Chair of Pharmacogenetics), the Wellcome Trust, MRC, EU-FP7 and the Wolfson Foundation for their support. MP is a NIHR Senior Investigator.

References

1 Pirmohamed M, James S, Meakin S, et al: Adverse drug reactions as cause of admission to hospital: prospective analysis of 18,820 patients. BMJ 2004; 329:15–19.

2 Davies EC, Green CF, Taylor S, Williamson PR, Mottram DR, Pirmohamed M: Adverse drug reactions in hospital in-patients: a prospective analysis of 3,695 patient-episodes. PLoS One 2009;4:e4439.

3 Davies EC, Green CF, Mottram DR, Pirmohamed M: Adverse drug reactions in hospitals: a narrative review. Curr Drug Saf 2007;2:79–87.

4 Lazarou J, Pomeranz BH, Corey PN: Incidence of adverse drug reactions in hospitalized patients: a meta-analysis of prospective studies. J Am Med Assoc 1998;279:1200–1205.

5 Rawlins MD, Thompson JW: Mechanisms of adverse drug reactions; in Davies DM, (ed): Textbook of Adverse Drug Reactions. Oxford, Oxford University Press, 1991, pp 18–45.

6 Wadelius M, Pirmohamed M: Pharmacogenetics of warfarin: current status and future challenges. Pharmacogenomics J 2007;7:99–111.

7 Alfirevic A, Pirmohamed M: Drug-induced hypersensitivity reactions and pharmacogenomics: past, present and future. Pharmacogenomics 2010;11: 497–499.

8 Voight BF, Scott LJ, Steinthorsdottir V, et al: Twelve type 2 diabetes susceptibility loci identified through large-scale association analysis. Nat Genet 2010;42: 579–589.

9 Roujeau JC, Stern RS: Severe adverse cutaneous reactions to drugs. New Engl J Med 1994;331: 1272–1285.

10 Rawlins MD: Pharmacovigilance: paradise lost, regained or postponed? J R Coll Physicians Lond 1995;29:41–49.

11 Pirmohamed M, Aithal GP, Behr E, Daly A, Roden D: The phenotype standardization project: improving pharmacogenetic studies of serious adverse drug reactions. Clin Pharmacol Ther 2011;89:784–785.
12 Pirmohamed M, Friedmann PS, Molokhia M, et al: Phenotype standardization for immune-mediated drug-induced skin injury. Clin Pharmacol Ther 2011;89:896–901.
13 Hindorff LA, Sethupathy P, Junkins HA, et al: Potential etiologic and functional implications of genome-wide association loci for human diseases and traits. Proc Natl Acad Sci USA 2009;106:9362–9367.
14 Daly AK: Genome-wide association studies in pharmacogenomics. Nat Rev Genet 2010;11:241–246.
15 Alfirevic A, Pirmohamed M: Drug induced hypersensitivity and the HLA complex. Pharmaceuticals 2011;4:69–90.
16 Hetherington S, Hughes AR, Mosteller M, et al: Genetic variations in HLA-B region and hypersensitivity reactions to abacavir. Lancet 2002;359: 1121–1122.
17 Hughes DA, Vilar FJ, Ward CC, Alfirevic A, Park BK, Pirmohamed M: Cost-effectiveness analysis of HLA B*5701 genotyping in preventing abacavir hypersensitivity. Pharmacogenetics 2004;14:335–342.
18 Mallal S, Nolan D, Witt C, et al: Association between presence of HLA-B*5701, HLA-DR7, and HLA-DQ3 and hypersensitivity to HIV-1 reverse-transcriptase inhibitor abacavir. Lancet 2002;359: 727–732.
19 Bodmer W, Bonilla C: Common and rare variants in multifactorial susceptibility to common diseases. Nat Genet 2008;40:695–701.
20 Pirmohamed M, Park BK: Genetic susceptibility to adverse drug reactions. Trends Pharmacol Sci 2001; 22:298–305.
21 Green VJ, Pirmohamed M, Kitteringham NR, et al: Genetic analysis of microsomal epoxide hydrolase in patients with carbamazepine hypersensitivity. Biochem Pharmacol 1995;50:1353–1359.
22 Sullivan JR, Shear NH: The drug hypersensitivity syndrome: what is the pathogenesis? Arch Dermatol 2001;137:357–364.
23 Pirmohamed M, Naisbitt DJ, Gordon F, Park BK: The danger hypothesis – potential role in idiosyncratic drug reactions. Toxicology 2002;181–182: 55– 63.
24 Naisbitt DJ, Britschgi M, Wong G, et al: Hypersensitivity reactions to carbamazepine: characterization of the specificity, phenotype, and cytokine profile of drug-specific T cell clones. Mol Pharmacol 2003;63:732–741.
25 Naisbitt DJ, Farrell J, Wong G, et al: Characterization of drug-specific T cells in lamotrigine hypersensitivity. J Allergy Clin Immunol 2003;111:1393–1403.
26 Pichler WJ, Adam J, Daubner B, Gentinetta T, Keller M, Yerly D: Drug hypersensitivity reactions: pathomechanism and clinical symptoms. Med Clin North Am 2010;94:645–664, xv.
27 Easterbrook PJ, Waters A, Murad S, et al: Epidemiological risk factors for hypersensitivity reactions to abacavir. HIV Med 2003;4:321–324.
28 Phillips EJ, Sullivan JR, Knowles SR, Shear NH: Utility of patch testing in patients with hypersensitivity syndromes associated with abacavir. AIDS 2002;16:2223–2225.
29 Kauf TL, Farkouh RA, Earnshaw SR, Watson ME, Maroudas P, Chambers MG: Economic efficiency of genetic screening to inform the use of abacavir sulfate in the treatment of HIV. Pharmacoeconomics 2010;28:1025–1039.
30 Nieves Calatrava D, Calle-Martin Ode L, Iribarren-Loyarte JA, et al: Cost-effectiveness analysis of HLA-B*5701 typing in the prevention of hypersensitivity to abacavir in HIV+ patients in Spain. Enferm Infecc Microbiol Clin 2010;28:590–595.
31 Schackman BR, Scott CA, Walensky RP, Losina E, Freedberg KA, Sax PE: The cost-effectiveness of HLA-B*5701 genetic screening to guide initial antiretroviral therapy for HIV. AIDS 2008;22:2025–2033.
32 Rauch A, Nolan D, Martin A, McKinnon E, Almeida C, Mallal S: Prospective genetic screening decreases the incidence of abacavir hypersensitivity reactions in the Western Australian HIV cohort study. Clin Infect Dis 2006;43:99–102.
33 Waters LJ, Mandalia S, Gazzard B, Nelson M: Prospective HLA-B*5701 screening and abacavir hypersensitivity: a single centre experience. AIDS 2007;21:2533–2534.
34 Zucman D, Truchis P, Majerholc C, Stegman S, Caillat-Zucman S: Prospective screening for human leukocyte antigen-B*5701 avoids abacavir hypersensitivity reaction in the ethnically mixed French HIV population. J Acquir Immune Defic Syndr 2007; 45:1–3.
35 Saag M, Balu R, Phillips E, et al: High sensitivity of human leukocyte antigen-b*5701 as a marker for immunologically confirmed abacavir hypersensitivity in white and black patients. Clin Infect Dis 2008; 46:1111–1118.
36 Mallal S, Phillips E, Carosi G, et al: HLA-B*5701 screening for hypersensitivity to abacavir. New Engl J Med 2008;358:568–579.
37 Colombo S, Rauch A, Rotger M, et al: The HCP5 single-nucleotide polymorphism: a simple screening tool for prediction of hypersensitivity reaction to abacavir. J Infect Dis 2008;198:864–867.

38 Dello Russo C, Lisi L, Lofaro A, et al: Novel sensitive, specific and rapid pharmacogenomic test for the prediction of abacavir hypersensitivity reaction: HLA-B*57:01 detection by real-time PCR. Pharmacogenomics 2011;12:567–576.
39 Kostenko L, Kjer-Nielsen L, Nicholson I, et al: Rapid screening for the detection of HLA-B57 and HLA-B58 in prevention of drug hypersensitivity. Tissue Antigens 2011;78:11–20.
40 Chessman D, Kostenko L, Lethborg T, et al: Human leukocyte antigen class I-restricted activation of CD8+ T cells provides the immunogenetic basis of a systemic drug hypersensitivity. Immunity 2008;28: 822–832.
41 Chung WH, Hung SI, Hong HS, et al: Medical genetics: a marker for Stevens-Johnson syndrome. Nature 2004;428:486.
42 Hung SI, Chung WH, Jee SH, et al: Genetic susceptibility to carbamazepine-induced cutaneous adverse drug reactions. Pharmacogenet Genomics 2006;16: 297–306.
43 Man CB, Kwan P, Baum L, et al: Association between HLA-B*1502 allele and antiepileptic drug-induced cutaneous reactions in Han Chinese. Epilepsia 2007; 48:1015–1018.
44 Locharernkul C, Loplumlert J, Limotai C, et al: Carbamazepine and phenytoin induced Stevens-Johnson syndrome is associated with HLA-B*1502 allele in Thai population. Epilepsia 2008;49: 2087–2091.
45 Tassaneeyakul W, Tiamkao S, Jantararoungtong T, et al: Association between HLA-B*1502 and carbamazepine-induced severe cutaneous adverse drug reactions in a Thai population. Epilepsia 2010; 51:926–930.
46 Ding WY, Lee CK, Choon SE: Cutaneous adverse drug reactions seen in a tertiary hospital in Johor, Malaysia. Int J Dermatol 2010;49:834–841.
47 Mehta TY, Prajapati LM, Mittal B, et al: Association of HLA-B*1502 allele and carbamazepine-induced Stevens-Johnson syndrome among Indians. Indian J Dermatol Venereol Leprol 2009;75:579–582.
48 Alfirevic A, Jorgensen AL, Williamson PR, Chadwick DW, Park BK, Pirmohamed M: HLA-B locus in Caucasian patients with carbamazepine hypersensitivity. Pharmacogenomics 2006;7:813–818.
49 Lonjou C, Borot N, Sekula P, et al: A European study of HLA-B in Stevens-Johnson syndrome and toxic epidermal necrolysis related to five high-risk drugs. Pharmacogenet Genomics 2008;18:99–107.
50 Lonjou C, Thomas L, Borot N, et al: A marker for Stevens-Johnson syndrome. . .: ethnicity matters. Pharmacogenomics J 2006;6:265–268.
51 Ikeda H, Takahashi Y, Yamazaki E, et al: HLA class I markers in Japanese patients with carbamazepine-induced cutaneous adverse reactions. Epilepsia 2010; 51:297–300.
52 Kaniwa N, Saito Y, Aihara M, et al: HLA-B locus in Japanese patients with anti-epileptics and allopurinol-related Stevens-Johnson syndrome and toxic epidermal necrolysis. Pharmacogenomics 2008; 9:1617–1622.
53 Romano A, Gueant-Rodriguez RM, Viola M, Gaeta F, Caruso C, Gueant JL: Cross-reactivity among drugs: clinical problems. Toxicology 2005;209: 169–179.
54 Chen YC, Chu CY, Hsiao CH: Oxcarbazepine-induced Stevens-Johnson syndrome in a patient with HLA-B*1502 genotype. J Eur Acad Dermatol Venereol 2009;23:702–703.
55 Chen P, Lin JJ, Lu CS, et al: Carbamazepine-induced toxic effects and HLA-B*1502 screening in Taiwan. New Engl J Med 2011;364:1126–1133.
56 McCormack M, Alfirevic A, Bourgeois S, et al: HLA-A*3101 and carbamazepine-induced hypersensitivity reactions in Europeans. New Engl J Med 2011;364:1134–1143.
57 Hung SI, Chung WH, Liou LB, et al: HLA-B*5801 allele as a genetic marker for severe cutaneous adverse reactions caused by allopurinol. Proc Natl Acad Sci USA 2005;102:4134–4139.
58 Tassaneeyakul W, Jantararoungtong T, Chen P, et al: Strong association between HLA-B*5801 and allopurinol-induced Stevens-Johnson syndrome and toxic epidermal necrolysis in a Thai population. Pharmacogenet Genomics 2009;19:704–709.
59 Kang HR, Jee YK, Kim YS, et al: Positive and negative associations of HLA class I alleles with allopurinol-induced SCARs in Koreans. Pharmacogenet Genomics 2011;21:303–307.
60 Lee MH, Stocker SL, Anderson J, et al: Initiating allopurinol therapy: do we need to know the patient's HLA status? Intern Med J 2011, Epub ahead of print.
61 Shen Y, Nicoletti P, Floratos A, et al: Genome-wide association study of serious blistering skin rash caused by drugs. Pharmacogenomics J 2011, Epub ahead of print.
62 Daly AK, Donaldson PT, Bhatnagar P, et al: HLA-B*5701 genotype is a major determinant of drug-induced liver injury due to flucloxacillin. Nat Genet 2009;41:816–819.
63 Lucena MI, Molokhia M, Shen Y, et al: Susceptibility to amoxicillin-clavulanate-induced liver injury is influenced by multiple HLA class I and II alleles. Gastroenterology 2011;141:338–347.

64 Spraggs CF, Budde LR, Briley LP, et al: HLA-DQA1*02:01 is a major risk factor for lapatinib-induced hepatotoxicity in women with advanced breast cancer. J Clin Oncol 2011;29:667–673.
65 Singer JB, Lewitzky S, Leroy E, et al: A genome-wide study identifies HLA alleles associated with lumiracoxib-related liver injury. Nat Genet 2010;42:711–714.
66 Kindmark A, Jawaid A, Harbron CG, et al: Genome-wide pharmacogenetic investigation of a hepatic adverse event without clinical signs of immunopathology suggests an underlying immune pathogenesis. Pharmacogenomics J 2008;8:186–195.
67 Pirmohamed M: Acceptance of biomarker-based tests for application in clinical practice: criteria and obstacles. Clin Pharmacol Ther 2010;88:862–866.
68 Ozeki T, Mushiroda T, Yowang A, et al: Genome-wide association study identifies HLA-A*3101 allele as a genetic risk factor for carbamazepine-induced cutaneous adverse drug reactions in Japanese population. Hum Mol Genet 2011;20:1034–1041.
69 Roujeau JC, Huynh TN, Bracq C, Guillaume JC, Revuz J, Touraine R: Genetic susceptibility to toxic epidermal necrolysis. Arch Dermatol 1987;123:1171–1173.
70 Roujeau JC, Bracq C, Huyn NT, Chaussalet E, Raffin C, Duedari N: HLA phenotypes and bullous cutaneous reactions to drugs. Tissue Antigens 1986;28:251–254.
71 Hughes AR, Mosteller M, Bansal AT, et al: Association of genetic variations in HLA-B region with hypersensitivity to abacavir in some, but not all, populations. Pharmacogenomics 2004;5:203–211.
72 Hughes AR, Brothers CH, Mosteller M, Spreen WR, Burns DK: Genetic association studies to detect adverse drug reactions: abacavir hypersensitivity as an example. Pharmacogenomics 2009;10:225–233.
73 Romano A, De Santis A, Romito A, et al: Delayed hypersensitivity to aminopenicillins is related to major histocompatibility complex genes. Ann Allergy Asthma Immunol 1998;80:433–437.
74 Martin AM, Nolan D, James I, et al: Predisposition to nevirapine hypersensitivity associated with HLA-DRB1*0101 and abrogated by low CD4 T-cell counts. AIDS 2005;19:97–99.
75 Vitezica ZG, Milpied B, Lonjou C, et al: HLA-DRB1*01 associated with cutaneous hypersensitivity induced by nevirapine and efavirenz. AIDS 2008;22:540–541.
76 Littera R, Carcassi C, Masala A, et al: HLA-dependent hypersensitivity to nevirapine in Sardinian HIV patients. AIDS 2006;20:1621–1626.
77 Gatanaga H, Yazaki H, Tanuma J, et al: HLA-Cw8 primarily associated with hypersensitivity to nevirapine. AIDS 2007;21:264–265.
78 Chantarangsu S, Mushiroda T, Mahasirimongkol S, et al: HLA-B*3505 allele is a strong predictor for nevirapine-induced skin adverse drug reactions in HIV-infected Thai patients. Pharmacogenet Genomics 2009;19:139–146.
79 Likanonsakul S, Rattanatham T, Feangvad S, et al: HLA-Cw*04 allele associated with nevirapine-induced rash in HIV-infected Thai patients. AIDS Res Ther 2009;6:22.
80 Kim SH, Choi JH, Lee KW, et al: The human leucocyte antigen-DRB1*1302-DQB1*0609-DPB1*0201 haplotype may be a strong genetic marker for aspirin-induced urticaria. Clin Exp Allergy 2005;35:339–344.
81 Palikhe NS, Kim SH, Park HS: What do we know about the genetics of aspirin intolerance? J Clin Pharm Ther 2008;33:465–472.
82 Torres MJ, Mayorga C, Cornejo-Garcia JA, et al: Monitoring non-immediate allergic reactions to iodine contrast media. Clin Exp Immunol 2008;152:233–238.
83 Rodriguez-Perez M, Gonzalez-Dominguez J, Mataran L, Garcia-Perez S, Salvatierra D: Association of HLA-DR5 with mucocutaneous lesions in patients with rheumatoid arthritis receiving gold sodium thiomalate. J Rheumatol 1994;21:41–43.
84 Kazeem GR, Cox C, Aponte J, et al: High-resolution HLA genotyping and severe cutaneous adverse reactions in lamotrigine-treated patients. Pharmacogenet Genomics 2009;19:661–665.
85 Ozkaya-Bayazit E, Akar U: Fixed drug eruption induced by trimethoprim-sulfamethoxazole: evidence for a link to HLA-A30 B13 Cw6 haplotype. J Am Acad Dermatol 2001;45:712–717.
86 Pellicano R, Lomuto M, Ciavarella G, Di Giorgio G, Gasparini P: Fixed drug eruptions with feprazone are linked to HLA-B22. J Am Acad Dermatol 1997;36:782–784.

Prof. Munir Pirmohamed
The Wolfson Centre for Personalised Medicine
Department of Molecular and Clinical Pharmacology, University of Liverpool
Block A: Waterhouse Buildings, 1–5 Brownlow Street
Liverpool L69 3GL (UK)
Tel. +44 151 794 5549, E-Mail munirp@liv.ac.uk

French LE (ed): Adverse Cutaneous Drug Eruptions.
Chem Immunol Allergy. Basel, Karger, 2012, vol 97, pp 32–46

Etiology and Pathogenesis of Adverse Drug Reactions

O. Hausmann · B. Schnyder · W.J. Pichler

Department of Rheumatology and Clinical Immunology/Allergology, Inselspital, University of Bern, Bern, Switzerland

Abstract

In clinical routine, adverse drug reactions (ADR) are common, and they should be included in the differential diagnosis in all patients undergoing drug treatment. Only part of those ADR are immune-mediated hypersensitivity reactions and thus true drug allergies. Far more common are non-immune-mediated ADR, e.g. due to the pharmacological properties of the drug or to the individual predisposition of the patient (enzymopathies, cytokine dysbalance, mast cell hyperreactivity). In true drug allergies, T cell- and immunoglobulin E (IgE)-mediated reactions dominate the clinical presentation. T cell-mediated ADR usually have a delayed appearance and include skin eruptions in most cases. Nevertheless, it should not be forgotten that they may involve systemic T cell activation and thus take a severe, sometimes lethal turn. Clinical danger signs are involvement of mucosal surfaces, blistering within the exanthematous skin areas and systemic symptoms, e.g. fever or malaise. Drug presentation via antigen-presenting cells to T cells can either involve the classical pathway of haptenization of endogenous proteins or be directly mediated via noncovalent binding to immune receptors (MHC molecules or T cell receptors), the so-called p-i concept. Flare-up reactions during the acute phase of T cell-mediated ADR should not be mistaken for true drug allergies, as they only occur in the setting of a highly activated T cell pool. IgE-mediated ADR are less frequent and involve mast cells and/or basophils as peripheral effector cells. Recent data suggest that certain patients with drug allergy have a preexistent sensitization although they have never been exposed to the culprit drug, probably due to cross-reactivity. Thus, allergic drug reactions on first encounter are possible. In general, the extent of cross-reactivity is higher in IgE- compared to T cell-mediated ADR. Based on a specific ethnic background and only for severe T cell-mediated ADR to certain drugs, a strong HLA association has been established recently.

Essentials in a Nutshell

- Type A adverse drug reactions (ADR) are due to a pharmacological property of the causative drug, considered as pharmacotoxicological effects, and thus predictable

- Type B ADR comprise about 10–15% of all ADR, and include enzymopathies, cytokine or mediator dysbalances, nonspecific mast cell degranulation and specific immune reactions (true drug allergies)
- The vast majority of true drug allergies are considered to be either Ig-E (type I) or T cell mediated (type IV)
- T cell-mediated hypersensitivity reactions may be explained by the hapten/prohapten concept and/or by a pharmacological interaction of drugs with immune receptors (p-i concept)
- The hapten/prohapten concept may be a valid explanation for contact dermatitis, whereas p-i concept may play a major role in the effector phase of ADR to systemically applied drugs
- Recent data suggest that certain drug-allergic patients have a preexisting sensitization, although they have never been exposed to the culprit drug; thus drug allergies on first encounter are possible
- For severe T cell-mediated hypersensitivity reactions to certain drugs, a strong HLA association has been established recently

Introduction

The World Health Organization defines an ADR as a noxious and unintended response to a drug that occurs at a dose normally used in man [1]. ADRs encompass all adverse events related to drug administration, regardless of etiology or pathogenetic mechanism. A new drug usually undergoes toxicological and pharmacological tests in animals, followed by clinical trials in humans before it is authorized for marketing by drug regulatory agencies for specific indication(s). However, the preclinical and clinical premarketing investigation of a new drug does not always reveal all possible effects, side effects or adverse reactions. Most drugs are studied in less than 4,000 patients before approval. Therefore, drug reactions that occur in less than 1 in 1,000 patients are difficult to detect. In addition, premarketing trials often exclude special populations such as women of childbearing age, and many adverse reactions can be detected only in the presence of multiple cofactors of real life. They may also occur during off-label drug use and inappropriate administrations.

In the clinical setting, ADRs are a common and important public health problem, and they always need to be included in the differential diagnosis of patients under treatment with drugs. There are different classifications of ADRs [2–5] (table 1). Currently, the classification which has been proposed by Rawlins and Thompson is the most commonly used [6]. It differentiates two major subtypes:

- type A reactions which are due to a pharmacological propriety of the causative drug, and are thus predictable
- type B reactions which occur only in predisposed individuals and which are thus hard to predict.

Table 1. Classification of ADR

Type A (pharmacological; 85–90%)	side effects		
	drug interactions		
	others		
Type B (hypersensitivity)	nonspecific mechanisms	defective or absent enzymes	
		cytokine dysbalance	
		dysbalance of inflammatory mediators	
		nonspecific mast cell degranulation	
	specific immune reactions (true allergies)	type I: IgE mediated	
		type II: IgG-mediated cytotoxicity	
		type III: immune complex deposition	
		type IV: T cell mediated:	(a) monocytic inflammation (b) eosinophilic inflammation (c) cytotoxic T cells (d) neutrophilic inflammation

Type B reactions comprise approximately 10–15% of all ADR and encompass idiosyncrasies, other non-immune-mediated and immune-mediated reactions. Hypersensitivity reactions may be immune mediated and non-immune mediated [7], even though a few authors use the term hypersensitivity reaction synonymously with drug allergy. It is often stated that type B reactions are not dose dependent and unpredictable. Both statements are however wrong. Although certain type B reactions are elicited by low drug doses, the possibility of drug desensitization has demonstrated a clear dose dependency for such reactions as well; unpredictability is also no longer true, as some immune-mediated ADR can be predicted by genetic markers (e.g. abacavir hypersensitivity and HLA B5701; cf. below 'Genetic Factors') and this is likely to be more frequently the case in the future.

Pathogenesis

Type A Reactions

Type A reactions include pharmacotoxicological effects resulting from medication errors such as e.g. overdose, exaggeration of a drug's normal pharmacological actions in sensitive patients, interactions with other drugs and/or underlying illness, impaired metabolism or excretion, and effects that are not directly related to the desired pharmacological action of the drug. For their recognition, a complete history is essential. Sometimes, a thorough search for precedent medical treatment also with hidden xenobiotics is needed. Pharmacotoxicological effects and possible interactions of a certain drug are described in a pertinent summary of product characteristics or monographs. The search for interactions can be supported by computer-based drug interaction checkers. Unfortunately, drug monographs frequently do not clearly differentiate between adverse event (any undesirable event experienced by a patient whilst taking a medicine), ADR (event that is suspected to be caused by the drug), and different causes of ADRs (e.g. pharmacotoxicological or immune mediated). Thus, the diagnosis of an ADR and its cause can often only be assumed by the constellation of exposure, timing, and clinical features including the pattern of organ manifestations.

Type B Reactions

Defective or Absent Enzymes

Idiosyncratic reactions may be caused by an enzymopathy, congenital or acquired. In the affected patients, symptoms may arise due to slower or absent metabolism of the involved drug, causing an accumulation of the drug itself or of other substances to be processed.

Nonspecific Cytokine Dysbalance

Most cytokines are produced locally and have a predominant local activity. Thus, for most cytokines, only the local concentration is relatively high [8, 9]. If the cytokine is administered as a systemic therapy, the situation is reversed, with comparatively high systemic concentrations as required in order to achieve a sufficient local concentration at the site of interest. Such high systemic cytokine concentrations may lead to severe side effects limiting their use, for example, flu-like symptoms during interferon-α therapy. A different situation arises if a monoclonal antibody is directed against a potentially stimulatory receptor like CD3 on T cells (OKT3, muromunab) or CD28 on T cells (TGN1412). Under certain circumstances, the target cell releases a high amount of different cytokines. If those cytokines reach high systemic levels, they may cause various, occasionally severe symptoms [10] referred to as cytokine release syndrome (or cytokine storm). In the phase 1 clinical trial of TGN1412, the previously mentioned anti-CD28 antibody, this principle led to a near-fatal cytokine storm in the first 6 healthy volunteers investigated. Prior animal trials failed to reveal this ADR as the T cells of the animals chosen lacked CD28 on their surface [11]. The product was withdrawn from further trials.

Nonspecific Dysbalance of Inflammatory Mediators

Reactions to nonsteroidal anti-inflammatory drugs (NSAIDs) may comprise approximately 20–25% of all hypersensitivity reactions to drugs [12]. Hypersensitivity to aspirin and other NSAIDs may manifest similar to an immunoglobulin E (IgE)-mediated reaction with cutaneous symptoms such as urticaria and angioedema and/or with respiratory symptoms such as bronchospasm. There is good evidence that most of these reactions to NSAIDs are not IgE mediated, but caused by inhibition of the enzyme cyclooxygenase-1 (COX-1) in the skin and/or airways of hypersensitive patients. The inhibition of the COX-1 diminishes the production of prostaglandin E2 (PGE2) and, as a consequence, the production of the sulfidoleukotrienes LTC4, LTD4, and LTE4 is increased [13]. In addition, there is evidence that leukotriene C4 synthase is overexpressed in the bronchial mucosa of patients with respiratory hypersensitivity to NSAIDs [14].

Angiotensin-converting enzyme (ACE) inhibitor-induced cough or angioedema is another example of nonimmune-mediated hypersensitivity reactions caused by a dysbalance of inflammatory mediators. Bradykinin is degraded by kininase II (= ACE), and thus ACE inhibition reduces the catabolism of bradykinin, which accumulates in tissues [15, 16]. More recently, low levels of aminopeptidase P and dipeptidyl peptidase IV, enzymes known to catabolize bradykinin, have been suggested to be predisposing factors for the development of angioedema in patients treated with ACE inhibitors [17, 18].

Nonspecific Mast Cell Degranulation

Hypersensitivity to opiates such as codeine and morphine are common and usually limited to the skin (urticaria). These reactions are again not IgE mediated but probably caused by interaction with the endorphin receptor on mast cells and subsequent release of histamine and other mediators. As this is only partially inhibited by opiate receptor antagonists, components independent of opiate receptor binding may be also involved [19, 20]. Human mast cell opiate sensitivity may also vary, since in vitro cutaneous mast cells release inflammatory mediators after stimulation by morphine, whereas mast cells residing in lung, heart, and gastrointestinal tissues do not [21].

Formerly, neuromuscular blocking agents (NMBAs) and radio contrast media (RCM) were also considered to induce a non-IgE-mediated mast cell degranulation [22]. However, more recently several investigators found positive skin tests in vivo and basophil activation tests in vitro in patients with hypersensitivity reactions after NMBAs and RCM exposure. The tests were often positive only for the incriminated NMBA and RCM, and negative for the others. These findings suggest the involvement of immune mechanisms in a substantial part of such reactions

[23–25]. Interestingly, approximately 50% of patients with positive skin tests were found to have reacted on primary exposure, which may be best explained by preexistent sensitization to drug-independent cross-reactive antigens (see section on cross-reactivity below).

Specific Immune Reactions (True Allergies)

Sensitization

To induce a specific immune response, antigens have to be recognized by T cells presented on appropriate major histocompatibility complexes (MHC) by antigen-presenting cells (APCs). Most pharmaceutical agents are molecules of low molecular weight and not able to bind per se to MHC. The hapten/prohapten concept is the common explanation for primary sensitizations: drugs or their reactive metabolites gain immunogenicity by forming stable hapten carrier compounds with human proteins, mostly albumin [26]. These compounds are taken up as neoantigens by dendritic cells, processed and transported to the local draining lymphoid tissue and presented there. They may induce sensitization, if they are recognized by specific naïve T cells. The event of sensitization is usually clinically inapparent. It may involve T cells alone or both T and B cells with consecutive differentiation and generation of specific antibodies with determined isotype, depending on the cytokine pattern of the involved T cells [27]. Upon renewed exposure, concerned specific T cells and/or antibodies may mediate allergic reactions which can be divided into 4 categories corresponding to type I–IV reactions according Gell and Coombs [28]. The vast majority of real drug allergies are considered to be either Ig-E (type I) or T cell mediated (type IV).

IgE-Mediated Allergic Reactions

If the primary sensitization leads to the formation of drug-specific Ig-E, most of the specific primed B cells differentiate into plasma cells and secrete IgE antibodies that bind to high-affinity receptors (e.g. FcεRI) on the surface of mast cells and basophils. Upon renewed exposure, the causative drug binds to the Fab part of the IgE molecule. A current paradigm postulates that the antigen must be presented in multivalent form to induce an allergic reaction: binding of two or more cell surface-bound IgE molecules (crosslinking) leading to activation of the mast cell and the release of factors such as histamine, leukotrienes, prostaglandins and cytokines. These released molecules elicit vasodilatation, increased vascular permeability, enhanced mucus production, bronchoconstriction and contribute to eosinophil recruitment. IgE-mediated reactions to drugs often result in urticaria or angioedema. But they may include gastrointestinal and respiratory symptoms, shock and severe cardiac complications as well. The IgE/mast cell system is extremely sensitive, and even very small amounts of a causative drug may induce generalized and severe symptoms.

IgG-Mediated Cytotoxicity (Type II)

Type II reactions are based on IgG molecules predominantly directed against erythrocytes, leukocytes, platelets and probably also hematopoietic precursor cells in the bone marrow, and subsequent complement-dependent cytotoxicity of these cells. The antibody (and complement)-coated cells will be sequestrated to the reticuloendothelial system in the liver and spleen by Fc or complement receptor binding or, more rarely – intravascular destruction may occur by complement-mediated lysis. Different pathways of antibody recognition of target cells have been proposed [29–31]:

- Structures of cell membranes are modified by the hapten and drug, respectively, inducing an immune response directed against these target structures. Such development of an IgG immune reaction against the hapten-carrier complex is rather rare, and occurs after longer drug exposure times at high-dose treatment. Some antibody reactivity may be directed to the carrier molecule itself (= autoantibodies). This autoimmune form is less abrupt, but longer lasting after cessation of the drug.
- The drug induces conformational changes in structures of cell membranes resulting in nonspecific adherence with naturally occurring autoantibodies. Such a reaction may only occur as long as the drug is present in soluble form.

Immune Complex Deposition (Type III)

Formation of immune complexes is a common event during a normal immune response and does normally not cause symptoms. In type III reactions, the immune complexes formed activate endothelial cells with complement activation in small vessels and deposition due to Fc-IgG R interaction. Why and under which exact circumstances an immune complex disease develops is at present not clear. Clinical symptoms of a type III reaction comprise serum sickness, drug-induced lupus erythematosus and/or vasculitis.

T Cell-Mediated, Delayed Drug Hypersensitivity Reactions (Type IV)

Based on a large body of experimental, immunohistochemical and clinical data, there is strong evidence that most delayed immune-mediated drug hypersensitivity reactions with skin involvement are T cell mediated [32]. T cell-mediated hypersensitivity may result in the release of different patterns of cytokines with distinct functions. They can be further sub-classified as follows [33] (cf. fig. 1):

- Predominance of cytokines and chemokines that preferentially activate and recruit monocytes (type IVa)
- Predominance of cytokines and chemokines that preferentially activate and recruit eosinophils (type IVb)
- Predominance of cytotoxic functions by either CD4+ or CD8+ T cells (type IVc)
- Predominance of cytokines and chemokines that preferentially activate and recruit neutrophils (type IVd).

Antibody (I–III) and T cell-orchestrated hypersensitivity reactions (IVa–d)

	Type I	Type II	Type III	Type IVa	Type IVb	Type IVc	Type IVd
Immune reactant	IgE	IgG	IgG	IFNγ, TNFα (T_H1 cells)	IL-5, IL-4/IL-13 (T_H2 cells)	Perforin/ granzymeB (CTL)	CXCL-8, IL-17 GM-CSF (T cells)
Antigen	Soluble antigen	Cell- or matrix-associated antigen	Soluble antigen	Antigen presented by cells or direct T cell stimulation	Antigen presented by cells or direct T cell stimulation	Cell-associated antigen or direct T cell stimulation	Soluble antigen presented by cells or direct T cell stimulation
Effector	Mast cell activation	FcR+ cells (phagocytes, NK cells)	FcR+ cells complement	Macrophage activation	Eosinophils	T cells	Neutrophils
Example of hypersensitivity reaction	Allergic rhinitis, asthma, systemic anaphylaxis	Hemolytic anemia, thrombocytopenia (e.g. penicillin)	Serum sickness, Arthus reaction	Tuberculin reaction, contact dermatitis (with IVc)	Chronic asthma, chronic allergic rhinitis Maculopapular exanthema with eosinophilia	Contact dermatitis Maculopapular and bullous exanthema hepatitis	AGEP Behçet disease

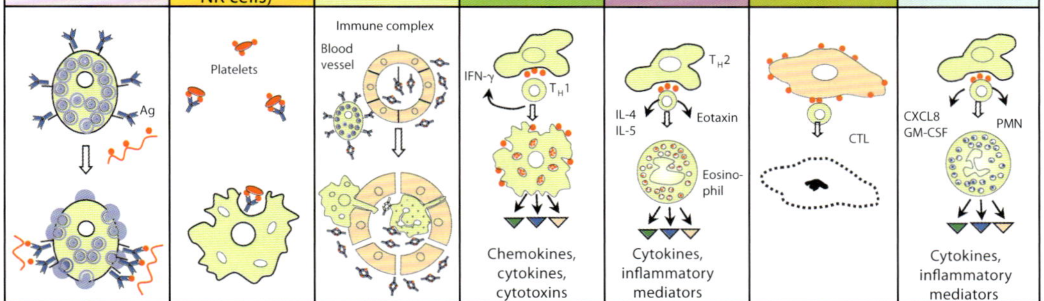

Fig. 1. Revised Gell and Coombs classification of drug reactions. Drugs can elicit all types of immune reactions. The effector function may rely mainly on antibody-mediated effector functions (type I–III) or more T cell/cytokine-dependent functions (type IVa–d). AGEP = Acute generalized exanthematous pustulosis; PMN = polymorphonuclear leukocyte; CTL = cytotoxic T lymphocytes; GM-CSF = granulocyte-macrophage colony-stimulating factor.

T cells react with the drug in two different ways. 'Immunologically', namely by 'recognizing' a hapten-modified peptide with their T cell receptor (TCR) in the frame of MHC molecules. This corresponds to a classical immune response and is highly relevant for contact dermatitis, and is due to haptens covalently bound to proteins and peptides. Alternatively, T cells may be stimulated 'pharmacologically' – the drug itself binds either directly to certain regions of the TCR, which results, together with MHC interaction, in a stimulation of this T cell with the particular T cell receptor, or the drug may modify MHC peptide complexes directly, making them immunogenic for T cells.

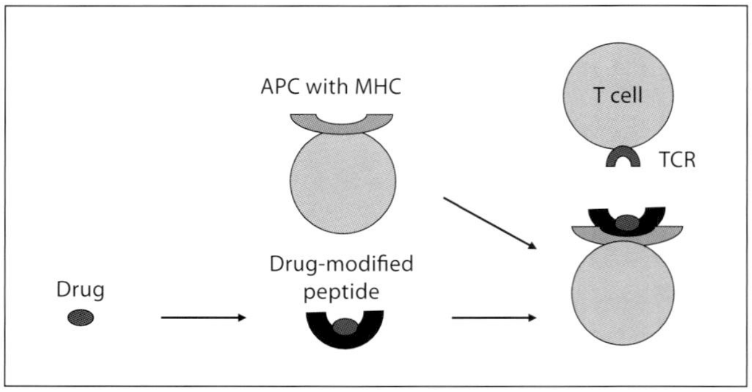

Fig. 2. Specific T cell recognition of drug carrier compounds (hapten/prohapten concept). Drug/drug metabolite carrier compounds are presented on APCs, where T cells with appropriate TCR recognize them.

Contact Dermatitis

Allergic contact dermatitis (ACD) is well investigated and can be explained by the hapten and prohapten concept [34, 35]. ACD is usually caused by molecules of low molecular weight (<500 Da). These small molecules can penetrate into the skin where they can interact with cutaneous proteins to form covalent adducts. However, many drugs (prohaptens) must first undergo metabolism (bioactivation) to become reactive metabolites (haptens) and to covalently bind to proteins to form hapten-carrier compounds. The hapten and prohapten concept postulates that even specifically primed T cells cannot recognize low molecular weight drugs unless they form stable hapten-carrier compounds which are presented by APCs on their MHC. Thus, the prohapten model attributes an important role in the effector phase to drug metabolism in the skin. Hapten-carrier complexes may be processed and presented on APCs in tissue residing APCs as well as in the lymph nodes (cf. fig. 2). There, they may restimulate primed T cells (TEff and TEM in the involved tissue or TCM in corresponding draining lymph nodes) [36, 37]. Upon systemic exposure to nickel, systemic contact dermatitis has also been observed in sensitive individuals [38].

Delayed-Type Hypersensitivity Reactions in the Skin after Systemic Drug Administration

A 'rash' is the most common manifestation of delayed-type hypersensitivity reactions after systemic drug administration. Such a reaction is hard to explain by the hapten/prohapten concept: Effector T cells (TEff and TEM) home to where the prohapten/hapten-carrier compounds derived from during primary sensitization [39, 40]. Drug derivatives will be predominantly presented at the site where they are applied (hapten-like drugs) or metabolized (prohapten drugs). Thus, the gastrointestinal tract (oral hapten drugs) or the liver (prohapten drugs) would be expected to be a preferred target organ for T cell-mediated allergies. Nevertheless, immune-meditated drug-induced gastroenteritis or hepatitis are rare events and much less frequent than would be predicted by the hapten/prohapten concept. Alternatively, delayed-type hypersensitivity reactions in the skin after systemic drug administration may be explained by pharmacological

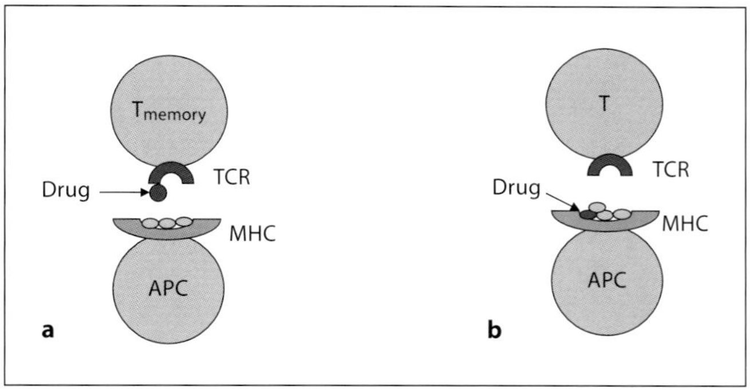

Fig. 3. Stimulation of specific T cells by a native drug (p-i concept). **a** T cells with a peptide specificity may be stimulated by an interaction of a native drug with the TCR, supplemented by the interaction with a fitting MHC molecule; preactivation of the T cell might be necessary to induce a reaction. **b** T cells recognize a drug-altered MHC-peptide complex: in contrast to the hapten concept, this modification is not due to covalent binding of the drug.

interactions of drugs with immune receptors (so-called p-i reaction). Most drugs exert their effects in tissues and organs into which they diffuse or were transported from the circulation. In contrast to classical protein antigens, they are not confined and concentrated in the lymph and lymphatic tissues, but are present throughout the body. If a sufficient drug concentration is reached in the tissue in vivo, drugs may not only fulfill their intended activity, e.g. block some receptor or enzyme activity, but also interact with the specific immune system, in particular with certain T cells with their highly polymorphous TCR. Actually, investigations of drug-specific human T cell clones (TCC) from drug allergic subjects have revealed specific reactivity against the causative drug in its native form without being processed or bound stably to a carrier molecule. Even chemically poorly reactive native drugs can reactivate TCC within minutes in the presence of both the inert drug and the APCs with the appropriate MHC [33, 41–44]. They are capable of transmitting specifically a stimulatory signal via the TCR, which activates specific T cells, resulting in proliferation, cytokine production and cytotoxicity (cf. fig. 3). To induce T cell activation via the p-i concept, the following conditions have to be fulfilled, if the stimulation occurs via drug binding to the TCR:

- The T cells express a TCR, into which the drug fits and can induce a stimulatory signal.
- The T cells have a low threshold for activation, which allows them to react to a 'minor' signal such as the drug binding to its TCR. Antigen-experienced, memory T cells (TEM) may have these properties.
- In addition to a sufficient drug concentration, APCs with an appropriate MHC are present. Thus, a dense network of T cells and APCs is favorable.

Recent findings indicate that such conditions are mainly found in the skin: TEM are highly concentrated in the skin [45], where they may act as 'sentinel' cells, rapidly stimulated by antigen penetrating the skin [45, 46]. In addition, the skin possesses a dense network of various dendritic cells acting as APCs – another feature which makes this organ predestined to become affected in hypersensitivity reactions due to the p-i concept.

However, the mechanism of TCR-dependent T cell sensitization by native drugs has not yet been elucidated. Memory T cells have a lower threshold for reactivation than naïve T cells [42, 47, 48]. Thus, it may be assumed that T cells which are preferentially reactivated by native drugs are memory cells (TEM or TCM) which have been previously primed by cross-reactive peptides from constantly present sources, e.g. herpes viruses.

Cross-Reactivity

Specific sensitization in drug-allergic patients may be induced not only by drug/drug metabolite carrier compounds but also by drug-independent cross-reactive antigens. The existence of such cross-reactivity is supported by recent findings: in 17 of 25 patients with cetuximab-induced anaphylaxis, IgE antibodies were found in pretreatment samples. The antibodies were shown to be specific for galactose-α-1,3-galactose [49], which is present on the Fab portion of the cetuximab heavy chain. Sensitization may have occurred via a tick bite. Another model is pholcodine, and anaphylaxis to NMBAs: patients exposed to pholcodine were shown to develop IgE antibodies towards pholcodine, which are cross-reactive with morphine and suxamethonium, which also carries a tertiary or quaternary ammonium group, and which is associated with allergy to NMBAs [50]. The fact that the cough sirup containing pholcodine was only marketed in Norway but not in Sweden elegantly explained the striking regional discrepancy in NMBA allergy.

Still unknown is the cross-reactive antigen in patients with IgE to iodinated contrast media: half of the patients with clinical hypersensitivity had a positive immediate skin test to iodinated contrast media and were found to have reacted on primary exposure without previous contact with contrast media in their history [51].

One could imagine that infectious antigens like viruses may lead to presentation of peptides which are cross-reactive with the TCR specific for certain drugs. Since chronic commensal viral infections are a persistent source of stimulation, cross-reactivity between drugs and such viruses might explain why drug-specific T cell reactivity can persist for a very long time even in the absence of the causative drug. A relationship between viral infections and the simultaneous or subsequent development of a drug rash has been observed in a number of distinct clinical situations, e.g. the detection of high levels of HHV6 DNA in severe T cell-mediated drug hypersensitivity syndrome [52].

Flare-Up Reactions

In patients with systemic drug allergies, e.g. drug rash with eosinophilia and systemic symptoms (DRESS/DIHS), the T cell compartment is extensively activated, similar to acute viral infections for which DRESS is sometimes mistaken. These patients seem to have a lower threshold to react to another, structurally unrelated drug. They might show a flare up of their rash to this second drug, which is often an antibiotic or virostatic drug administered in an attempt to treat the DRESS patient for an underlying infection. The patient is then labeled allergic to the initial and the second drug, but testing after remission might reveal an exclusive sensitization to the initial one. Provocation tests performed with the second drug at a time when the acute symptoms of drug allergy and the associated immune stimulation have resolved are negative in the vast majority of cases [pers. observ.].

The clinical observation of a flare-up reaction, and the previously mentioned cofactors for drug hypersensitivity reactions such as viral infections etc., suggest that an efficient stimulation of T cells by a drug is the sum of drug-TCR affinity and 'readiness' of the cell to react. Quite a few TCRs may have the ability to interact with drugs, probably with different affinities. If the immune system is resting, only drug-TCR interactions of high affinity may be able to stimulate T cells sufficiently to cause T cell expansion. But even such a high affinity interaction may remain 'silent' if too few cells are stimulated. If the immune system is activated and the readiness to react is increased (lower threshold), even drug-TCR interactions of relatively low affinity might suffice to activate many T cells, thus resulting in a symptomatic reaction. When the costimulatory conditions are no longer present, the low-affinity binding drug remains negative in skin tests and is later well tolerated. This hypothesis might also explain the transient nature of many exanthemas caused by antibiotics in childhood as the viral cofactors are missing during later testing and provocation.

Genetic Factors

The incidence of hypersensitivity varies between different ethnic groups. In addition, there are case reports with familial clustering of drug hypersensitivity, suggesting a genetic predisposition. In immune-mediated drug hypersensitivity, the most significant genetic associations have been identified for the MHC. Recent findings show a strong genetic association between HLA alleles and the susceptibility to drug-specific immune-mediated hypersensitivity: HLAB*5701 is associated with abacavir hypersensitivity, HLA-B*5801 with allopurinol-induced severe cutaneous adverse reactions including DRESS, SJS, and TEN, and HLA-B*1502 with carbamazepine-induced SJS and TEN, but not with maculopapular exanthema. Carbamazepine-SJS/TEN associated with B*1502 is seen in Southeast Asians but not in Caucasians [53]. A single gene may contribute to the risk of developing the hypersensitivity reaction, but each individual gene may be neither necessary nor sufficient by itself to cause the reaction.

Conclusion

Only a fraction of drug hypersensitivity reactions are mediated by a specific immune response and thus are true drug allergies. Most of these truly allergic reactions to drugs are T cell mediated. They are probably due to a multifactorial process and dependent on a complex interaction between genetic background and the environment. Drug allergies often have a bizarre clinical picture, possibly due to an unusual and not well-coordinated stimulation of the immune system, bypassing many rules and immunological 'checkpoints'. This situation is reminiscent of secondary syphilis. With the rise of effective antibiotic treatment for syphilis, drug hypersensitivity may have replaced this old human plague as the 'great imitator' of disease. The immune system is faced with a man-made challenge for which it was not trained during evolution – as the extensive use of drugs as foreign substances (xenobiotics) did not occur previously. The better understanding of these puzzling diseases in recent years has opened up the possibility of preventing many of them in the near future, as has been well demonstrated for abacavir and carbamazepine-induced reactions, where typing for immunogenetic markers dramatically reduced the incidence of severe forms of allergy to these drugs.

References

1 International drug monitoring: the role of national centres. Report of a WHO meeting. World Health Organ Tech Rep Ser 1972;498:1–25.

2 Edwards IR, Aronson JK: Adverse drug reactions: definitions, diagnosis, and management. Lancet 2000; 356:1255–1259.

3 Meyboom RH, Lindquist M, Egberts AC: An ABC of drug-related problems. Drug Saf 2000;22:415–423.

4 Aronson JK, Ferner RE: Joining the DoTS: new approach to classifying adverse drug reactions. BMJ 2003;327:1222–1225.

5 Nebeker JR, Barach P, Samore MH: Clarifying adverse drug events: a clinician's guide to terminology, documentation, and reporting. Ann Intern Med 2004;140:795–801.

6 Rawlins MD, Thompson JW: Pathogenesis of adverse drug reactions. In: Davies DM (ed) Textbook of adverse drug reactions. Oxford: Oxford University Press, 1977, pp 10–17.

7 Johansson SG, Bieber T, Dahl R, Friedmann PS, Lanier BQ, Lockey RF, et al: Revised nomenclature for allergy for global use: Report of the Nomenclature Review Committee of the World Allergy Organization, October 2003. J Allergy Clin Immunol 2004;113:832–836.

8 Abbas AK, Lichtman AH: Cellular and Molecular Immunology, 6th updated ed. Philadelphia: Saunders, 2009.

9 Desgeorges A, Gabay C, Silacci P, Novick D, Roux-Lombard P, Grau G, et al: Concentrations and origins of soluble interleukin 6 receptor-alpha in serum and synovial fluid. J Rheumatol 1997;24:1510–1516.

10 Vasquez EM, Fabrega AJ, Pollak R: OKT3-induced cytokine-release syndrome: occurrence beyond the second dose and association with rejection severity. Transplant Proc 1995;27:873–874.

11 Suntharalingam G, Perry MR, Ward S, Brett SJ, Castello-Cortes A, Brunner MD, et al: Cytokine storm in a phase 1 trial of the anti-CD28 monoclonal antibody TGN1412. N Engl J Med 2006;355: 1018–1028.

12 Faich GA: Adverse-drug-reaction monitoring. N Engl J Med 1986;314:1589–1592.

13 Szczeklik A, Stevenson DD: Aspirin-induced asthma: advances in pathogenesis, diagnosis, and management. J Allergy Clin Immunol 2003;111: 913–921, quiz 922.

14 Cowburn AS, Sladek K, Soja J, Adamek L, Nizankowska E, Szczeklik A, et al: Overexpression of leukotriene C4 synthase in bronchial biopsies from patients with aspirin-intolerant asthma. J Clin Invest 1998;101:834–846.

15 Israili ZH, Hall WD: Cough and angioneurotic edema associated with angiotensin-converting enzyme inhibitor therapy. A review of the literature and pathophysiology. Ann Intern Med 1992;117: 234–242.

16 Nussberger J, Cugno M, Amstutz C, Cicardi M, Pellacani A, Agostoni A: Plasma bradykinin in angio-oedema. Lancet 1998;351:1693–1697.
17 Adam A, Cugno M, Molinaro G, Perez M, Lepage Y, Agostoni A: Aminopeptidase P in individuals with a history of angio-oedema on ACE inhibitors. Lancet 2002;359:2088–2089.
18 Lefebvre J, Murphey LJ, Hartert TV, Jiao Shan R, Simmons WH, Brown NJ: Dipeptidyl peptidase IV activity in patients with ACE-inhibitor-associated angioedema. Hypertension 2002;39:460–464.
19 Casale TB, Bowman S, Kaliner M: Induction of human cutaneous mast cell degranulation by opiates and endogenous opioid peptides: evidence for opiate and nonopiate receptor participation. J Allergy Clin Immunol 1984;73:775–781.
20 Blunk JA, Schmelz M, Zeck S, Skov P, Likar R, Koppert W: Opioid-induced mast cell activation and vascular responses is not mediated by mu-opioid receptors: an in vivo microdialysis study in human skin. Anesth Analg 2004;98:364–370.
21 Tharp MD, Kagey-Sobotka A, Fox CC, Marone G, Lichtenstein LM, Sullivan TJ: Functional heterogeneity of human mast cells from different anatomic sites: in vitro responses to morphine sulfate. J Allergy Clin Immunol 1987;79:646–653.
22 Lagunoff D, Martin TW, Read G: Agents that release histamine from mast cells. Annu Rev Pharmacol Toxicol 1983;23:331–351.
23 Brockow K, Romano A, Aberer W, Bircher AJ, Barbaud A, Bonadonna P, et al: Skin testing in patients with hypersensitivity reactions to iodinated contrast media – a European multicenter study. Allergy 2009;64:234–241.
24 Ebo DG, Bridts CH, Hagendorens MM, Mertens CH, De Clerck LS, Stevens WJ: Flow-assisted diagnostic management of anaphylaxis from rocuronium bromide. Allergy 2006;61:935–939.
25 Mertes PM, Laxenaire MC: Allergic reactions occurring during anaesthesia. Eur J Anaesthesiol 2002;19: 240–262.
26 Riley RJ, Leeder JS: In vitro analysis of metabolic predisposition to drug hypersensitivity reactions. Clin Exp Immunol 1995;99:1–6.
27 Stavnezer J, Amemiya CT: Evolution of isotype switching. Semin Immunol 2004;16:257–275.
28 Gerber BO, Pichler WJ: Cellular mechanisms of T cell mediated drug hypersensitivity. Curr Opin Immunol 2004;16:732–737.
29 Aster RH: Drug-induced immune cytopenias. Toxicology 2005;209:149–153.
30 Reese JA, Li X, Hauben M, Aster RH, Bougie DW, Curtis BR, et al: Identifying drugs that cause acute thrombocytopenia: an analysis using 3 distinct methods. Blood 116:2127–2133.
31 Warkentin TE, Levine MN, Hirsh J, Horsewood P, Roberts RS, Gent M, et al: Heparin-induced thrombocytopenia in patients treated with low-molecular-weight heparin or unfractionated heparin. N Engl J Med 1995;332:1330–1335.
32 Roychowdhury S, Svensson CK: Mechanisms of drug-induced delayed-type hypersensitivity reactions in the skin. AAPS J 2005;7:E834–E846.
33 Pichler WJ: Delayed drug hypersensitivity reactions. Ann Intern Med 2003;139:683–693.
34 Gorbachev AV, Fairchild RL: Induction and regulation of T-cell priming for contact hypersensitivity. Crit Rev Immunol 2001;21:451–472.
35 Saint-Mezard P, Krasteva M, Chavagnac C, Bosset S, Akiba H, Kehren J, et al: Afferent and efferent phases of allergic contact dermatitis (ACD) can be induced after a single skin contact with haptens: evidence using a mouse model of primary ACD. J Invest Dermatol 2003;120:641–647.
36 Budinger L, Hertl M: Immunologic mechanisms in hypersensitivity reactions to metal ions: an overview. Allergy 2000;55:108–115.
37 Naisbitt DJ, Gordon SF, Pirmohamed M, Park BK: Immunological principles of adverse drug reactions: the initiation and propagation of immune responses elicited by drug treatment. Drug Saf 2000;23: 483–507.
38 Jensen CS, Lisby S, Larsen JK, Veien NK, Menne T: Characterization of lymphocyte subpopulations and cytokine profiles in peripheral blood of nickel-sensitive individuals with systemic contact dermatitis after oral nickel exposure. Contact Dermatitis 2004; 50:31–38.
39 Ebert LM, Schaerli P, Moser B: Chemokine-mediated control of T cell traffic in lymphoid and peripheral tissues. Mol Immunol 2005;42:799–809.
40 Mora JR, von Andrian UH: T-cell homing specificity and plasticity: new concepts and future challenges. Trends Immunol 2006;27:235–243.
41 Posadas SJ, Pichler WJ: Delayed drug hypersensitivity reactions – new concepts. Clin Exp Allergy 2007; 37:989–999.
42 Schmid DA, Depta JP, Luthi M, Pichler WJ: Transfection of drug-specific T-cell receptors into hybridoma cells: tools to monitor drug interaction with T-cell receptors and evaluate cross-reactivity to related compounds. Mol Pharmacol 2006;70:356–365.
43 Schnyder B, Mauri-Hellweg D, Zanni M, Bettens F, Pichler WJ: Direct, MHC-dependent presentation of the drug sulfamethoxazole to human alphabeta T cell clones. J Clin Invest 1997;100:136–141.

44 Zanni MP, von Greyerz S, Schnyder B, Brander KA, Frutig K, Hari Y, et al: HLA-restricted, processing- and metabolism-independent pathway of drug recognition by human alpha beta T lymphocytes. J Clin Invest 1998;102:1591–1598.
45 Clark RA, Chong B, Mirchandani N, Brinster NK, Yamanaka K, Dowgiert RK, et al: The vast majority of CLA+ T cells are resident in normal skin. J Immunol 2006;176:4431–4439.
46 Schaerli P, Moser B: Chemokines: control of primary and memory T-cell traffic. Immunol Res 2005;31:57–74.
47 Croft M: Activation of naive, memory and effector T cells. Curr Opin Immunol 1994;6:431–437.
48 Rogers PR, Dubey C, Swain SL: Qualitative changes accompany memory T cell generation: faster, more effective responses at lower doses of antigen. J Immunol 2000;164:2338–2346.
49 Chung CH, Mirakhur B, Chan E, Le QT, Berlin J, Morse M, et al: Cetuximab-induced anaphylaxis and IgE specific for galactose-alpha-1,3-galactose. N Engl J Med 2008;358:1109–1117.
50 Harboe T, Johansson SG, Florvaag E, Oman H: Pholcodine exposure raises serum IgE in patients with previous anaphylaxis to neuromuscular blocking agents. Allergy 2007;62:1445–1450.
51 Kvedariene V, Martins P, Rouanet L, Demoly P: Diagnosis of iodinated contrast media hypersensitivity: results of a 6-year period. Clin Exp Allergy 2006;36:1072–1077.
52 Descamps V, Valance A, Edlinger C, Fillet AM, Grossin M, Lebrun-Vignes B, et al: Association of human herpesvirus 6 infection with drug reaction with eosinophilia and systemic symptoms. Arch Dermatol 2001;137:301–304.
53 Chung WH, Hung SI, Chen YT: Human leukocyte antigens and drug hypersensitivity. Curr Opin Allergy Clin Immunol 2007;7:317–323.

Prof. Dr. Werner J. Pichler
Department of Rheumatology and Clinical Immunology/Allergology
Inselspital, University of Bern
CH–3010 Bern (Switzerland)
Tel. +41 31 632 2264, E-Mail werner.pichler@insel.ch

French LE (ed): Adverse Cutaneous Drug Eruptions.
Chem Immunol Allergy. Basel, Karger, 2012, vol 97, pp 47–60

Diagnostic Approach to Drug Allergy

Thomas Harr

Department of Dermatology, University Hospital Zurich, Zurich, Switzerland

Abstract

The approach to drug hypersensitivity always comprises a clinical and a diagnostic workup. About 15% of drug side effects are due to hypersensitivity reactions. All types of immunological reactions can be induced by drugs, but type I and type IV reactions are seen most often. The initial judgment of the skin symptoms is therefore one of the key factors besides a stringent history of drug intake for a further diagnostic workup. The goal of a diagnostic workup is not only to identify the culprit drug, but also to defer the patient from similar drugs in order to prevent a second episode. In the case of missing alternatives and unidentified drug sensitivity, reexposure to the previous drug must be discussed; however, in severe cutaneous reactions this should generally be avoided.

Essentials in a Nutshell

- Different diagnostic approaches including skin and as well laboratory tests exist to identify causative substances in drug hypersensitivity reactions
- Identification of the causative drug may help prevent patients from having recurrent potentially more severe reactions also to crossreactive drugs

Introduction

The first step in the diagnostic approach to drug allergy is to suspect a hypersensitivity reaction to an applied drug. Next, the suspicion must be substantiated by history, clinical picture, skin and laboratory testing and sometimes drug provocation.

A useful diagnostic approach always starts with a history of drug exposure (dosage, time of intake, interval between beginning or stop of intake and start of skin or other clinical manifestations). However, a careful history must also be taken for previous drug exposure due to the fact that with earlier intake a sensitization is possible, and for potential cross-reactive drugs given to a patient with a known history to

Table 1. Indications and sensitivity of diagnostic tests in drug allergy

Tests (method)	Indications	Sensitivity	Limitations/remarks
Prick test	Type I reaction	Low	Only immediate read-out
Prick/scratch test	Type I reaction	Higher compared to prick test	Frequent skin irritation, difficult interpretation
Intradermal test	Type I reaction/ type IV reaction	Higher compared to prick test	Immediate and late read-out Irritation (immediate read-out), only sterile preparations of drugs approved for human use
Scratch/patch test Patch test	Type IV reaction		Only late read-out AGEP: consider read-out after 96 h or longer!
BAT (flow cytometry)	Type I reaction		
LTT	Type IV reaction (type I–III, less sensitive)	Highest for DRESS, low for bullous exanthema	
Cytotoxicity assay	Bullous drug reactions	Possibly higher sensitivity compared to LTT	Experimental, technique under evaluation

DRESS = Drug reaction with eosinophilia and systemic symptoms.

drug allergy to similar medications. Reexposure must also always be suspected given the increased usage of generic medications with the same ingredients but different brand names. The assessment of the actual clinical picture is a second mainstay in the approach to the diagnosis of drug allergy. A careful skin examination should always be performed as these symptoms can give a hint what type of drug hypersensitivity might be involved (type I–IV) and directs future diagnostic workup. Furthermore, peripheral lymph nodes and mucosal membranes should be inspected. The diagnostic workup should also include a complete blood count, liver function tests, the measurement of body temperature, and in the case of severe or unknown skin signs a skin biopsy, optionally with direct immunofluorescence. Only confronting all these investigations together with the history give the physicians the adequate tools to make an assessment of the severity of the disease, to narrow in the diagnosis for drug allergy, and to decide if selected drugs should be discontinued.

The further diagnostic work-up of a suspected culprit involved drug is usually done after cessation of clinical symptoms. Skin tests, if available, are often a primary approach in identifying a potential causative drug. Skin prick and scratch tests are used for immediate type reactions, whereas patch tests are used for delayed type reactions. Intradermal testing can be used in both above-mentioned reaction types (table 1).

Lymphocyte transformation (LTT) and basophil activation tests (BAT) are the most frequently used ex vivo/in vitro test systems. Whereas LTT mainly focuses on the detection of drug-specific T lymphocytes, the BAT attempts to indirectly detect drug-specific IgE bound to receptors of basophil cells. Unfortunately, drug-specific IgE only exist for a few drugs such as e.g. penicillins and amoxicillin.

Diagnostic Approach for Selected Types of Adverse Cutaneous Drug Reactions

Stevens-Johnson Syndrome/Toxic Epidermal Necrolysis (Lyell Syndrome)

Toxic epidermal necrolysis (TEN) and Stevens-Johnson syndrome (SJS) are severe adverse cutaneous drug reactions that predominantly involve the skin and mucous membranes. A detailed drug history is very important to identify the culprit drug in SJS/TEN. In some cases, several drugs are possible candidates, and allergological testing can be helpful in identifying the most likely candidate. Although two case reports describe intradermal testing without triggering a second episode of TEN [1, 2], in principle, the severity of SJS and TEN does not allow rechallenge and intradermal testing with the culprit drugs due to the risk of re-inducing a second episode of SJS/TEN. Induction of SJS/TEN has, however, been documented following local eye treatment [3, 4]. Patch testing might be an option, but not routine to date. Data from Wolkenstein et al. [5] have shown that low sensitivity is however a problem with patch testing in SJS/TEN, as only 2 of 22 tested patients had a relevant positive patch test. In this study patch testing did not trigger severe cutaneous reactions. Due to the low sensitivity and a lack of larger safety studies patch testing cannot be recommended up to date.

Currently, allergy testing in SJS/TEN focuses on ex vivo/in vitro tests. The LTT, measuring the proliferation of T cells to a drug in vitro, has a sensitivity of 60–70% for patients allergic to beta-lactam antibiotics [6]. Unfortunately, the sensitivity of the LTT is low in SJS/TEN even if performed within one week after onset of the disease [7]. Another recently reported approach analyzes upregulation of CD69 on T lymphocytes as a sign of drug hypersensitivity 2 days after lymphocyte stimulation in vitro [8]. However, published data show similar sensitivity to the LTT.

Recently, Zawodniak et al. [9] introduced a new modified cytotoxicity test. This test aims at identifying specific cytotoxic lymphocytes using an ELISPOT for the measurement of granzyme B release and flow cytometry for the detection of upregulation of the degranulation marker CD107. In a small series, this test showed promising results. Thus, it might be an interesting additional test in the future, especially as it does not rely on proliferation [10].

Acute Generalized Exanthematous Pustulosis

Acute generalized exanthematous pustulosis (AGEP) is an acute febrile, generalized rash with small uniform noninfectious, nonfollicular associated pustules with typical involvement of intertriginous and flexural regions, and a predilection for females. In the vast majority of cases, AGEP is induced by drugs, mainly by anti-infectives (antibiotics, antimalarials and antifungals).

The diagnostic procedures include in vivo diagnostics with patch testing and ex vivo LTT in order to identify drug-specific T cells, either indirectly by performing patch tests, or by monitoring proliferation of specific T cells (directly and indirectly) ex vivo. Patch testing in order to identify the culprit drug has an intermediate sensitivity (approximately 50%). Therefore, in addition to classical readings after 48 and 72 h, readouts either at 96 or 120 h are advised in order to increase sensitivity. Like in acute AGEP, pustule formation can be observed at the patch test site. The test should be done as early as one month after resolution of the exanthema. The sensitivity of patch testing for the identification of the culprit drug was 50% in a small case series [5]. The possibility of induction of AGEP due to patch-testing is generally considered to be low.

As a further tool besides patch tests, LTT or interferon-γ release tests can be performed in the case of negative or nonconclusive patch tests in order to increase sensitivity of diagnostic procedures [6, 11, 12].

Fixed Drug Eruption

Fixed drug eruption (FDE) represents a late type hypersensitivity reaction against a single drug or a combination of different, structurally related drugs [13]. The typical clinical features are sharply defined livid plaques with a site preference on the face/lips, hands and genital area. In the case of manifestation with multiple plaques, the clinical picture might resemble erythema multiforme and may be difficult to distinguish even with the use of histology [14]. Recurrence of FDE after intake of the culprit drug typically occurs at the same site, suggesting a local allergic phenomenon. Unfortunately, the typical skin hyperpigmentation is infrequent. According to Ozkaya-Bayazit et al. [15], a correlation between the type of the culprit drug and the involved areas could only be established for tetracycline, naproxen and metamizol. As to the frequency of involved drugs, regional differences were found: whereas in France paracetamol/acetaminophen seems to be the most common substance inducing FDE, followed by NSAIDs [16], a Turkish study found sulfamethoxazole/trimethoprim followed by naproxen, dyprone, dimenhydrinate and paracetamol to be the most frequent drugs [15].

Classical patch testing is considered the mainstay of diagnostic procedure. However, in FDE patch testing should be done on previously affected skin. A modified form of patch testing in formerly affected skin, the open topical provocation test, showed a higher sensitivity compared to the read out of the patch test or open topical test in formerly unaffected skin [17]. In order to increase the permeability through the skin, DMSO was used as an additional vehicle and showed a higher sensitivity for sulfamethoxazole/trimethoprime [17]. Similar results were found in the study of Ozkaya-Bayazit et al. [18], where 27 patients with known FDE after oral provocation with sulfamthoxazole/trimethoprime underwent skin testing. Open testing with sulfamethoxazole/trimethoprim in DMSO (10–20% in the genital area, 50% on the skin) showed a positive reaction at the former reaction site in 25 out of 27 patients, whereas only one patient showed a positive reaction in formerly unaffected skin.

Diagnostic Approach in Hypersensitivity Reactions to Selected Substances

Excipients and Stabilizers

Although in the vast majority of cases the culprit drug itself is the cause for the adverse reaction, sometimes excipients and stabilizers can also be the cause of the adverse reaction. The identification of these molecules as causative agents is inevitable in order not to prevent patients from using important and well-tolerated drugs, and also to prevent secondary events due to the involvement of excipients/stabilizers in other structurally nonrelated drug preparations.

Immediate-type reactions are well documented for carboxymethylcellulose (CMC) and macrogol/polyethyleneglycol. Therefore, it is advisable to screen all preparations for possible allergens beside the active molecule. CMC is typically used in many injectable glucocorticosteroid preparations [19]. Injectable glucosteroid preparations are often used in combination with local anesthetics for infiltration in orthopedic and rheumatological procedures. Several case reports and small case series were able to identify CMC as the single causative agent in the anaphylactic event to glucocorticoid preparations and not the suspected glucocorticoid itself [20–24].

CMC should therefore always be tested separately. Besides prick testing, it is advisable to perform intradermal testing with diluted CMC in different concentrations. CMC is also available for basophil activation testing. In addition, specific IgE can be measured, but the usefulness of a positive reaction is doubtful due to high prevalence of CMC-specific IgE in the normal unaffected population [25]. Whereas most CMC allergic patients tolerate CMC by oral route [26], there are single case reports of near-fatal immediate type reactions after a diagnostic procedure of barium enema [27].

Macrogol/polyethyleneglycol is used in food, cosmetics and medications. It can be the causative agent for immediate-type reactions not only with parenteral application, but also with oral or topical application. Besides case reports of anaphylactic reactions after parenteral macrogol containig glucocorticoid preparations [28], there are case reports for evacuant solutions [29], macrogol-containing penicillin tablets, fluoride tablets and cetomacrogol-containing cream [30]. Interestingly, all of these affected patients tolerated macrogol-containing food. In addition to skin prick testing, the diagnostic workup includes scratch testing and if available intradermal sterile macrogol testing in serial dilution. Oral challenge should only be discussed in the case of negative testing, and the need to identify Macrogol as an allergen due to lack of alternative medications or repeated events of recurrent immediate-type reactions without having identified other allergens.

Iodine-Containing Preparations

Iodine-containing contrast media (ICM) can induce pseudoallergic and allergic reactions. Due to the structure of ICM, immediate or late-type reactions are reported already at the first application. Pseudoallergic immediate-type reactions can be triggered by unspecific mast cell liberation and can lead to pruritus, urticaria, angioedema, respiratory and gastrointestinal symptoms and shock [31]. Late-type pseudoallergic reactions might be triggered by a direct interaction of the molecule with the MHC-II complex of an antigen-presenting cell and the T cell receptor inducing a T cell-specific response with a maculopapular rash (p-i concept) [32]. Apart from the above-mentioned unspecific reactions, all types of hypersensitivity mechanisms can be seen after application of ICM. Approaches to identify a sensitivity towards an ICM are difficult, because the actual tests have only a modest sensitivity, and the clinical symptoms do not always allow to discriminate between pseudoallergic and allergic reactions.

The diagnostic approach hence starts with a careful skin examination in order to rule out a cutaneous mastocytosis that might be the reason for an urticarial rash, due to the mast cell-liberating properties of ICM. Additionally, serum tryptase level should be determined. Serum tryptase within the normal range excludes systemic mastocytosis to a large extent. In a second-step skin testing, especially intradermal testing is a feasible approach. The European Network of Drug Allergy has collected data of several centers and concluded that skin testing has a very high specificity, but a low to intermediate sensitivity for immediate-type (50%) and late-type (47%) reactions. Interestingly, cross-reactivity among the different groups of ICM was higher in patients with late-type reactions. However, the question why certain patients are skin test positive already after a single application of ICM is still under investigation [31]. The additional use of LTT is also still under investigation. Thereby, it has to be kept in mind that due to the structure of ICM (p-i concept, unspecific discrete proliferation) the proliferation response has to be stronger for a positive result (stimulation index positive >2, ICM >4) [10]. Most cases of hypersensitivity reactions to ICM show that the ICM is the culprit drug and not iodine [33]. Rechallenge should only be discussed with skin test-negative ICM which are structurally different (monomer – dimer, ionic – non-ionic). Rechallenge has to be avoided in all patients with severe cutaneous adverse reactions such as SJS/TEN.

Antineoplastic Drugs

Antineoplastic drugs are a common and rising cause for drug hypersensitivity due to their increasing use, new agents and repeated use in the context of cycles of chemotherapy or complex therapeutic modalities after relapse. Additionally, patients with neoplasia, such as lymphoma, or patients with cranial irradiation have a higher probability of developing severe adverse drug reactions. Thus, major problems in identifying a drug hypersensitivity and the culprit drug are the polymedication, repeated use (chemotherapeutic cycles) and concomitant immunosuppression leading to higher infection rates. A careful history of drug intake and onset of the skin or other reactions must be precisely documented. In certain cases, skin biopsies are a useful tool discriminating allergic from nonallergic reactions. Reactions should be distinguished according to time of occurrence, i.e. during the infusion or shortly after (max. 1 h), and hours to days later. Careful examination of the skin is advisable in some cases over several days in order not to miss potentially life-threatening cutaneous manifestations such as erythema multiforme, SJS and TEN (Lyell's syndrome). Only after initial assessment of these facts does allergic diagnostic workup make sense. As cancer is a potentially life-threatening disease, therapeutic options must be as wide as possible. On the other hand, rechallenge of an unidentified allergen in cancer patients can be fatal, especially in those with a history of severe anaphylaxis or SJS/TEN. As an alternative to rechallenge (with or without antiallergic medication, infusion time alteration), desensitization can be discussed in patients with a clinical immediate-type reaction and a negative skin test for late reactions.

Although drug hypersensitivity has been described for many antineoplastic drugs and successful desensitization protocols exist for a wide variety of different antineoplastic drugs, including rituximab [34], platinum salts (carboplatin, cisplatin, oxaliplatin) are often in the center of interest for suspected drug allergy. Platinum salt-containing chemotherapies for ovarian, lung, head and neck and colorectal cancer are often identified as hypersensitivity-causing drugs.

The incidence of cross-sensitization among the different platinum salts, carboplatin, cisplatin, and oxaliplatin is still unclear [35]. Skin tests with carboplatin might identify patients who are in danger or will tolerate rechallenge with carboplatin. Whereas certain reports were able to predict safe rechallenges with skin tests, other reports question this. Therefore, it is advisable in skin test-positive and skin test-negative patients after immediate-type reactions to use desensitization protocols upon rechallenge with the same platinum preparation. An alternative strategy might be to switch to another skin test-negative platinum and rechallenge it with or without desensitization [36–45].

Neuromuscular Blocking Agents

Neuromuscular blocking agents (NMBA) are potent unspecific mast cell liberators, often causing urticarial reactions without a drug sensitization. Nevertheless, specific sensitization to NMBA has been described, and this poses a serious problem in anesthetics due to almost exclusively immediate-type reactions leading to anaphylaxis in severe cases. The primary approach to the patient with suspected NMBA pseudo-allergy/allergy is a thorough skin examination to rule out cutaneous mastocytosis. Serum tryptase levels should be measured to rule out systemic mastocytosis. In a next step, intradermal skin tests should be performed by using different concentrations of usual NMBA in order to identify the causative drug and to get an overview of potential cross-sensitization between different NMBA. The major problem of skin testing is false positive results due to unspecific mast cell release with high concentrations of NMBA leading to inappropriate diagnoses of NMBA allergy.

Newer NMBAs as for example rocuronium and cisatracurium have either no metabolites (rocuronium) or only very low levels of metabolites (cisatracurium). Therefore, skin testing can be performed with the active drugs without missing potential allergic effects due to unknown or not testable metabolites [46]. In a French study, false positive results were found with dilutions lower than 1:100, but rocuronium and mivacurium should only be used up to a concentration of 1:200 [47], although a Norwegian study showed in some cases positive results at 1:1,000 dilution for rocuronium and cisatracurium [48]. Other approaches to evade the skin testing problems and to increase the sensitivity of detection of the culprit drug, but also to get more precise knowledge about potential cross-sensitization among NMBA, are conventional or flow cytometry-assisted BAT and specific IgEs against suxamethonium, rocuronium, morphine, pholcodine and quaternary ammonium morphine [49–52].

Betalactams

Penicillins, cephalosporins, carbapenems and monobactams are typical representatives of betalactam antibiotics. Maculopapular rash, a late-type skin reaction is the most frequent manifestation for all betalactam antibiotic allergies, followed by immediate-type reactions, as e.g. urticaria and anaphylaxis. Betalactam hypersensitivity is the best-studied drug allergy, and a diagnostic workup is more or less standardized, in contrast to almost all other drug groups. The European Network on Drug Allergy has also published position papers on how to identify possible betalactam-allergic patients.

The diagnosis of late- and immediate-type reactions to betalactam antibiotics comprises skin tests, specific IgE and ex vivo tests (LTT, BAT). The main goal of the diagnostic workup is not only to identify a betalactam allergy, but also to assess potential cross-reactivities within the betalactam antibiotic group.

The diagnostic approach to immediate-type reactions, mainly to penicillins and cephalosphorins, is always a combination of skin and ex vivo tests. Besides testing the whole intact molecule (penicillin, amoxicillin, cephalosporins, etc.) with skin prick and intradermal testing and performing readouts within 20–30 min, penicilloyl-polylysine (PPL) and minor determinant mixtures (MDM) are tested additionally. Serological tests for the detection of IgE against penicillin and amoxicillin are marketed. A cellular-based BAT can be used to get more information about a possible IgE-mediated betalactam allergy. Bousquet et al. [53] report a sensitivity of 46% to PPL and MDM. Whereas PPL and MDM have a clear role in the detection of immediate-type reactions to penicillins, the additional use of amoxicilloic acid and diketopiperazine besides amoxicillin in skin tests to potential amoxicillin-allergic patients did not increase the sensitivity of the skin test [54]. However, the use of serological tests to identify specific IgE to benzylpenicilloyl and amoxicilloyl increased the sensitivity not only for penicillin- but also for amoxicillin-allergic patients, when used in combination with skin tests [55]. However, in one study 27% of patients with both skin test and IgE negative to penicillins, were rechallenged with benzylpenicillin and amoxicillin. Fifty-five percent of the rechallenged patients showed an immediate type reaction towards the applied penicillin [56]. BAT should be used in patients with a high suspicion of immediate-type betalactam allergy and negative skin tests in order to increase the sensitivity, and minimize false negative results and consecutively endangering patients when penicillin is readministered [57, 58].

A major goal besides the identification of immediate-type sensitization to penicillin, is to evaluate patients for potential cross-reactivity to other betalactams, in order not to withhold important medications in severe infections. Romano et al. [59] identified cross-sensitivity between penicillins and cephalosporins among penicillin-allergic patients in 10.9% of cases by skin testing with cephalosporins. All patients with negative skin testing to cephalosporins underwent provocation tests, and all of them tolerated the applied cephalosporins, rendering skin tests a useful screening test before drug challenge.

The potential cross-reactivity in immediate-type reactions between penicillins and carbapenems are considered to be low, and could be confirmed with skin tests and negative graded drug challenges in different studies in children and adults (ca. 1%) [60–62]. One study rechallenged the immediate-type penicillin-allergic patients directly without skin testing with the carbapenem meropenem, without any adverse reaction in any of the patients [63].

The monobactam aztreonam is tolerated in IgE-positive betalactam antibiotic allergic patients, although a skin prick test with a negative result with aztreonam should be required before application [64].

So far, only patients with immediate-type reactions to the cephalosporin ceftazidime are considered to have potential cross-sensitivity to the monobactam aztreonam due to similar side chains [60].

Cross-sensitivity among penicillin and cephalosporins in immediate-type reactions are in the majority probably due to side chain-specific immune reactions [65, 66]. Among the two side chain positions, the side chain directly linked to the thiazolidin ring (R1) plays the more important role in cross-reactivity than the betalactam structure among penicillins and cephalosporins [67]. Even among different cephalosporins, the side chain R1 is important in recognizing the molecule as an antigen. Interestingly, 2/3 of patients with immediate-type cephalosporin reactions are only positive to the incriminated cephalosporin, and not to other ones [67]. Furthermore, negative skin tests to penicillin in cephalosporin-positive patients predict penicillin tolerability [67].

Non-immediate-type, or late-type reactions in betalactam antibiotics are prone to patch testing or intradermal testing with read out after 24–48 h. Although intradermal testing tends to have a higher sensitivity compared to patch testing, intradermal testing might also have a slightly higher false positive rate [68]. However, the sensitivity for both delayed-type tests is low for benzylpenicillin, amoxicillin and cephalosporins [69–71].

In delayed-type reactions, LTT should be considered in test-negative patients. The sensitivity of the LTT for potential betalactam allergy in well-documented and in severe cases is significantly higher compared to the intradermal and patch tests. Furthermore, a very high specificity is shown; however, the disadvantage of the LTT is time consumption, the need for laboratory skills and radioactivity [10].

Cross-reactivity in delayed-type hypersensitivity between aminopenicillin and cephalosporins without an aminobenzyl side chain is very low, and even between aminopenicillin and benzylpenicillin, 72% of patients tolerated benzylpenicillin [71].

Cross-sensitization in delayed-type reactions between penicillin and carbapenems are reported in 0% (meropenem) [63], 5.5% (imipenem-cilastin) [72] and 9.2% (meropenem or imipenem/cilastin) of cases [73].

In delayed-type allergy to betalactam antibiotics, all monobactam aztreonam-challenged patients tolerated the drug [74]; however, none of these patients were known to be allergic or tested to ceftazidim.

Biologicals

Biologicals are a heterogeneous group of human and chimeric proteins with different structures and different molecular targets. Side effects were recently classified into 5 classes: alpha (cytokine associated), beta (classical hypersensitivity, typically immediate and late type), gamma (immune and cytokine imbalance), delta (cross-reactivity) and epsilon (nonimmunological side effects) [75, 76]. In this context, Benucci et al. [77] analyzed data of classical hypersensitivity adverse reactions to biologicals in terms of the frequency in atopic patients, and were able to show that there is no increased risk in atopic patients. The diagnostic approach to this heterogeneous group of biologicals requires a thorough clinical workup. A neurodermitis-like clinical presentation can be due to a cytokine imbalance mediated by TNF-α inhibitors as a class effect, and does not reflect a drug hypersensitivity, whereas acute urticaria and rhinitis after adalimumab application can be a possible presentation of a classical drug hypersensitivity [78]. In this case, intradermal testing was positive, and a rechallenge with a desensitization scheme could be performed successfully [78]. However, general symptoms and urticaria are also reported for other TNF-α antagonists as e.g. infliximab, but in a case report a clear-type sensitization was not identified either in skin or in BAT, but confirmed upon rechallenge. A class effect was ruled out by tolerated rechallenge with adalimumab [79]. The reliability of intradermal testing for the identification of typical immediate type reactions with biologicals remains unclear. Bircher and Scherer [80] investigated 6 patients with anaphylactoid reactions to etanercept or infliximab with intradermal testing and LTT. Only one out of 6 patients was positive in the intradermal test. LTT was positive in some exposed and nonexposed controls.

In conclusion, the value of skin tests, basophil activation and LTT for the investigation of possible adverse cutaneous reactions to biologicals is unclear, and larger case series are needed.

References

1 Romano A, Di Fonso M, Pocobelli D, Giannarini L, Venuti A, Garcovich A: Two cases of toxic epidermal necrolysis caused by delayed hypersensitivity to beta-lactam antibiotics. J Investig Allergol Clin Immunol 1993;3:53–55.

2 Tagami H, Tatsuta K, Iwatski K, Yamada M: Delayed hypersensitivity in ampicillin-induced toxic epidermal necrolysis. Arch Dermatol 1983;119:910–913.

3 Asensio-Sanchez VM: Toxic epidermal necrolysis following dorzolamide eyedrops (in Spanish). An Med Interna 2008;25:47–48.

4 Schmutz JL, Barbaud A, Trechot P: Polymorphous bullous erythema and trihexiphenidyl (or why police questioning is not always the most productive method) (in French). Ann Dermatol Venereol 2007;134:899.

5 Wolkenstein P, Chosidow O, Flechet ML, Robbiola O, Paul M, Dume L, Revuz J, Roujeau JC: Patch testing in severe cutaneous adverse drug reactions, including Stevens-Johnson syndrome and toxic epidermal necrolysis. Contact Dermatitis 1996;35:234–236.

6 Pichler WJ, Tilch J: The lymphocyte transformation test in the diagnosis of drug hypersensitivity. Allergy 2004;59:809–820.

7 Kano Y, Hirahara K, Mitsuyama Y, Takahashi R, Shiohara T: Utility of the lymphocyte transformation test in the diagnosis of drug sensitivity: dependence on its timing and the type of drug eruption. Allergy 2007;62:1439–1444.

8 Beeler A, Zaccaria L, Kawabata T, Gerber BO, Pichler WJ: CD69 upregulation on T cells as an in vitro marker for delayed-type drug hypersensitivity. Allergy 2008;63:181–188.

9 Zawodniak A, Lochmatter P, Yerly D, Kawabata T, Lerch M, Yawalkar N, Pichler WJ: In vitro detection of cytotoxic T and NK cells in peripheral blood of patients with various drug-induced skin diseases. Allergy 2010;65:376–384.

10 Porebski G, Gschwend-Zawodniak A, Pichler WJ: In vitro diagnosis of T cell-mediated drug allergy. Clin Exp Allergy 2011;41:461–470.

11 Halevy S: Acute generalized exanthematous pustulosis. Curr Opin Allergy Clin Immunol 2009;9:322–328.

12 Halevy S, Cohen A, Livni E: Acute generalized exanthematous pustulosis associated with polysensitivity to paracetamol and bromhexine: the diagnostic role of in vitro interferon-gamma release test. Clin Exp Dermatol 2000;25:652–654.

13 Tham SN, Kwok YK, Chan HL: Cross-reactivity in fixed drug eruptions to tetracyclines. Arch Dermatol 1996;132:1134–1135.
14 Ozkaya E: Fixed drug eruption: state of the art. J Dtsch Dermatol Ges 2008;6:181–188.
15 Ozkaya-Bayazit E, Bayazit H, Ozarmagan G: Drug related clinical pattern in fixed drug eruption. Eur J Dermatol 2000;10:288–291.
16 Brahimi N, Routier E, Raison-Peyron N, Tronquoy AF, Pouget-Jasson C, Amarger S, Machet L, Amsler E, Claeys A, Sassolas B, et al: A three-year-analysis of fixed drug eruptions in hospital settings in France. Eur J Dermatol 2010;20:461–464.
17 Alanko K, Stubb S, Reitamo S: Topical provocation of fixed drug eruption. Br J Dermatol 1987;116: 561–567.
18 Ozkaya-Bayazit E, Bayazit H, Ozarmagan G: Topical provocation in 27 cases of cotrimoxazole-induced fixed drug eruption. Contact Dermatitis 1999;41: 185–189.
19 Oppliger R, Hauser C: Anaphylaxis after injection of corticosteroid preparations –carboxymethylcellulose as a hidden allergen (in German). J Dtsch Dermatol Ges 2004;2:928–930.
20 Garcia-Ortega P, Corominas M, Badia M: Carboxymethylcellulose allergy as a cause of suspected corticosteroid anaphylaxis. Ann Allergy Asthma Immunol 2003;91:421.
21 Murrieta-Aguttes M, Michelen V, Leynadier F, Duarte-Risselin C, Halpern GM, Dry J: Systemic allergic reactions to corticosteroids. J Asthma 1991; 28:329–339.
22 Patterson DL, Yunginger JW, Dunn WF, Jones RT, Hunt LW: Anaphylaxis induced by the carboxymethylcellulose component of injectable triamcinolone acetonide suspension (Kenalog). Ann Allergy Asthma Immunol 1995;74:163–166.
23 Venturini M, Lobera T, del Pozo MD, Gonzalez I, Blasco A: Immediate hypersensitivity to corticosteroids. J Investig Allergol Clin Immunol 2006;16:51–56.
24 Bigliardi PL, Izakovic J, Weber JM, Bircher AJ: Anaphylaxis to the carbohydrate carboxymethylcellulose in parenteral corticosteroid preparations. Dermatology 2003;207:100–103.
25 Muroi N, Mori S, Ono S, Takahashi HK, Fujii T, Hosoi S, Henmi K, Nishibori M: Allergy to carboxymethylcellulose. Allergy 2002;57:1212–1213.
26 Rival-Tringali AL, Gunera-Saad N, Berard F, Chambost V, Roziere A, Guillot-Pouget I, Nicolas JF: Tolerability of oral administration of carboxymethylcellulose in two patients presenting anaphylactic reaction after carboxymethylcellulose injection (in French). Ann Dermatol Venereol 2008;135:402–406.
27 Dumond P, Franck P, Morisset M, Sainte Laudy J, Kanny G, Moneret-Vautrin DA: Pre-lethal anaphylaxis to carboxymethylcellulose confirmed by identification of specific IgE – review of the literature. Eur Ann Allergy Clin Immunol 2009;41:171–176.
28 Dewachter P, Mouton-Faivre C: Anaphylaxis to macrogol 4000 after a parenteral corticoid injection. Allergy 2005;60:705–706.
29 Anton Girones M, Roan Roan J, de la Hoz B, Sanchez Cano M: Immediate allergic reactions by polyethylene glycol 4000: two cases. Allergol Immunopathol (Madr) 2008;36:110–112.
30 Hyry H, Vuorio A, Varjonen E, Skytta J, Makinen-Kiljunen S: Two cases of anaphylaxis to macrogol 6000 after ingestion of drug tablets. Allergy 2006; 61:1021.
31 Brockow K, Romano A, Aberer W, Bircher AJ, Barbaud A, Bonadonna P, Faria E, Kanny G, Lerch M, Pichler WJ, et al: Skin testing in patients with hypersensitivity reactions to iodinated contrast media – a European multicenter study. Allergy 2009;64:234–241.
32 Lerch M, Keller M, Britschgi M, Kanny G, Tache V, Schmid DA, Beeler A, Gerber BO, Luethi M, Bircher AJ, et al: Cross-reactivity patterns of T cells specific for iodinated contrast media. J Allergy Clin Immunol 2007;119:1529–1536.
33 Scherer K, Harr T, Bach S, Bircher AJ: The role of iodine in hypersensitivity reactions to radio contrast media. Clin Exp Allergy 2010;40:468–475.
34 Castells MC: Hypersensitivity to antineoplastic agents. Curr Pharm Des 2008;14:2892–2901.
35 Leguy-Seguin V, Jolimoy G, Coudert B, Pernot C, Dalac S, Vabres P, Collet E: Diagnostic and predictive value of skin testing in platinum salt hypersensitivity. J Allergy Clin Immunol 2007;119:726–730.
36 Abe A, Ikawa H, Ikawa S: Desensitization treatment with cisplatin after carboplatin hypersensitivity reaction in gynecologic cancer. J Med Invest 2010; 57:163–167.
37 Castells M: Rapid desensitization of hypersensitivity reactions to chemotherapy agents. Curr Drug Saf 2006;1:243–251.
38 Confino-Cohen R, Fishman A, Altaras M, Goldberg A: Successful carboplatin desensitization in patients with proven carboplatin allergy. Cancer 2005;104: 640–643.
39 Gomez R, Harter P, Luck HJ, Traut A, Kommoss S, Kandel M, du Bois A: Carboplatin hypersensitivity: does introduction of skin test and desensitization reliably predict and avoid the problem? A prospective single-center study. Int J Gynecol Cancer 2009; 19:1284–1287.

40 Hesterberg PE, Banerji A, Oren E, Penson RT, Krasner CN, Seiden MV, Wong JT: Risk stratification for desensitization of patients with carboplatin hypersensitivity: clinical presentation and management. J Allergy Clin Immunol 2009;123:1262–1267, e1.
41 Lee CW, Matulonis UA, Castells MC: Carboplatin hypersensitivity: a 6-h 12-step protocol effective in 35 desensitizations in patients with gynecological malignancies and mast cell/IgE-mediated reactions. Gynecol Oncol 2004;95:370–376.
42 Limsuwan T, Castells MC: Outcomes and safety of rapid desensitization for chemotherapy hypersensitivity. Expert Opin Drug Saf 2010;9:39–53.
43 Markman M, Zanotti K, Peterson G, Kulp B, Webster K, Belinson J: Expanded experience with an intradermal skin test to predict for the presence or absence of carboplatin hypersensitivity. J Clin Oncol 2003;21:4611–4614.
44 Zanotti KM, Rybicki LA, Kennedy AW, Belinson JL, Webster KD, Kulp B, Peterson G, Markman M: Carboplatin skin testing: a skin-testing protocol for predicting hypersensitivity to carboplatin chemotherapy. J Clin Oncol 2001;19:3126–3129.
45 Syrigou E, Makrilia N, Vassias A, Nikolaidis I, Xyla V, Manolopoulos L, Syrigos K: Administration of cisplatin in three patients with carboplatin hypersensitivity: is skin testing useful? Anticancer Drugs 2010;21:333–338.
46 Mirakhur RK, McCourt KC, Kumar N: Use of intermediate acting muscle relaxants by infusion: the future. Acta Anaesthesiol Belg 1997;48:29–34.
47 Mertes PM, Guttormsen AB, Harboe T, Johansson SG, Florvaag E, Husum B, Garvey LH, Kroigaard M, Gramstad L, Kvande KT, et al: Can spontaneous adverse event reporting systems really be used to compare rates of adverse events between drugs? Anesth Analg 2007;104:471–472.
48 Berg CM, Heier T, Wilhelmsen V, Florvaag E: Rocuronium and cisatracurium-positive skin tests in non-allergic volunteers: determination of drug concentration thresholds using a dilution titration technique. Acta Anaesthesiol Scand 2003;47: 576–582.
49 Ebo DG, Bridts CH, Hagendorens MM, Mertens CH, De Clerck LS, Stevens WJ: Flow-assisted diagnostic management of anaphylaxis from rocuronium bromide. Allergy 2006;61:935–939.
50 Ebo DG, Venemalm L, Bridts CH, Degerbeck F, Hagberg H, De Clerck LS, Stevens WJ: Immunoglobulin E antibodies to rocuronium: a new diagnostic tool. Anesthesiology 2007;107: 253–259.
51 Laroche D, Chollet-Martin S, Leturgie P, Malzac L, Vergnaud MC, Neukirch C, Venemalm L, Gueant JL, Roland PN: Evaluation of a new routine diagnostic test for immunoglobulin E sensitization to neuromuscular blocking agents. Anesthesiology 2011;114:91–97.
52 Laxenaire MC, Gastin I, Moneret-Vautrin DA, Widmer S, Gueant JL: Cross-reactivity of rocuronium with other neuromuscular blocking agents. Eur J Anaesthesiol Suppl 1995;11:55–64.
53 Bousquet PJ, Co-Minh HB, Arnoux B, Daures JP, Demoly P: Importance of mixture of minor determinants and benzylpenicilloyl poly-L-lysine skin testing in the diagnosis of beta-lactam allergy. J Allergy Clin Immunol 2005;115:1314–1316.
54 Torres MJ, Ariza A, Fernandez J, Moreno E, Laguna JJ, Montanez MI, Ruiz-Sanchez AJ, Blanca M: Role of minor determinants of amoxicillin in the diagnosis of immediate allergic reactions to amoxicillin. Allergy 2010;65:590–596.
55 Blanca M, Mayorga C, Torres MJ, Reche M, Moya MC, Rodriguez JL, Romano A, Juarez C: Clinical evaluation of Pharmacia CAP System RAST FEIA amoxicilloyl and benzylpenicilloyl in patients with penicillin allergy. Allergy 2001;56:862–870.
56 Torres MJ, Mayorga C, Leyva L, Guzman AE, Cornejo-Garcia JA, Juarez C, Blanca M: Controlled administration of penicillin to patients with a positive history but negative skin and specific serum IgE tests. Clin Exp Allergy 2002;32:270–276.
57 Abuaf N, Rostane H, Rajoely B, Gaouar H, Autegarden JE, Leynadier F, Girot R: Comparison of two basophil activation markers CD63 and CD203c in the diagnosis of amoxicillin allergy. Clin Exp Allergy 2008;38:921–928.
58 Gamboa PM, Garcia-Aviles MC, Urrutia I, Antepara I, Esparza R, Sanz ML: Basophil activation and sulfidoleukotriene production in patients with immediate allergy to betalactam antibiotics and negative skin tests. J Investig Allergol Clin Immunol 2004;14: 278–283.
59 Romano A, Gueant-Rodriguez RM, Viola M, Pettinato R, Gueant JL: Cross-reactivity and tolerability of cephalosporins in patients with immediate hypersensitivity to penicillins. Ann Intern Med 2004; 141:16–22.
60 Frumin J, Gallagher JC: Allergic cross-sensitivity between penicillin, carbapenem, and monobactam antibiotics: what are the chances? Ann Pharmacother 2009;43:304–315.
61 Atanaskovic-Markovic M, Gaeta F, Medjo B, Viola M, Nestorovic B, Romano A: Tolerability of meropenem in children with IgE-mediated hypersensitivity to penicillins. Allergy 2008;63:237–240.

62 Romano A, Viola M, Gueant-Rodriguez RM, Gaeta F, Valluzzi R, Gueant JL: Brief communication: tolerability of meropenem in patients with IgE-mediated hypersensitivity to penicillins. Ann Intern Med 2007;146:266–269.
63 Cunha BA, Hamid NS, Krol V, Eisenstein L: Safety of meropenem in patients reporting penicillin allergy: lack of allergic cross reactions. J Chemother 2008;20:233–237.
64 Patriarca G, Schiavino D, Lombardo C, Altomonte G, De Cinti M, Buonomo A, Nucera E: Tolerability of aztreonam in patients with IgE-mediated hypersensitivity to beta-lactams. Int J Immunopathol Pharmacol 2008;21:375–379.
65 Audicana M, Bernaola G, Urrutia I, Echechipia S, Gastaminza G, Munoz D, Fernandez E, Fernandez de Corres L: Allergic reactions to betalactams: studies in a group of patients allergic to penicillin and evaluation of cross-reactivity with cephalosporin. Allergy 1994;49:108–113.
66 Sastre J, Quijano LD, Novalbos A, Hernandez G, Cuesta J, de las Heras M, Lluch M, Fernandez M: Clinical cross-reactivity between amoxicillin and cephadroxil in patients allergic to amoxicillin and with good tolerance of penicillin. Allergy 1996;51: 383–386.
67 Antunez C, Blanca-Lopez N, Torres MJ, Mayorga C, Perez-Inestrosa E, Montanez MI, Fernandez T, Blanca M: Immediate allergic reactions to cephalosporins: evaluation of cross-reactivity with a panel of penicillins and cephalosporins. J Allergy Clin Immunol 2006;117:404–410.
68 Romano A, Viola M, Mondino C, Pettinato R, Di Fonso M, Papa G, Venuti A, Montuschi P: Diagnosing nonimmediate reactions to penicillins by in vivo tests. Int Arch Allergy Immunol 2002; 129:169–174.
69 Lammintausta K, Kortekangas-Savolainen O: The usefulness of skin tests to prove drug hypersensitivity. Br J Dermatol 2005;152:968–974.
70 Romano A, Gaeta F, Valluzzi RL, Alonzi C, Viola M, Bousquet PJ: Diagnosing hypersensitivity reactions to cephalosporins in children. Pediatrics 2008;122: 521–527.
71 Trcka J, Seitz CS, Brocker EB, Gross GE, Trautmann A: Aminopenicillin-induced exanthema allows treatment with certain cephalosporins or phenoxymethyl penicillin. J Antimicrob Chemother 2007;60:107–111.
72 Schiavino D, Nucera E, Lombardo C, Decinti M, Pascolini L, Altomonte G, Buonomo A, Patriarca G: Cross-reactivity and tolerability of imipenem in patients with delayed-type, cell-mediated hypersensitivity to beta-lactams. Allergy 2009;64:1644–1648.
73 Sodhi M, Axtell SS, Callahan J, Shekar R: Is it safe to use carbapenems in patients with a history of allergy to penicillin? J Antimicrob Chemother 2004;54: 1155–1157.
74 Buonomo A, Nucera E, De Pasquale T, Pecora V, Lombardo C, Sabato V, Colagiovanni A, Rizzi A, Aruanno A, Pascolini L, et al: Tolerability of aztreonam in patients with cell-mediated allergy to beta-lactams. Int Arch Allergy Immunol 2010;155: 155–159.
75 Hausmann OV, Seitz M, Villiger PM, Pichler WJ: The complex clinical picture of side effects to biologicals. Med Clin North Am 2010;94:791–804, xi–xii.
76 Pichler WJ: Adverse side-effects to biological agents. Allergy 2006;61:912–920.
77 Benucci M, Manfredi M, Saviola G, Baiardi P, Campi P: Correlation between atopy and hypersensitivity reactions during therapy with three different TNF-alpha blocking agents in rheumatoid arthritis. Clin Exp Rheumatol 2009;27:333–336.
78 Rodriguez-Jimenez B, Dominguez-Ortega J, Gonzalez-Herrada C, Kindelan-Recarte C, Loribo-Bueno P, Garrido-Peno N: Successful adalimumab desensitization after generalized urticaria and rhinitis. J Investig Allergol Clin Immunol 2009;19:246–247.
79 Manso L, Polo B, Fernandez-Nieto M, Sastre LB, del Pozo V, Sastre J: Basophil activation test in a case of systemic hypersensitivity reaction to infliximab with good tolerance to another anti-TNF-alpha agent (adalimumab). J Investig Allergol Clin Immunol 2010;20:537–538.
80 Bircher AJ, Scherer k: Arzneimittelhypersensitivität – unerwünschte Arzneimittelreaktionen durch Biologika. Kongress der DGAKI und AEDA Erfurt, Dustri, 2009.

Dr. Thomas Harr
Department of Dermatology, University Hospital Zurich
Gloriastrasse 31
CH–8091 Zurich (Switzerland)
Tel. +41 44 255 25 50, E-Mail th.harr@gmail.com

French LE (ed): Adverse Cutaneous Drug Eruptions.
Chem Immunol Allergy. Basel, Karger, 2012, vol 97, pp 61–78

Histopathological Patterns Indicative of Distinct Adverse Drug Reactions

Katrin Kerl

Dermatopathology, Department of Dermatology, University Hospital Zurich, Zurich, Switzerland

Abstract

Histologically, drug eruptions may present virtually all patterns of inflammation in the skin, including spongiotic, lichenoid and psoriasiform dermatitis as well as vasculitis or panniculitis. Drug reactions may mimic specific skin diseases such as lupus erythematosus, lichen planus or lymphoma. While a single drug may cause a wide range of reaction patterns, no reaction pattern is specific for a certain drug. Nevertheless, some reactions are quite characteristic for certain drugs as for example psoriasiform dermatitis for anti-TNF agents or folliculitis for epidermal growth factor receptor antagonists. Heightened awareness to the possible mimicry of other skin diseases as well as integration of clinical data is pivotal for the appropriate histological diagnosis of drug reactions in the skin. For practical reasons and in the aim of helping clinicians, the different drug reactions described in this chapter are classified according to the main histological reaction pattern present. Nevertheless, this classification may be somewhat artificial in some cases as drug reactions often reveal a coexistence of different reaction patterns.

Essentials in a Nutshell

- The histological spectrum of cutaneous adverse drug reactions is very broad and heterogeneous (table 1, 2)
- Histological changes are often nonspecific
- No histological pattern is specific for a certain drug; one drug can cause a variety of different patterns
- Histopathological clues for the diagnosis of a drug reaction are:
  - Mixed histological patterns in one specimen (e.g. lichenoid and spongiotic)
  - Presence of eosinophils (although not mandatory!)
  - Apoptotic keratinocytes

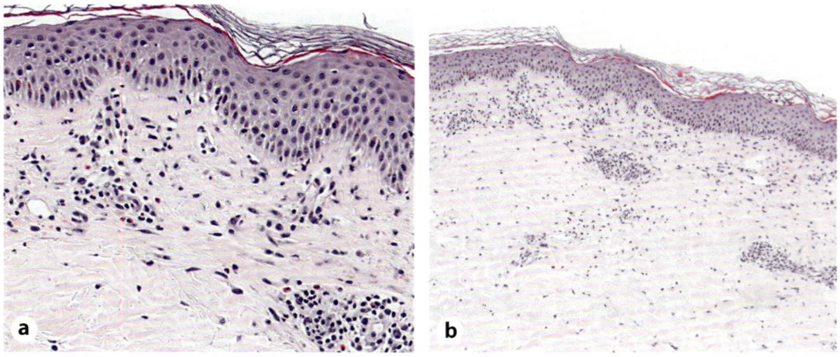

Fig. 1. a, **b** Maculopapular drug eruption. Perivascular lymphohistiocytic infiltrate with eosinophils.

Drug Reactions with Superficial and Deep Dermal Infiltrates

Maculopapular Drug Reaction

This most frequent manifestation of drug hypersensitivity is histologically characterized by a superficial and deep, perivascular inflammatory infiltrate, mainly lymphocytic, with some eosinophils and rarely plasma cells (fig. 1). Occasionally, scattered apoptotic keratinocytes and a discrete interface dermatitis with vacuolar alteration of the basal keratinocytes may be present. It should be noted however that viral exanthemas may exhibit identical changes and may therefore be histologically undistinguishable from drug-induced exanthemas.

Urticarial Drug Reaction

Similarly to the clinical presentation, the histological presentation of urticaria induced by a drug is indistinguishable from urticaria of other causes (viral, etc.). Urticaria in general presents with dermal edema and a mixed interstitial infiltrate essentially composed of neutrophils and eosinophils.

Lymphomatoid (Pseudolymphomatous) Drug Reaction

Drugs can mimic the clinical as well as histological presentation of cutaneous lymphomas of T or B cell type. Patients with lymphomatoid drug reactions present clinically with isolated or generalized papules, plaques, nodules or even erythroderma.

In the case of T cell pseudolymphomas, a band-like, lichenoid lymphocytic infiltrate, sometimes with epidermotropism, mimicking mycosis fungoides is characteristic.

In contrast to true mycosis fungoides, the epidermal lymphocytes are smaller and less atypical than the dermal ones. Sometimes diffuse or nodular deep lymphocytic infiltrates with some eosinophils are present.

B cell pseudolymphomas mimic either follicle center lymphoma or marginal zone lymphoma, though reactive germinal centers, a mixed infiltrate with eosinophils and the presence macrophages in germinal centers (tingible body macrophages) are indicators of a lymphomatoid drug reaction.

Assessment of clonality, though often helpful, may give confusing results, as in certain cases pseudolymphomas may be clonal, and inversely certain cases of lymphoma, especially early-stage mycosis fungoides or low-grade cutaneous B cell lymphomas, may lack evidence of clonality.

Close correlation of histological, immunohistological, molecular and clinical data including the evolution of lesions over time are mandatory here for the establishment of a correct diagnosis.

Drug Reaction with Eosinophilia and Systemic Symptoms

Drug reaction with eosinophilia and systemic symptoms (DRESS), also referred to as DIHS (drug-induced hypersensitivity syndrome) in Japan, is characterized by the clinical concomitance of a drug-induced rash with facial edema and systemic symptoms (fever, hepatotoxicity, eosinophilia and lymphadenopathy). Latent herpesvirus 6, 7 and EBV infections have been implicated in the pathogenesis.

Histopathologically, DRESS is characterized by dermal edema with a dense pseudolymphomatous perivascular infiltrate, or diffuse lymphocytic infiltrates. Eosinophils are usually present. Emperipolesis (phagocytosis of leukocytes) may be observed (fig. 2).

Photoallergic Reactions

An erythematous skin eruption on the face, the dorsa of hands, the neck and presternal area with a sharp cutoff at the clothing margins is the typical clinical presentation of a photoallergic reaction.

Histological features are superficial and deep perivascular lymphocytic infiltrates (sometimes with eosinophils), and edema of the papillary dermis with spongiosis and focal parakeratosis of the epidermis.

Drug-Induced Lupus Erythematosus

Histologically, drug-induced systemic, subacute and discoid lupus erythematosus (LE) are indistinguishable from idiopathic LE.

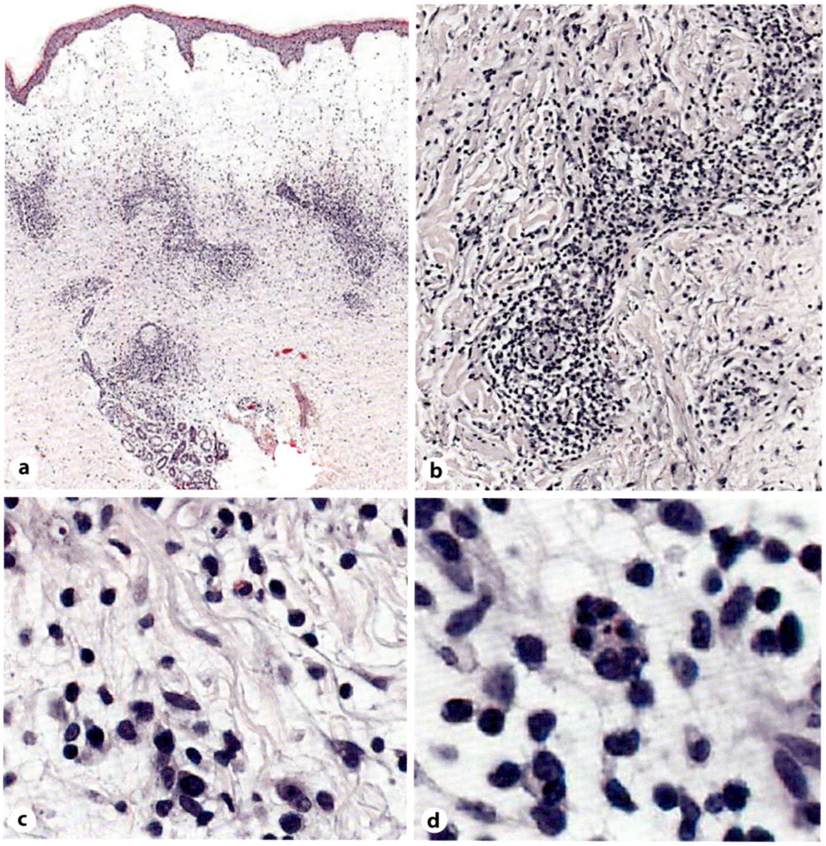

Fig. 2. DRESS. **a**, **b** Marked dermal edema and deep perivascular and interstitial lymphocytic infiltrate. **c** Sparse eosinophils. **d** Emperipolesis.

Drug Reactions with Predominant Cytotoxic Epidermal Changes

Erythema Multiforme/Fixed Drug Eruption

Targetoid maculae are the typical lesions in EM. Fixed drug eruption (FDE) clinically presents with violaceous patches and plaques, leaving a postinflammatory hyperpigmentation and recurring in the same location after reexposure to the offending drug.

Histologically, EM and FDE are both characterized by the presence of scattered and clustered apoptotic keratinocytes in different layers of the epidermis, interface dermatitis with vacuolar changes at the dermoepidermal junction, occasional subepidermal blistering, and a mixed inflammatory infiltrate with some eosinophils and plasma cells too. Subepidermal and intraepidermal blistering may occur (fig. 3). Whereas the infiltrate is usually superficial in EM, it tends to be deeper and contains more melanophages in FDE. In the chronic stage of FDE, only melanophages are present.

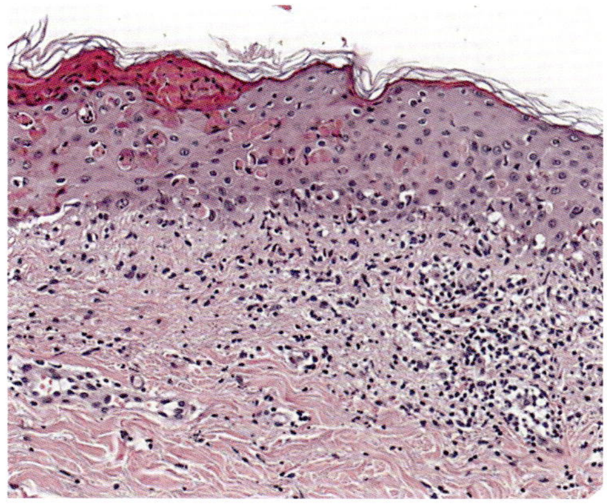

Fig. 3. EM. Scattered apoptotic keratinocytes in different layers of the epidermis and mixed inflammatory infiltrate.

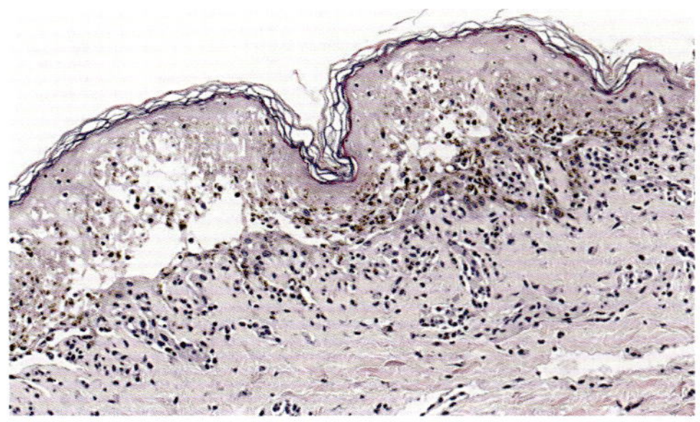

Fig. 4. TEN (LS). Subepidermal blister with whole-thickness necrosis of the epidermis.

Stevens-Johnson/Toxic Epidermal Necrolysis

These entities represent a spectrum of severe, potentially lethal, skin diseases characterized by different degrees of skin detachment. In the majority of cases, the mucosal epithelia are involved.

Histology shows subepidermal blistering with confluent apoptosis of keratinocytes subsequently leading to a full-thickness necrosis of the epidermis. The accompanying lymphohistiocytic infiltrates can be sparse and contain only few eosinophils (fig. 4).

Stevens-Johnson syndrome (SJS), toxic epidermal necrolysis (TEN), EM and early-stage FDE may be impossible to distinguish histologically.

Phototoxic Reactions

They clinically resemble severe sunburn, and occur after exposure to a photosensitizing drug and light.

Histological features are characterized by spongiosis and apoptotic and ballooned keratinocytes. In addition to edema of the papillary dermis, a superficial perivascular mainly lymphocytic infiltrate can be observed.

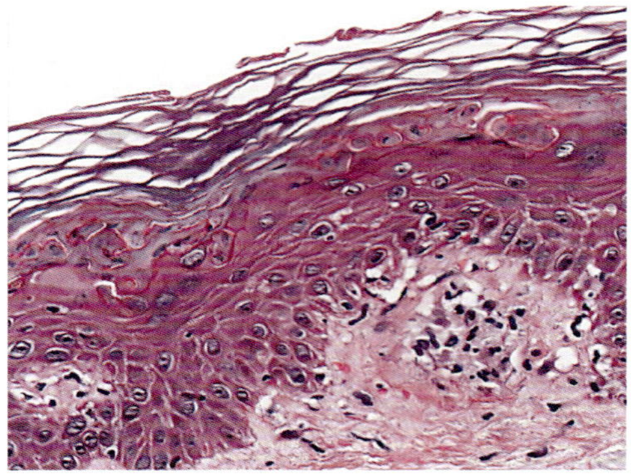

Fig. 5. Epidermal dysmaturation. Atypical keratinocytes, dyskeratosis and apoptosis within the epidermis.

Chemotherapy-Induced Cytotoxic Reactions: Epidermal Dysmaturation and Acral Erythema

The term epidermal dysmaturation refers to the presence of large atypical keratinocytes with pleomorphic nuclei, mitosis, dyskeratosis and apoptosis within the epidermis (fig. 5). These are characteristic histopathological features observed after chemotherapy or stem cell transplantation. Clinically a nonspecific maculopapular rash may be present.

Acral erythema is a frequent side effect of various chemotherapeutic agents, probably due to higher excretion of cytotoxic drugs via eccrine units in this localization. Histologically the features of epidermal dysmaturation with interface dermatitis of the epidermis, follicles and eccrine ducts, are usually present.

Radiation Recall Dermatitis

Radiation recall dermatitis occurs in previously irradiated fields when chemotherapy or other drugs are introduced. Clinical features are erythematous patches and plaques with vesicles and sometimes ulceration.

On histology, keratinocyte necrosis, subepidermal blistering and a mixed inflammatory infiltrate are observed.

Lichenoid Pattern – Lichen Planus-Like Reactions

The term lichenoid is applied here to describe the presence of a band-like subepidermal infiltrate as the predominant histopathological feature. Overlaps with the above-mentioned cytotoxic reactions characterized by vacuolar degeneration of the epidermis do exist.

Table 1. Pattern-based classification of drug-induced skin diseases and main histopathological features

A. Superficial and deep dermal infiltrates – Maculopapular exanthema – Urticaria – Lymphomatoid (pseudolymphomatous) drug reaction – DRESS – Photoallergic reactions – Drug-induced LE
B. Cytotoxic epidermal changes – EM – Fixed drug eruption – SJS/LS – Phototoxic reactions – Epidermal dysmaturation – Acral erythema – Radiation recall dermatitis
C. Lichenoid pattern – Lichenoid drug eruption
D. Spongiotic pattern – Pityriasis rosea-like drug reactions – Baboon syndrome
E. Granulomatous pattern – Interstitial granulomatous dermatitis
F. Vasculitic pattern – Hypersensitivity vasculitis
G. Psoriasiform pattern – Psoriasis induced by drugs – AGEP
H. Neutrophilic drug reactions – Sweet's syndrome/pyoderma gangrenosum – NEH – Halogenodermas
I. Vesiculobullous pattern – Linear IgA dermatosis-like drug reaction – Drug-induced pemphigus – Drug induced bullous pemphigoid – Drug-induced pseudoporphyria cutanea tarda
J. Panniculitis induced by drugs – Panniculitis secondary to drugs injected into the skin – Drug-induced erythema nodosum – Panniculitis secondary to chemotherapy

Table 1. Continued

K.	Folliculitis
–	Acneiform drug eruptions
–	Drug-induced eosinophilic pustular dermatosis
L.	Sclerodermoid drug reactions

Lichenoid drug reactions are clinically and histologically imitators of LP. Unlike idiopathic LP, drug-induced LP is clinically characterized by a more extensive or generalized eruption of violaceous papules. Photodistribution may occur.

Histologically, drug induced LP-like reactions are characterized by the typical features of lichen planus with band-like subepidermal lymphocytic infiltrates, basal keratinocyte vacuolar degeneration and apoptotic keratinocytes. Clues for a drug-induced process are the presence of parakeratosis, transepidermal necrotic keratinocytes, and deeper inflammatory infiltrates with eosinophils. Epidermal acanthosis and wedge-shaped hypergranulosis are usually less pronounced than in LP.

Spongiotic Pattern

Spongiotic changes of the epidermis may accompany virtually all other types of drug-induced reaction patterns. Spongiosis is a common feature in maculopapular exanthema and photoallergic reactions.

Pityriasis rosea-Like Drug Eruption

The absence of a herald patch, atypical distribution of lesions, fever, eosinophilia, and severe pruritus are features that distinguish drug-induced PR from the idiopathic form. The histological changes are very similar though, including focal spongiosis, slight epidermal hyperplasia, papillary edema, extravasation of erythrocytes, a mild superficial perivascuar lymphocytic infiltrate and mounds of parakeratosis. The only indicator, but not the proof of drug-induced etiology may be the presence of eosinophils.

Baboon Syndrome

Baboon syndrome, also named SDRIFE (symmetrical drug-related intertriginous and flexural exanthema), is the designation for a distinct form of systemic contact dermatitis or FDE, presenting with sharply demarcated erythema in the flexural area with nonspecific spongiotic dermatitis on histology.

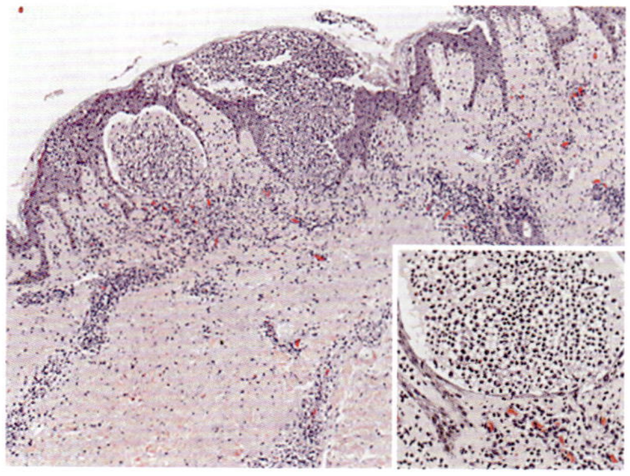

Fig. 6. AGEP. Epidermal hyperplasia with intraepidermal pustules and a mixed cell infiltrate containing eosinophils.

Granulomatous Pattern

Drug reactions characterized by a granulomatous reaction pattern are rare. They are defined by a predominance of histiocytes in the inflammatory infiltrate.

Interstitial Granulomatous Drug Eruption

This histological pattern presents clinically as erythematous or violaceous papules and plaques in annular array, localized preferentially over skin folds.

Histopathology reveals an interstitial dermal infiltrate of histiocytes and lymphocytes, sometimes associated with a vacuolar interface dermatitis.

The same pattern can also be observed in the interstitial variant of granuloma annulare, borreliosis, and in the context of autoimmune disease. The presence of vacuolar alteration at the dermoepidermal junction should be a clue for a drug-induced interstitial granulomatous dermatitis.

Vasculitic Pattern

Hypersensitivity vasculitis

About 20–30% of all vasculitides can be attributed to drug ingestion. They usually present clinically as purpuric papules.

The most frequent histological variant of vasculitis is leukocytoclastic vasculitis. Besides inflammation of small cutaneous vessels with deposition of fibrin and extravasation of erythrocytes, a predominantly neutrophilic infiltrate around and inside of the vessel walls is present. Usually, eosinophils can be found. Leukocytoclasia refers to the presence of small particles of 'broken' leukocytes.

Table 2. Main histopathological features of adverse cutaneous drug eruptions

Maculopapular rash
- superficial and deep perivascular and interstitial predominantly lymphohistiocytic infiltrate
- some eosinophils, rarely plasma cells
- sometimes necrotic keratinocytes/basal cell vacuolization/interface dermatitis

DD: viral infection

Urticarial drug eruption
- dermal edema
- interstitial infiltrates of neutrophils and eosinophils

DD: urticaria of other genesis (e.g. viral) histopathologically indistinguishable

Lymphomatoid drug reaction T type
- band-like superficial or nodular/diffuse deep lymphocytic infiltrates
- sometimes epidermotropism
- sometimes eosinophils
- only slight lymphocytic atypia

DD: mycosis fungoides, polymorphous light eruption, LE

Lymphomatoid drug reaction B type
- diffuse and nodular superficial and deep lymphocytic infiltrates
- reactive germinal centers with tingible body macrophages, apoptotic cells and high proliferation rate
- high percentage of reactive T cells
- sometimes eosinophils

DD: borreliosis, follicle center lymphoma, marginal zone lymphoma

DRESS/DIHS
- dermal edema
- dense perivascular and/or diffuse pseudolymphomatous lymphocytic infiltrates
- often eosinophils
- sometimes emperipolesis

DD: lymphoma, photoallergic reaction

Photoallergic reactions
- spongiosis and focal parakeratosis
- superficial (sometimes deep) mixed infiltrates with eosinophils
- edema of the papillary dermis

DD: allergic contact dermatitis, urticaria, DRESS

Drug-induced LE
- varying degrees of interface dermatitis with vacuolar changes of basal keratinocytes
- deep perivascular and perifollicular lymphocytic infiltrates
- anti-histone antibodies frequently positive

DD: idiopathic LE histologically indistinguishable

EM
- apoptotic keratinocytes, individually and in clusters, within different layers of the epidermis, follicular and eccrine epithelia

Table 2. Continued

- vacuolar changes of basal keratinocytes
- moderate to dense superficial mainly lymphocytic infiltrate in the papillary dermis and along the dermoepidermal junction
- eosinophils
- superficial dermal edema
- sometimes subepidermal and intraepidermal blister formation

DD: Fixed drug reaction, SJS, LS, phototoxic reaction

Fixed drug eruption

- apoptotic keratinocytes, individually and in clusters, within different layers of the epidermis, follicular and eccrine epithelia
- vacuolar changes of basal keratinocytes
- prominent pigment incontinence
- subepidermal and intraepidermal blister formation
- superficial and deep perivascular and interstitial lymphocytic infiltrate
- eosinophils
- superficial dermal oedema

Later stages:

- melanophages in the papillary dermis

DD: EM, SJS, LS, phototoxic reaction

SJS/TEN

- confluent apoptosis of keratinocytes – full-thickness epidermal necrosis
- sparse superficial lymphocytic infiltrate
- eosinophils rarely

DD: EM, fixed drug reaction, SJS, LS, phototoxic reaction

Phototoxic reactions

- Apoptotic keratinocytes within the epidermis
- Spongiosis with vesicle formation
- Vacuolization of keratinocytes within the basal layer
- Superficial perivascular mixed cell infiltrates with lymphocytes and few neutrophils
- Papillary edema

Later stages

- epidermal necrosis
- subepidermal blistering

Epidermal dysmaturation

- interface dermatitis with vacuolar changes of basal keratinocytes
- apoptotic and dyskeratotic keratinocytes
- keratinocytes with large pleomorphic nuclei and mitotic figures

DD: Bowen's disease

Acral erythema

- interface dermatitis with vacuolar changes of basal keratinocytes
- variable keratinocyte necrosis
- dilation of the superficial vascular plexus
- sparse superficial inflammatory infiltrate

DD: EM

Table 2. Continued

Radiation recall dermatitis – necrotic keratinocytes with mitotic figures – keratinocyte atypia – superficial perivascular mixed inflammatory infiltrate
Lichenoid drug eruption – superficial band-like and deep lymphohistiocytic infiltrate with eosinophils – focal parakeratosis – vacuolar changes of basal keratinocytes – scattered individual apoptotic keratinocytes DD: Lichen planus
Pityriasis rosea-like drug reactions – focal spongiosis and mounds of parakeratosis – slight epidermal hyperplasia – papillary edema – extravasations of erythrocytes – mild superficial perivascuar lymphocytic infiltrate with some eosinophils DD: viral infections, eczema
Baboon syndrome/SDRIFE – spongiosis with parakeratosis – superficial and mid dermal perivascular inflammatory infiltrates with eosinophils DD: viral infections, eczema
Interstitial granulomatous drug eruption – interstitial lymphohistiocytic infiltrate in the dermis – sometimes eosinophils DD: interstitial granulomatous dermatitis with connective tissue disease, granuloma anulare, erythema chronicum migrans
Hypersensitivity vasculitis – inflammation of small vessels (postcapillary venules) with endothelial cell swelling and neutrophilic invasion of blood vessel walls – disrupted neutrophils (leukocytoclasia) – extravasations of red blood cells – fibrinoid necrosis of the blood vessels walls DD: Henoch-Schönlein purpura, septic vasculitis, urticarial vasculitis
Psoriasis induced by drugs Histology identical to psoriasis and variants – epidermal hyperplasia with elongation of rete ridges and papillomatosis – hypogranulosis – spongiosis – superficial perivascular mixed cell infiltrate, sometimes with eosinophils
AGEP – intraepidermal spongiotic pustules – some apoptotic keratinocytes – superficial perivascular infiltrate with eosinophils DD: psoriasis, IgA pemphigus, fungus

Table 2. Continued

NEH – neutrophilic infiltrates around sweat glands – necrosis of sweat gland epithelial cells
Eccrine squamous syringometaplasia – squamous cells with intercellular bridges within eccrine epithelia – apoptosis and occasional mitosis within eccrine epithelia
Halogenoderma – pseudocarcinomatous epidermal hyperplasia – intraepidermal, dermal and follicular neutrophilic abscesses
Linear IgA dermatosis-like drug reaction Histology identical to idiopathic variant – subepidermal blistering – neutrophilic infiltrate with some eosinophils along the dermoepidermal junction – microabscesses in the dermal papillae occasionally – direct immunofluorescence: linear deposits of IgA, IgG and C3 along the dermoepidermal junction
Drug-induced pemphigus Histology identical to idiopathic variant – Intraepidermal acantholysis – mixed cell infiltrate with eosinophils – direct immunofluorescence: intercellular IgA and C3 deposits
Drug-induced bullous pemphigoid Histology identical to idiopathic variant – subepidermal clefting – many eosinophils in the inflammatory infiltrate – direct immunofluorescence: linear IgG and C3 deposits along the dermoepidermal junction
Drug-induced pseudoporphyria cutanea tarda – subepidermal blistering – no or few inflammation – preserved dermal papillae (festooning) – PAS-positive, homogenous eosinophilic deposits around blood vessels
Drug-induced panniculitis No specific histological features – septal (erythema nodosum) or lobular panniculitis
Acneiform drug eruptions – necrotizing folliculitis with neutrophilic infiltrates
Drug-induced eosinophilic pustular dermatosis – spongiosis of the follicular epithelium – intra- and perifollicular lymphohistiocytic infiltrate with many eosinophils

Table 2. Continued

Sclerodermoid drug reactions
Histology identical to idiopathic variant
– thickened collagen bundles
– rarefaction of adnexal structures
DD = Differential diagnosis.

Leukocytoclastic vasculitis may be due to drugs as well as infectious agents or underlying systemic disease. The different etiologies of leukocytoclastic vasculitis cannot be determined histologically.

Rarely, drug-induced vasculitis may be polyarteritis nodosa like, presenting with inflammation of middle-sized arteries, or pustular.

Psoriasiform Pattern

The term psoriasiform summarizes histological changes such as confluent parakeratosis, neutrophils in the epidermis, regular epidermal hyperplasia with elongation of rete ridges and papillomatosis, dilated vessels in the papillary dermis and a mixed inflammatory infiltrate. Depending on the age of the psoriatic skin lesion as well as the subtype (such as plaque type, acute, pustular psoriasis) the various features may be present or absent. Only the presence of eosinophils or occasionally of apoptotic keratinocytes may be indicative of a drug implicated in the disease.

Psoriasis Induced by Drugs

Drugs such as lithium or beta-blockers are well-known triggers of psoriasis in patients with a preexisting genetic predisposition. In these cases, histology reveals no particular histological features besides that of classical psoriasis and its variants.

As a paradoxical phenomenon, papular eruptions with psoriasiform features can develop in the course of a therapy with biologics (TNF-α inhibitors). Histology in these cases resembles that of early-stage psoriasis.

Acute Generalized Exanthematous Pustulosis

Clinically, a scarlatiniform exanthema is followed by rapidly evolving, widespread non-follicular pustules, often in association with fever. In general, the lesions resolve rapidly after withdrawing the offending drug.

Biopsies show features of pustular psoriasis with collections of neutrophils (usually subcorneal) in a spongiotic epidermis. In addition, apoptotic keratinocytes and a mixed infiltrate with eosinophils may be observed (fig. 6).

Neutrophilic Drug Reactions

Neutrophilic dermatoses such as Sweet's syndrome or pyoderma gangrenosum may be triggered by certain drugs such as carbamazepine and oral contraceptives.

Neutrophilic Eccrine Hidradenitis

Chemotherapy-induced cases present clinically with erythematous macules, papules, plaques, or vesicles, which may be generalized or localized to the intertriginous areas, or the palms and soles. Histologically, dense neutrophilic infiltrates around sweat glands and necrosis of sweat gland epithelial cells can be observed.

Eccrine squamous syringometaplasia is another chemotherapy-associated disorder of sweat glands with similar clinical features as neutrophilic eccrine hidradenitis (NEH). It is characterized histologically by transformation of the eccrine cuboidal epithelium into two or more layers of squamous cells with intercellular bridges, apoptosis, and occasional mitoses. It differs from NEH by the absence of neutrophils.

Halogenodermas

Halogenodermas develop after ingestion of bromide (bromoderma), iodines (iododerma) and fluorides (fluoroderma). Clinically, they are characterized by ulcerated, crusted, vegetative plaques, nodules and sometimes pustules, imitating deep fungal infection.

On histopathology, lesions show pseudocarcinomatous epidermal hyperplasia, and intraepidermal, dermal and follicular abscesses.

The main differential diagnosis is an infectious process including deep mycosis, sporotrichosis, atypical mycobacterial infection and blastomycosis-like pyoderma.

Vesiculobullous Drug Reactions

Linear IgA Dermatosis-Like Drug Reaction

Drug-induced and idiopathic linear IgA dermatoses are histologically characterized by subepidermal blistering and a neutrophilic infiltrate with some eosinophils along the dermoepidermal junction. Microabcesses in the dermal papillae may be observed. Direct immunofluorescence investigation reveals linear deposits of IgA, IgG and C3 in the basement membrane zone. Recent studies indicate that the probability of drug induction is higher if only deposits IgA and not IgG are found (reference). Furthermore, circulating anti-basement membrane IgA antibodies are less frequently found in the drug-induced cases.

Severe cases of drug-induced linear IgA dermatosis mimicking Lyell's syndrome (LS)/TEN have been reported, especially in association with vancomycin.

Drug-Induced Pemphigus

Acantholysis located in the epidermis, as well as in follicular or eccrine epithelia is the histological hallmark of all diseases of the pemphigus group, and can be found in drug-induced as well as in non-drug-induced cases. Also, immunofluorescence findings are identical, showing intercellular IgG and C3 deposits, though circulating antibodies are less often found in drug-induced cases.

Drug-Induced Bullous Pemphigoid

Like idiopathic bullous pemphigoid, drug-induced cases are characterized histologically by subepidermal clefting with numerous eosinophils in the inflammatory infiltrate and a direct immunofluorescence revealing linear IgG and C3 deposits along the dermoepidermal junction.

Drug-Induced Pseudoporphyria Cutanea Tarda

Pseudoporphyria is a bullous reaction clinically and histologically resembling porphyria cutanea tarda but without evident abnormalities in porphyrin metabolism. Besides hemodialysis, drugs may cause pseudoporphyria.

Typically, histology shows subepidermal blistering, with no or very few inflammatory cells. The dermal papillae maintain preserved ('festooning'). PAS-positive homogenous eosinophilic deposits are found around small blood vessels. Sclerosis of the collagen is present in old lesions.

Panniculitis Induced by Drugs

Panniculitis can either be caused by direct injection of certain drugs such as apomorphine, glatiramer or phosphatidylcholine, or as a systemic effect.

The most frequent type of panniculitis is erythema nodosum, which may be caused by many and varied agents, and one of them are drugs. Histologically, erythema nodosum is the prototype of a septal panniculitis with a lymphohistiocytic infiltrate and multinucleate giant cells.

Panniculitis induced by chemotherapy is most often a lobular panniculitis. Cases of lobular panniculitis with mixed or predominantly neutrophilic infiltrates have been reported for tyrosine kinase antagonists.

Folliculitis

Acneiform Drug Eruptions

Drug-induced acneiform eruptions and acne vulgaris both present with papules and pustules predominantly on the face and upper trunk. In contrast to acne vulgaris, drug-induced acneiform eruptions are more monomorphic and lack comedones. Drugs responsible for acneiform eruptions include antibiotics, immunosuppressive agents, anti-epileptics, corticosteroids, androgens, oral contraceptives and epidermal growth factor receptor inhibitors (EGFR-I). In the context of antitumor treatments, the acneiform eruption is an expected side effect of EGFR-Is. The rash is considered to be predictive of a better response to the EGFR-I.

Histologically, depending on the age of the lesion, a necrotizing folliculitis with a neutrophilic or lymphohistiocytic infiltrate is found.

Drug-Induced Eosinophilic Pustular Dermatosis

Drug-induced EPF presents clinically with pruritic follicular papules and pustules on face, scalp, trunk and arms.

Histologically, classical and drug-induced EPF are identical, presenting with spongiosis of the follicular epithelium and an intra- and perifollicular lymphohistiocytic infiltrate with numerous eosinophils, forming microabscesses within the follicular epithelium.

Sclerodermoid Drug Reactions

The term sclerodermoid refers to thickened collagen fibers and hardening of the skin. It can be a localized or systemic process. Clinically, hyperpigmented indurated plaques appear affecting often the upper and lower extremities. On histology, thickened collagen bundles, rarefaction of adnexae and displacement of the dermohypodermal junction is observed.

Several drugs have been implicated in sclerodermoid skin reactions; one of the most frequently associated is bleomycin. Bleomycin-induced fibroblast stimulation not only results in cutaneous sclerosis but also in pulmonary fibrosis. Taxanes and ergot alkaloids are other medications that may cause sclerodermoid skin reactions.

In conclusion, drug eruptions may histologically mimic virtually all patterns of inflammation in the skin, including spongiotic, lichenoid and psoriasiform dermatitis as well as vasculitis or panniculitis. Drug reactions may mimic specific skin diseases such as LE, lichen planus or lymphoma. While a single drug may cause a wide range of reaction patterns, no reaction pattern is specific for a certain drug. Nevertheless, some reactions are quite characteristic for certain drugs as for example psoriasiform dermatitis for anti-TNF agents, or folliculitis for EGFR antagonists. In this chapter, drug reactions have been classified according to the main histological reaction pattern present in order to help clinicians suspect these when confronting the histological and clinical signs in a patient in order to appropriately diagnose him/her with adverse cutaneous drug reactions [1–4].

References

1 Weedeon D: Weedon's Skin Pathology, ed 3. Amsterdam, Elsevier, 2010.

2 Ackerman AB, Boer A, Bennin B, Gottlieb GJ: Histologic Diagnosis of Inflammatory Skin Diseases: An Algorithmic Method Based on Pattern Analysis. New York, Ardor Scribendi, 2005.

3 Ramdial PK, Naidoo DK: Drug-induced cutaneous pathology. J Clin Pathol 2009;62:493–504.

4 Justiniano H, Berlingeri-Ramos AC, Sánchez JL: Pattern analysis of drug-induced skin diseases. Am J Dermatopathol 2008;30:352–369.

Dr. Katrin Kerl
Department of Dermatology, University Hospital Zurich
Gloriastrasse 31
CH–8031 Zurich (Switzerland)
Tel. +41 44 255 25 64, E-Mail katrin.kerl@uzh.ch

French LE (ed): Adverse Cutaneous Drug Eruptions.
Chem Immunol Allergy. Basel, Karger, 2012, vol 97, pp 79–97

Uncomplicated Drug-Induced Disseminated Exanthemas

Andreas J. Bircher

Allergy Unit, Dermatology Clinic, University Hospital, Basel, Switzerland

Abstract

Exanthematous reactions with various morphological and localization patterns are the most frequently encountered adverse drug reactions involving the skin. The time course of benign exanthemas typically encompasses a few days to some weeks. They are not complicated by severe systemic symptoms or internal organ involvement. They manifest themselves in a polymorphous manner with primary efflorescences including macules, papules, and more rarely limited pustules, vesicles or bullae, followed by secondary lesions such as scales, and more rarely erosions and hemorrhage. Due to the limited inflammatory reaction pattern of the skin, these exanthemas may mimic other discrete skin disorders and infectious exanthemas. Rarely, typical skin disorders such as lichen planus or psoriasis are imitated or inflammatory reaction patterns such as Sweet's syndrome and erythema nodosum are observed. The most common groups of eliciting drugs include antibiotics, anti-infectious drugs, tuberculostatic drugs, anticonvulsant and antihypertensive agents. On the other hand, there are some drugs that have been very rarely associated with an adverse cutaneous reaction. Immunological effector mechanisms often include T cells and various chemokines and cytokines. Diagnosis is based on a detailed history, an exact morphological diagnosis and an accurate evaluation of the chronology. Histology may support the clinical diagnosis. After complete healing and within an interval of 6 weeks to 6 months, diagnostic skin and some in vitro tests are recommended. The treatment includes early withdrawal of the suspected culprit drugs, application of topical corticosteroids, systemic antihistamines and, if necessary, systemic corticosteroids.

Essentials in a Nutshell

- Benign uncomplicated exanthemas without systemic symptoms and signs are the most common drug-induced cutaneous adverse reactions
- The inflammatory reaction patterns of the skin result in polymorphic clinical manifestations, sometimes imitating discrete skin diseases
- Even mild skin signs may herald systemic hypersensitivity reactions and internal organ involvement

- Diagnosis requires a detailed history and clinical description, and exact assessment of chronology

Introduction

Adverse drug reactions (ADR) commonly involve the skin, and the integument may be the only affected organ. On the other hand, cutaneous manifestations may herald the involvement of internal organs such as the liver, kidneys or lungs [1]. Since many drug hypersensitivity reactions are systemic immune reactions not only involving the skin, a thorough investigation is recommended to reveal internal organ involvement.

ADR affect a considerable number of patients. It is estimated that between 10 and 15% of treated patients have an unwanted drug reaction, 2–5% of them have to be hospitalized, and in 1–3% of these mortality may result [2]. The scale of the problem and the epidemiology is dealt with elsewhere in this book. The majority of ADR consist of uncomplicated exanthemas without systemic signs. The usual practice is to permanently avoid the culprit drug and to use a structurally different, non-cross-reacting drug for future treatment. The severe forms of ADR and syndromes that also present exanthematous cutaneous signs, as well as the 'immediate-type reactions' manifesting themselves as anaphylaxis, urticaria and angioedema are covered in other chapters.

Exanthematous drug reactions are the most common delayed hypersensitivity reactions and have been reported to occur in approx. 2% of hospitalized patients and complicate 3 per 1,000 courses of drug therapy [3]. Therefore, they represent the majority (31–90%) of drug-induced skin manifestations [4, 5].

Benign exanthematous drug reactions are often insufficiently designated as drug rashes, drug eruptions or somewhat more accurately pooled under the term maculopapular exanthemas. In Dermatology, this latter notion refers to the disseminated appearance of identical or varied types of primary and later secondary efflorescences. However, the term rash as well as the Latin word 'eruptio' indicating an outbreak, and the Greek term 'exanthema' meaning to flourish, just imply the appearance of any – mostly inflammatory skin lesions – without any further specification. Therefore, for a distinct clinical diagnosis these terms are not sufficient.

In many cases of (maculopapular) exanthema, a T cell-mediated pathogenesis is attributable [6, 7]. However, this can be supported or confirmed by further diagnostic means only, including skin patch or intradermal tests, histopathology, or in vitro techniques such as lymphocyte stimulation assays or the generation of T cell clones [8]. The chronology of onset and evolution of the skin lesions allows an approximate estimation of the type of pathomechanism that may be involved.

As it has been learnt from ADR to biologicals [9], manifold immunological and other pathomechanisms may be involved, resulting in varied symptoms ranging from isolated pruritus to eczema, full skin necrosis and anaphylaxis. So-called nonspecific reactions such as xeroderma, and elicitation or exacerbation of preexisting skin diseases, often lack a well-defined pathogenesis. Apart from the well-defined immunological pathways that are often involved, alternative mechanisms such as interaction with metabolic pathways generating skin lipids with potential disruption of the epidermal barrier [10] and resulting in dry skin with eczematous exanthema [11] in the absence of a specific immunological pathomechanism can be involved. Although most of these skin manifestations are not severe or life threatening, they may considerably influence the quality of life of affected patients.

Pruritus is a common symptom accompanying many skin diseases and particularly hyperergic reactions. Itching is present in most uncomplicated exanthemas, and may even be the only manifestation of drug hypersensitivity. It is mainly caused by histamine in immediate-type reactions and most probably inflammatory cytokines in delayed-type reactions. Isolated pruritus from drugs has also been described, for example for analgesics and NSAIDs, many antibiotics, cardiovascular drugs, opiates, radio-contrast media, vitamin A derivatives and hydroxyethyl starch.

The skin possesses a limited variety of inflammatory reaction patterns. Similar lesions may represent several distinct types of skin disease, e.g. physical urticarias, psoriasis or lichen planus. For this reason, the term 'the great imitator' initially coined for the manifold cutaneous and organ manifestations of syphilis, has also been attributed to drug hypersensitivity reactions, because they can also imitate a large number of other diseases [12]. Therefore, the correct identification and morphological diagnosis of skin lesions is paramount in the diagnosis of drug-induced hypersensitivity. In everyday clinical situations, cutaneous ADR often present a considerable challenge in the morphological differential diagnosis. In addition, in the absence of a sound clinical-morphological diagnosis, the selection of appropriate and meaningful diagnostic tests is difficult.

Morphology

The typical lesions of drug-induced exanthemas may encompass a wide variety of so-called primary and secondary efflorescences (fig. 1, 2). In Dermatology, these descriptive terms are used to describe lesions to make a clinical diagnosis and/or to attribute them to a putative pathophysiological process. Uncomplicated drug-induced exanthemas may consist of macules (fig. 3), papules, more rarely vesicles and pustules (table 1). Often, they are combined, i.e. maculopapular (fig. 4) or maculovesicular or papulopustular (fig. 5) lesions, and later secondary lesions may develop (fig. 1, 2). The wheal and flare reactions *(urtica)* are virtually pathognomonic for urticaria; swellings of the deeper skin layers with a pale appearance are characteristic of angioedema. These two conditions are discussed elsewhere in this book.

The size of primary efflorescences is typically between 5 and 10 mm. They start as single lesions, may be grouped and often become confluent. Secondary lesions encountered include erosions from scratching or due to the spontaneous rupture

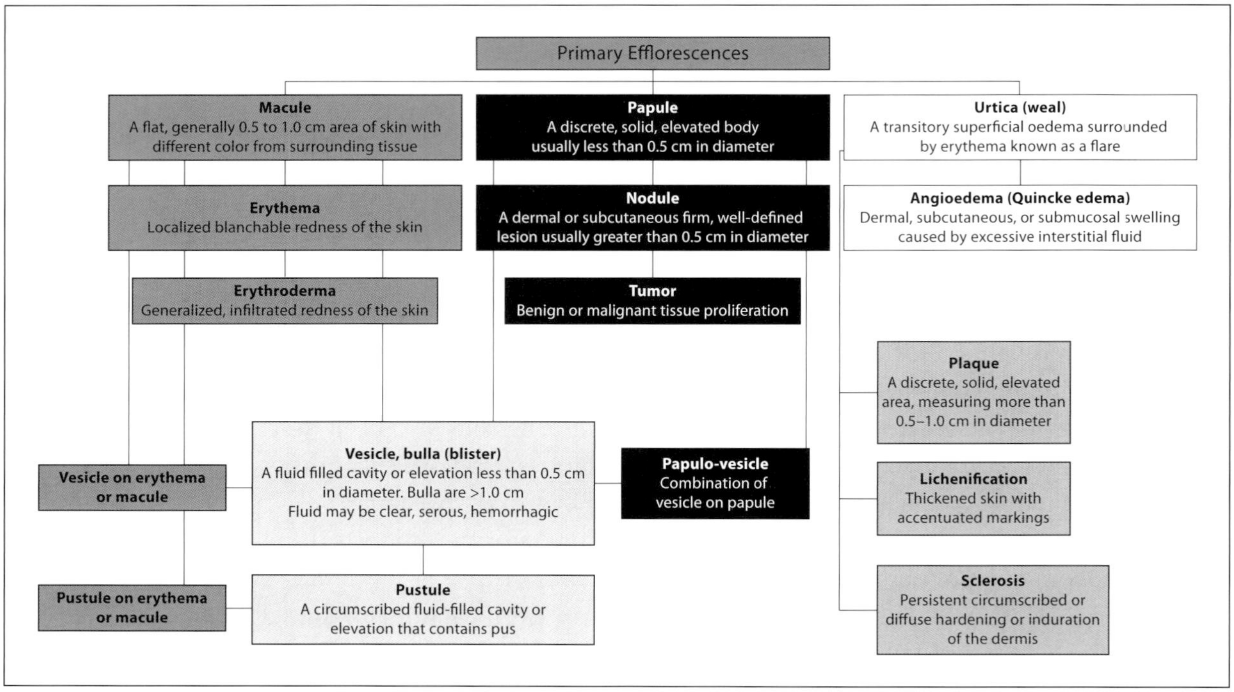

Fig. 1. Description of primary efflorescences, their potential relationships and evolution.

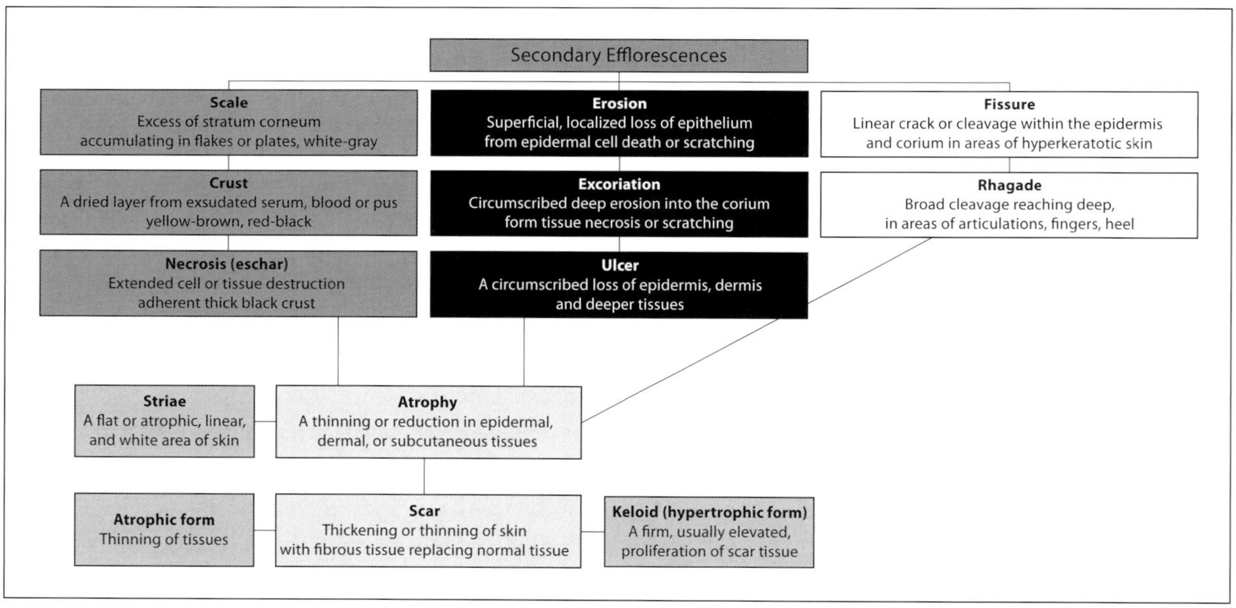

Fig. 2. Description of secondary efflorescences, their potential relationships and evolution.

Table 1. Drug-induced mucocutaneous efflorescences

Pruritus
Efflorescences primary
Erythema
Maculopapular exanthema
Vesicles
Pustules → AGEP
Bullae → SJS, TEN, vasculitis
Efflorescences secondary
Erosions → SJS, TEN
Ulcerations → vasculitis
Necrosis → vasculitis, SJS, TEN
Hemorrhage → vasculitis
Scales
Mucosae
Erythema
Edema
Erosions
Aphthous lesions
Large ulcerations → SJS, TEN
Necrosis → SJS, TEN
Descriptive terms
Lichenoid
Psoriasiform
Pityriasiform
Pseudolymphomatous
Exfoliative
Erythroderma

Modified from Bircher [1] and Bircher and Scherer [15]. AGEP = Acute generalized exanthematous pustulosis; SJS = Stevens-Johnson Syndrome; TEN = toxic epidermal necrolysis.

of vesicles and pustules. In gravity-dependent localizations, such as the legs, or in patients taking anticoagulants, maculopapules with a purpuric or hemorrhagic aspect may be seen. In vasculitic lesions, full-thickness epidermal necrosis with eschar formation and small ulcerations is present.

In the aftermath of more pronounced inflammatory lesions, desquamation of the keratinocyte layer manifesting as fine to extensive scaling may be seen (table 1).

The distribution pattern and combination of drug-induced efflorescences may mimic distinct skin diseases such as eczema, psoriasis or lichen planus. This has led to the descriptive terms of eczematoid, psoriasiform or lichenoid drug eruptions.

In rare instances, infiltrated plaque-like lesions, or nodules resembling cutaneous lymphoma, and widespread erythematous infiltration of large areas of the integument called erythroderma may develop. The formation of these latter lesions involves an extended time period of weeks to months.

Already a careful analysis of single lesions may help to point towards the etiology of an exanthema. For example, in children, purely macular or purely papular and maculopustular lesions are more likely to be associated with a drug etiology, as opposed to maculopapular lesions with petechiae or maculovesicular lesions which are more often seen in infectious disorders [13].

Localization, Distribution, and Evolution

Of further importance are the distribution and localization of the exanthemas, which most often affect the ventral and dorsal aspects of the trunk, followed by centrifugal expansion to the proximal extremities (fig. 3–5). In some exanthemas, particularly papular ones, a very sparse distribution starting on the extremities is possible. Other ones affect the large body folds and the intertriginous, perigenital and perianal area, and spare the central aspects of the trunk. This particular pattern is observed in the so-called symmetrical drug-related intertriginous and flexural exanthema (SDRIFE or so-called Baboon syndrome; fig. 6, 7) [14]. In uncomplicated exanthemas, usually the face, scalp, palms and soles and the mucosal surfaces of the oral cavity, the genital and perianal area are spared (fig. 7). Throughout the evolution of a drug exanthema, initial macules or papules may be followed by maculopapular, pustular or vesicular lesions increasing in size leading to confluence of lesions and spreading in a centrifugal manner. At this stage, the presence of so-called danger signals, heralding the evolution towards severe drug-induced syndromes should be carefully evaluated and observed (table 2).

Chronology

Another significant issue in the clinical diagnosis of drug-induced exanthemas is the chronology, i.e. the pattern of onset and evolution of the reaction [15]. In a nonsensitized patient, the first lesions may occur the earliest after a sensitization phase of at least 5–7 days, typically around the 8–10th day after the start of treatment. About one week is required for the expansion of drug-reactive cells and development of symptoms subsequent to initial drug exposure. In previously exposed and sensitized patients, where a T cell mechanism is involved, the typical latency period between renewed drug exposure and development of first skin lesions lies between 6–12 h extending up to 2 days. First clinical signs such as a discrete erythema may appear after a few hours; thereafter, single lesions develop over a time period of several days, and these may become confluent and fade within 7–14 days after discontinuation of the drug. In some instances, despite discontinuation of therapy, and up to 2 or

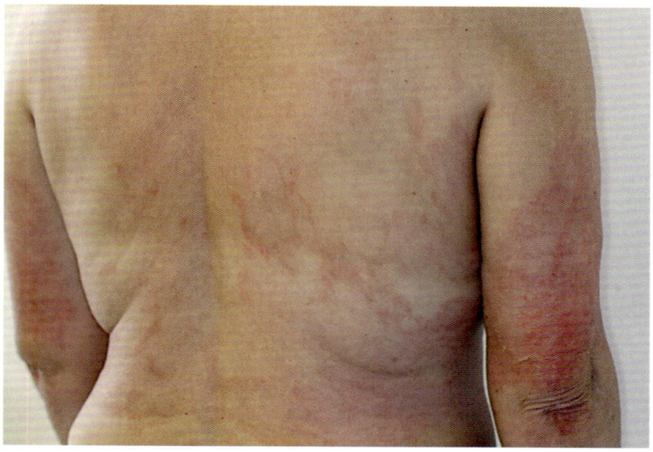

Fig. 3. Confluent drug-induced exanthema with large macular areas.

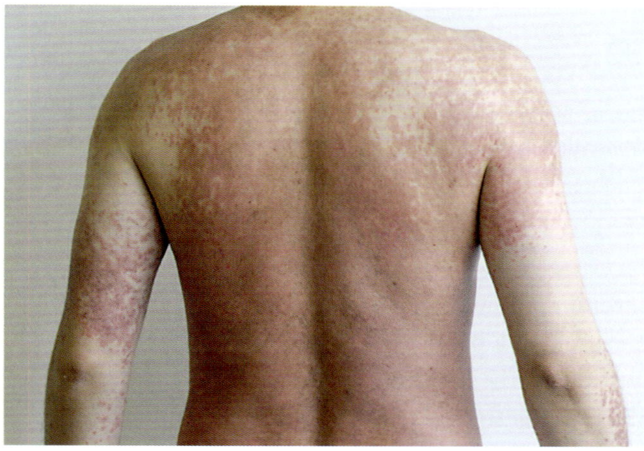

Fig. 4. Confluent macular and papular drug-induced exanthema.

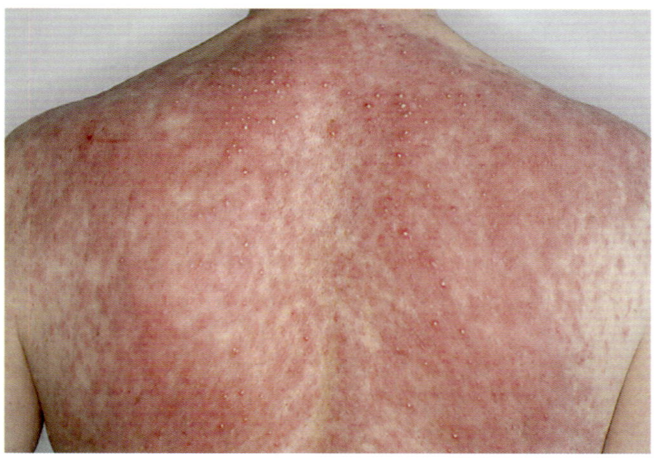

Fig. 5. Confluent papular drug-induced exanthema with few pustules.

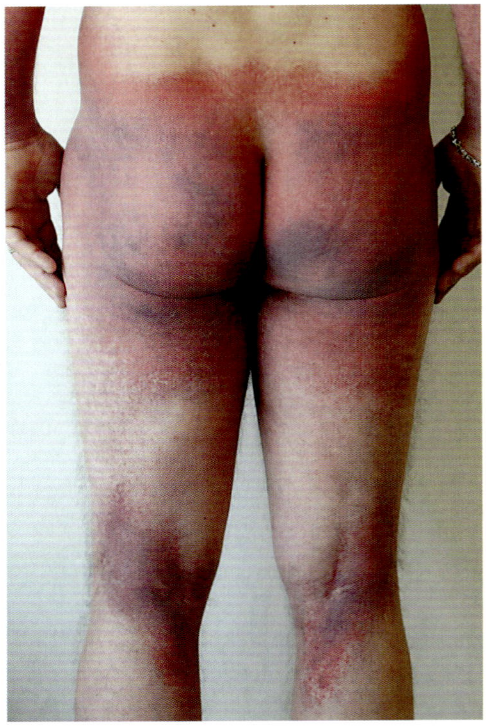

Fig. 6. SDRIFE with circumscribed sharply delineated localization on bottom and knee folds.

several days later, a drug-induced exanthema may still appear. If several drugs have been taken, a precise chronological assessment may help to single out the most suspect drugs. In urticaria and anaphylaxis, the elicitation phase is much shorter, usually ranging from a few minutes to hours, whereas in some types of exanthemas such as in drug hypersensitivity syndrome also referred to as drug rash with eosinophilia with systemic symptoms, and in lichenoid and pseudolymphomatous exanthemas, this latency or elicitation phase may last several weeks or months (fig. 8). Given this wide variability, the separation of the latency period into immediate and nonimmediate reactions with a cutoff situated at 1 h appears oversimplified [1, 15].

Etiology

A large number of drugs may induce an adverse cutaneous reaction. Some are immunologically mediated, for others the pathomechanism remains unknown. Some xenobiotics are primarily reactive, act as haptens, bind to macromolecules, and become full antigens. Examples are penicillins, cephalosporins, and chemical agents bearing a sulfhydryl group. Also, biological drugs, including murine, chimeric, humanized or human antibodies may primarily induce specific immune reactions [9]. In the case of certain other xenobiotics, biotransformation is necessary, and reactive metabolites are

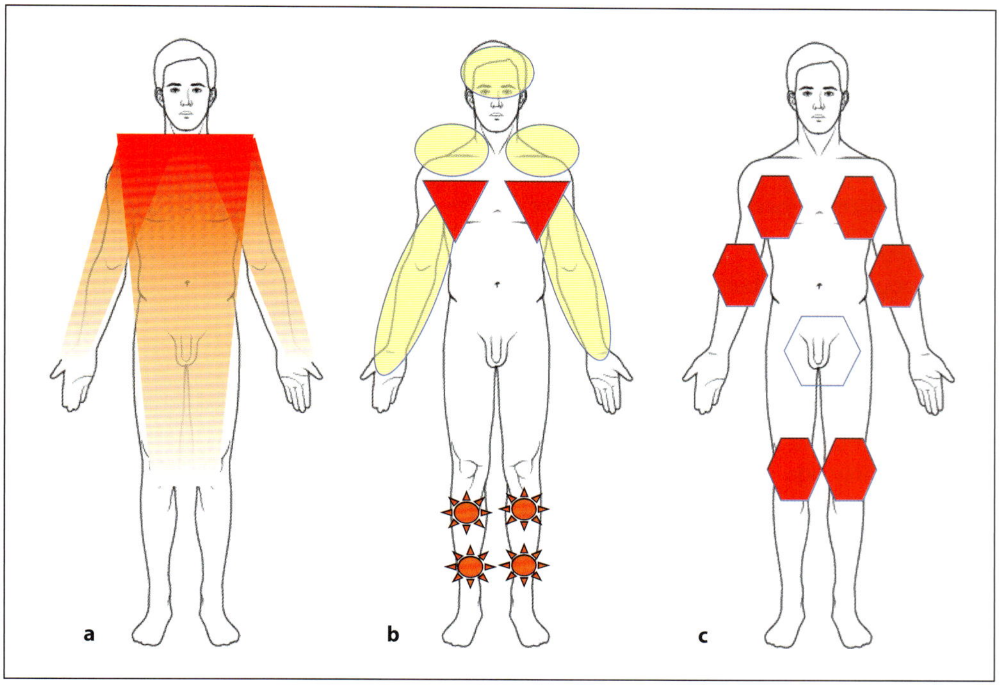

Fig. 7. Distribution and localization patterns. Modified from Bircher and Scherer [15], with permission. **a** Localization of macular, papular, pityriasiform, psoriasiform, lichenoid exanthemas. **b** Exanthemas with particular distribution patterns: ▼ interstitial granulomatous reaction (axillae), ⬭ Sweet's syndrome (head, face, upper extremities), ✸ erythema nodosum (pretibial). **c** ⬢ Localization of SDRIFE perigenital and perianal, large folds.

subsequently formed. Examples of such xenobiotics are the sulfonamides, anticonvulsant drugs, such as carbamazepine and phenytoin, and also some NSAIDs and paracetamol. This may also apply to reverse transcriptase inhibitors, such as nevirapine and abacavir, although the exact pathomechanisms are not completely understood [16].

Concerning the potential or likelihood that a given drug has elicited an adverse cutaneous reaction, regularly updated textbooks or online versions thereof including Litt's drug eruption reference manual [17] provide relevant information concerning the most frequently reported types of exanthemas for each drug, and the approximate frequency of an adverse cutaneous reaction to a given drug.

Pharmacogenetic issues based on the allele frequency of selected HLA antigens, such as HLA-B*1502 and HLA-B*5801, have been associated with a higher risk of developing an adverse cutaneous reaction to a given drug, particularly in severe drug-induced hypersensitivity reactions, such as Stevens-Johnson syndrome (SJS) and toxic epidermal necrolysis (TEN). This was shown for drugs such as carbamazepine, allopurinol and abacavir. In the future, this approach may further help to identify patients with high adverse cutaneous reaction susceptibility prior to a pharmacotherapy.

Table 2. Danger signals in delayed-type reactions heralding progression towards a more severe manifestation

Course
Rapid onset and dissemination
Protracted progression after stopping the offending drug
Recurrence without reexposure to offending or cross-reactive drug
Skin und mucosa
Spontaneous painful or burning skin, tender skin upon touch
Involvement of large body surfaces, erythroderma
Centrofacial erythema and edema (diffuse erythematous swelling)
Dusky red or grayish color of skin lesions (macules, papules)
Target lesions, particularly atypical forms
Vesicular and bullous lesions
Positive Nikolsky sign
Detachment of skin (epidermolysis)
Mucositis of oral cavity, eyes, nose, genitals, anal region (especially when affecting more than one mucosal site)
Purpura
Hemorrhagic lesions (except if under anticoagulation)
Necrotizing lesions
General signs
High fever
General malaise
Lymphadenopathy
Arthritis, arthralgia
Laboratory assessments
Eosinophilia $>1.5 \times 10^9$ cells/l
Cytopenia (granulocytopenia, lymphopenia, thromobopenia, anemia)
Internal organ involvement (liver, kidney, lung, heart, CNS)

Modified from Scherer and Bircher [43] and Bircher [44].

Drugs that are commonly used and have been very rarely implicated in eliciting exanthemas include antihistamines, digoxin, local anesthetics, steroid hormones (estrogens, androgens, corticosteroids), acetylsalicylic acid, paracetamol and coumarins [3, 4, 12].

Pathophysiology

Drug-induced exanthemas are often considered as immunologically mediated hypersensitivity reactions, although such a mechanism can be demonstrated in a minority of the adverse reactions only, depending on the type of the exanthema and the eliciting

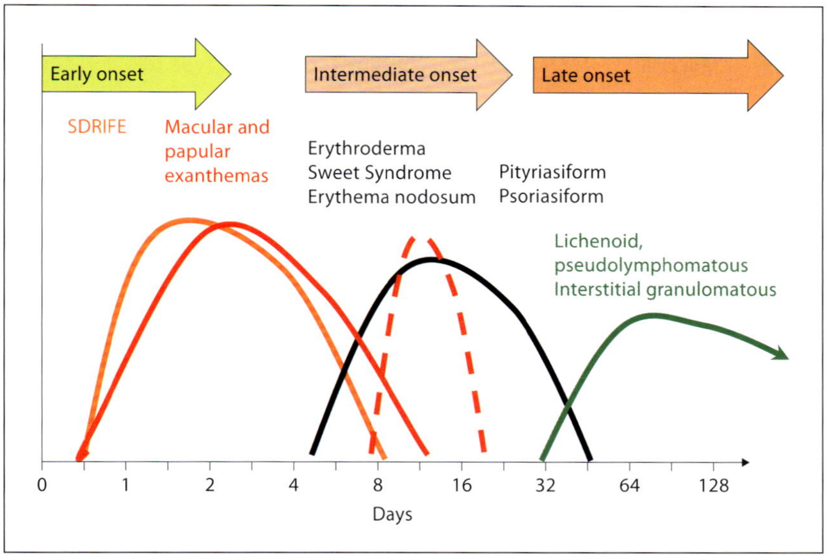

Fig. 8. Approximate onset and evolution of uncomplicated drug-induced exanthemas with probable T cell-mediated pathophysiology in previously sensitized individuals. The height of the lines reflects acuity, their ends the approximate duration. In newly sensitized individuals typically mild exanthemas develop between the 8 and 12th day (red dashed line).

drug. The pathophysiology is variable; in many cases an immunological pathomechanism is involved, particularly type IV hypersensitivity, according to Coombs and Gell. Recently, a further subclassification of type IV hypersensitivity reactions into types IVa–d has been proposed (table 3) [8]. Type IVa corresponds to a Th1 type immune reaction comprising macrophages as major effector cells which secrete interferon-γ and stimulate a proinflammatory response via TNF-α and IL-12. Type IVb corresponds to a Th2 type immune response involving particularly cytokines IL-4, IL-13 and IL-5, which promote B cell expansion and finally plasma cell activation with the production of IgE and IgG4. These pathomechanisms explain the eosinophil-rich inflammation that may be seen in many but by far not all drug-induced exanthemas.

In type IVc reactions, the T cells themselves are the effector cells. Direct cytotoxicity is mediated by granzyme B, granulysin and FAS ligand, the latter in cells expressing FAS. This may be seen as well in maculopapular but more often in bullous drug-induced exanthemas. Type IVd reactions mediated by CXCL8 (IL-8) and granulocyte-macrophage colony-stimulating factor (GM-CSF) producing T cells, which recruit particularly neutrophilic granulocytes and prevent their apoptosis. This pathomechanism appears to play a major role in acute generalized exanthematic pustulosis.

The main effector cells in drug-induced exanthemas are drug-specific cytotoxic T cells (CD4 positive, CD8 positive). These T cells are highly activated as manifested by the expression of CD25 and HLA-DR antigens. Endothelial cells are also activated and express adhesion molecules, such as E- and P-selectin, platelet endothelin,

Table 3. Classification of drug hypersensitivity

	Type I	Type II	Type III	Type IVa	Type IVb	Type IVc	Type IVd
	Antibody mediated			Cell mediated			
Immune reactant	IgE	IgG	IgG	IFN-γ TNF-α (T_H1-cells)	IL-5, IL-4/IL-13, (T_H2-cells)	perforin/ granzyme B (CTL)	CXCL8, IL-17, GM-CSF (T cells)
Antigen	soluble antigen	cell- or matrix-associated antigen	soluble antigen	antigen presented by cells or direct T cell stimulation		cell-associated antigen or direct T cell stimulation	soluble antigen presented by cells or direct T cell stimulation
Effector	mast cell activation	FcR+ cells (phagocytes, NK cells)	FcR+ cells, complement	macrophage activation	eosinophils	T cells	neutrophils
Example of hypersensitivity reaction	anaphylaxis, broncho-constriction	hemolytic anemia, thrombo-cytopenia (e.g. penicillin)	serum sickness, Arthus reaction	tuberculin reaction, allergic contact dermatitis (with IVc)	maculopapular exanthema with eosinophilia internal organ involvement (DRESS)	contact dermatitis, maculopapular and bullous exanthema, hepatitis	AGEP

Adapted from Pichler et al. [8] and Pichler [45].

cell adhesion molecule 1, and intracellular adhesion molecule [6]. Keratinocytes and dendritic cells of the epidermis play an important role too. As opposed to TEN, increased expression of perforin and granzyme B are present in maculopapular exanthemas, but not of FAS ligand. It appears that cytotoxic T cells also play a crucial role in the generation of vesicles in many drug-induced exanthemas. In maculopapular exanthema, perforin-positive and granzyme B-positive CD4+ T cells kill activated keratinocytes, while a large number of cytotoxic CD8+ T cells in the epidermis are associated with formation of vesicles and bullae. Cytokines may also play a major role, particularly Th1 cytokines such as interferon-γ and TNF-α, and also Th2 type cytokines such as IL-5. Various chemokines have also been shown to play a role in drug exanthemas [6]. The involvement of T cells is supported by positive responses in patch tests, delayed-read intradermal tests and lymphocyte transformation or activation tests.

Cofactors in the elicitation of exanthemas include concomitant viral infections, particularly with representatives of the herpes group such as EBV, CMV and human herpes virus-6 (HHV-6) [18], and HIV. Patients with some autoimmune disorders, such as systemic lupus, also have a higher incidence of exanthemas [19].

A different pathogenesis has been postulated for eczematiform exanthemas [11], psoriasis and ichthyosis [20] due to lipid-lowering drugs, particularly statins [21]. The desired systemic interference with cholesterol synthesis may result in an altered lipid composition in the stratum corneum and a change in skin barrier function [11]. This leads to xeroderma, eczematiform changes of the skin and can initiate psoriasis and acquired ichthyosis. In some studies of the above drugs, nonspecified 'skin rashes' have been reported in 1–4% of patients; however, with regard to the common use of statins clinical practice suggests that such adverse effects are rare [11].

In hydroxyethyl starch-induced pruritus, deposition of starch prominently in macrophages seems to be the relevant pathomechanism. Itch appears with a delay of several weeks, is generally refractory to treatment and can persist for up to a year [22].

Special Manifestations of Benign or Uncomplicated Drug Exanthemas

Symmetrical Drug-Related Intertriginous and Flexural Exanthema

Rarely, a drug-related exanthema appears in a symmetrical distribution concentrated in the flexural areas. It has been initially called Baboon syndrome [14]. To delineate this particular drug reaction from systemic contact dermatitis due to systemically eliciting contact allergens such as mercury or nickel, the neutral acronym SDRIFE has been proposed [14]. SDRIFE stands for the mnemonic acronym symmetrical drug-related intertriginous and flexural exanthema. In contrast to most other drug exanthemas, males are more often affected than females. A sharply delineated erythema of the perigenital and perianal area (fig. 6) is associated with the involvement of the large body folds, such as the axilla, the elbows and the knees. Although the exanthema in SDRIFE typically consists of large erythematous patches and plaques, rarely papules, pustules or vesicles may be present. High fever, malaise and internal organ involvement are absent. The exanthema may later result in considerable desquamation. This particular type of drug reaction is most often elicited by aminopenicillins, but other drugs have also been implicated [14]. The literature is controversial concerning the exact chronology of SDRIFE development, i.e. rather long reaction times from up to 7 days between drug intake and onset of lesions have been reported, indicating a new sensitization. Most cases of SDRIFE appear to involve a T cell-mediated pathomechanism and follow the above-mentioned chronology (fig. 8).

Pityriasiform Exanthemas

Pityriasis rosea is a common probably infectious skin disorder that has been suggested to be associated with HHV type 6 and 7 [23], and more recently with HHV-

8 [24] infection or reactivation. Typically, it starts with a solitary, erythematous slightly elevated patch with fine scaling borders, the 'herald patch' located on the trunk, more rarely an extremity. After 10–14 days, an acute dissemination consisting of 10- to 20-mm large oval macules with discrete peripheral scales develops. The symmetrical orientation of these lesions along the cleavage lines (Christmas tree distribution) is highly suggestive of pityriasis rosea. Many drugs have been incriminated as possible triggers of pityriasis rosea-like eruptions, including gold, captopril, tyrosine kinase inhibitors, and nonsteroidal anti-inflammatory agents among many others. Also an association with vaccines such as for diphteria, smallpox, pneumococcus, hepatitis B, and BCG has been reported. However, drug-induced pityriasis rosea often has an atypical clinical presentation, and in histopathology an interface dermatitis with eosinophils is found. Lichen planus-like changes may follow, leaving marked hyperpigmentation [23].

Psoriasiform Exanthemas

A number of drugs have been implicated in the elicitation or exacerbation of psoriasis [25]. The strongest evidence exists for lithium, beta-blockers and antimalarials. It may take several weeks to months until the psoriatic lesions appear [26]. The paradoxal elicitation or exacerbation of psoriasis has been well documented in patients receiving monoclonal antibodies particularly TNF antagonists for psoriasis [27] and sorafenib, an RAF and tyrosine kinase inhibitor [28]. It should be kept in mind that in psoriasis, the Koebner phenomenon may play a confounding role. In patients with a psoriatic background, an initially macular or papular drug-induced exanthema may evolve into psoriatic lesions. Withdrawal of the culprit drug may result in a complete healing. However, it may still be difficult to differentiate between a koebnerized drug exanthema and a drug-induced psoriasis. Also tuberculostatic medications have been implicated in psoriasiform exanthemas [29].

Erythroderma

Any drug-induced exanthemas may show confluence of lesions and progress towards an eczematiform involvement of a large proportion of the skin surface. Particularly in older individuals, the preexistence of xeroderma may favor the development of eczematous lesions after a drug-induced exanthema. The other causes of erythroderma are manifold including atopic dermatitis, psoriasis, contact dermatitis and lymphoma, and these should be excluded if possible. Allopurinol, sulfonamides and anticonvulsant drugs have been most frequently incriminated in drug-induced erythroderma.

Lichenoid and Pseudolymphomatous Forms

Lichen planus or lichen planus-like reactions to drugs have been reported [30]. The skin lesions are small, shiny, polygonal papules with the characteristic Wickham's keratosis. The oral mucosa may also be affected. In terms of location, morphology and histology, lichen planus and drug-induced lichenoid eruptions are identical. Most often gold, antimalarials, methyldopa, beta-blockers and lithium salts have been incriminated [30]. Also biologicals can elicit lichen planus in rare cases [31].

Initial macules may slowly proceed into very pruritic infiltrated nodules and plaques with the clinicohistological presentation of a pseudolymphoma [26]. They have a slower and more protracted time course, obscuring the relation to the eliciting drug. Carbamazepine, phenytoin [32], ACE inhibitors and quinidine have been reported to induce pseudolymphomatous drug eruptions [33]. Histology is in such cases mandatory to exclude cutaneous lymphoma.

Interstitial Granulomatous Drug Reaction

Interstitial granulomatous drug reaction is a rare drug-related reaction pattern. It is characterized by erythematous and violaceous, nonpruritic sometimes painful plaques and nodules in intertriginous areas [26]. It appears very late within a time frame of weeks to months. Eliciting drugs include biologicals such as anakinra, adalimumab and TNF-α antagonists [34], gancyclovir, ACE inhibitors, furosemide, calcium antagonists, beta-blockers, sennosides, herbal medicines, antihistamines, anticonvulsants and antidepressants [35, 36].

Erythema Nodosum

Erythema nodosum-like drug reactions, histologically a septal panniculitis, have been observed to sulfonamides, oral contraceptives, salicylates and azathioprine [26]. Clinically painful pretibial inflammatory nodules and plaques are present. From a clinical and histopathological point of view, the etiology cannot be differentiated.

Acute Febrile Neutrophilic Dermatosis (Sweet's Syndrome)

Sweet's syndrome comprises a symptom complex including fever, neutrophilia, and tender erythematous papules, nodules, and plaques located on the face, neck, chest, and extremities [15]. Three forms are distinguished: classical (idiopathic), malignancy-associated and drug-induced Sweet's syndrome [37]. For the diagnosis of the drug-induced variant, five criteria are required: (A) abrupt onset of painful erythematous plaques or nodules, (B) a dense neutrophilic infiltrate without evidence of leukocytoclastic vasculitis, (C) fever >38°C, (D) a temporal relationship between drug ingestion and manifestation, OR temporally related recurrence after reexposure, and (E) temporally related resolution of lesions after drug withdrawal or treatment with systemic corticosteroids [37]. A large number of drugs have been implicated; however, best evidence exists for GM-CSF, all-trans-retinoic acid, vaccines and probably minocycline [38]. Other reported drugs include bortezomib, azathioprine and sulfonamides.

Differential Diagnosis

The differential diagnosis of drug-induced exanthemas should first be approached from a morphological and then from an etiological point of view. In the former, particular infectious exanthemas such as viral exanthemas (e.g. EBV, HHV-6, CMV, enterovirus, adenovirus, parvovirus B19 and HIV) should be considered [6]. The classical viral infections rubella and measles have a typical clinical appearance and should not be confounded with a drug-induced exanthema. The similarity of the confluent macular lesions has led to the old terms 'morbilliform' and 'rubeoliform' applied to drug-induced exanthemas. As previously mentioned, in children the detailed analysis of the single lesions may help distinguish an infectious or drug-related etiology [13]. Virus-induced exanthemas such as disseminated herpes simplex infections or varicella zoster infections are usually not confounded with drug exanthemas due to their typical clinical manifestations. However, in the initial phase they may have a macular appearance and, particularly in immune-suppressed patients, the skin lesions may be atypical. On the other hand, purpuric gloves and socks syndrome most often associated with parvovirus B19, has been reported as a consequence of cotrimoxazol with a positive reexposure test [39].

Exanthemas associated with bacterial infections manifest more likely with pustular lesions, and may be associated with higher fever and systemic symptoms. The most important differential diagnosis is acute generalized exanthematous pustulosis, a typical drug-induced exanthema discussed elsewhere in this book. A classical imitator of many skin disorders is syphilis, a disease that must not be missed, atypical manifestations thereof have been confounded with drug exanthemas. Also parasitic skin disorders particularly scabies has been confounded with drug exanthemas.

In some patients, skin lesions which are typical for a distinct skin disorder are present, such as psoriasis, lichen planus, pityriasis rosea and others. Here, the personal history, the pattern of distribution of the lesions and histopathology may be helpful in differentiating these skin disorders from drug-induced variants. It should be kept in mind that particularly psoriasis and lichen planus may present with the Koebner phenomenon, which means that slight trauma or inflammation may induce specific skin lesions in patients with a corresponding genetic background. This means that in a patient with psoriasis, first a drug-induced exanthema may occur which later turns into typical disseminated psoriatic lesions. The same phenomenon is possible in lichen planus.

Diagnostic Procedures

Diagnostic steps depend on the phase of the reaction. In an acutely ill patient, the detailed history, accurate clinical analysis of ten skin lesions and histological examination of a lesional skin biopsy (helpful but not specific) are the only steps available. Later on, after the complete healing of the reaction, preferentially in a time window ranging between 6 weeks and 6 months, an allergological workup including skin tests (prick, intradermal with immediate and late readings, as well as patch tests) is recommended. After 6 months, the sensitivity of the tests decreases.

Lymphocyte transformation tests are sometimes recommended as a diagnostic in vitro tool depending on the type of skin reaction, particularly if the involvement of T cells is suspected. Depending on the culprit drug and the laboratory technique used, very variable results have been reported. The specificity in uncomplicated macular or maculopapular exanthemas is low and lies approximately between 30 and 50% depending on the drug [7, 40].

Provocation tests are typically used to identify an alternative drug to be recommended for future pharmacotherapeutic treatments. They are the gold standard; however, even a negative test does not completely exclude the drug in question [41]. The absence of particular cofactors, such as coinfection or, ultraviolet irradiation in phototoxic reactions etc., could result in such false negative tests.

Therapeutic Options

Treatment is aimed at the control of inflammation and troubling symptoms. First, the offending agent should be stopped as rapidly as possible. Here, particularly the precise consideration of the chronology of the induction and elicitation phases may be helpful in patients who take several drugs. Drugs that have been introduced within a time frame of 3–4 weeks previous to onset of skin lesions are more likely to be involved than drugs that have been taken for months or years, at least when taken in a continuous manner. Depending on signs and symptoms, topical corticosteroids and systemic antihistamines can be helpful. In severe reactions, treatment with systemic corticosteroids may be indicated. In some cases, the patient may be treated despite a mild exanthema, particularly when the medical indication for treatment is life-threatening and no alternative drug is available. 'Treating through' is the continuation of a drug treatment in the presence of a developing or established drug hypersensitivity reaction. In rare situations, patients have been treated through, sometimes under cover of antiallergic medication such as corticosteroids and antihistamines. However, the continuation of an eliciting drug may potentially result in a more severe and widespread manifestation of the drug exanthema. The exact risk of developing a severe bullous reaction, such as SJS or TEN, is not known.

Finally, desensitization may be an option in certain cases; however, this is well established for immediate-type hypersensitivity reactions [42], and less for delayed-type cutaneous hypersensitivity reactions. However, there is increasing evidence suggesting that particularly in patients that are in repeated need of a particular drug, such as sulfonamides (cotrimoxazol) in HIV patients, or antibiotic courses in patients with cystic fibrosis, tolerance induction may be an option.

References

1 Bircher AJ: Approach to the patient with a drug hypersensitivity reaction – clinical perspectives; in Pichler W (ed): Drug Hypersensitivity. Basel, Karger, 2007, pp 352–365.

2 Demoly P, Hillaire-Buys D: Classification and epidemiology of hypersensitivity drug reactions. Immunol Allergy Clin North Am 2004;24:345–356.

3 Bigby M, Jick S, Jick H, Arndt K: Drug-induced cutaneous reactions. A report from the Boston Collaborative Drug Surveillance Program on 15,438 consecutive inpatients, 1975 to 1982. JAMA 1986; 256:3358–3363.

4 Bigby M: Rates of cutaneous reactions to drugs. Arch Dermatol 2001;137:765–770.

5 Nigen S, Knowles SR, Shear NH: Drug eruptions: approaching the diagnosis of drug-induced skin diseases. J Drugs Dermatol 2003;2:278–299.

6 Yawalkar N: Maculopapular drug eruptions; in Pichler WJ (ed): Drug Hypersensitivity. Basel, Karger, 2007, pp 242–250.

7 Schnyder B: Approach to the patient with drug allergy. Med Clin North Am 2010;94:665–679, xv.

8 Pichler WJ, Adam J, Daubner B, Gentinetta T, Keller M, Yerly D: Drug Hypersensitivity Reactions: Pathomechanism and Clinical Symptoms; in Pichler WJ, Glover R (eds): Drug Hypersensitivity: Medical Clinics of North America. Philadelphia, Saunders, 2010, vol 94, pp 645–664.

9 Scherer K, Spoerl D, Bircher AJ: Adverse drug reactions to biologics. J Dtsch Dermatol Ges 2010;8: 411–426.

10 Sparsa A, Boulinguez S, Le Brun V, Roux C, Bonnetblanc JM, Bedane C: Acquired ichthyosis with pravastatin. J Eur Acad Dermatol Venereol 2007;21:549–550.

11 Krasovec M, Elsner P, Burg G: Generalized eczematous skin rash possibly due to HMG-CoA reductase inhibitors. Dermatology 1993;186:248–252.

12 Bircher AJ: Arzneimittelallergie und Haut. Stuttgart, Thieme, 1996.

13 Drago F, Rampini P, Rampini E, Rebora A: Atypical exanthems: morphology and laboratory investigations may lead to an aetiological diagnosis in about 70% of cases. Br J Dermatol 2002;147:255–260.

14 Hausermann P, Harr T, Bircher AJ: Baboon syndrome resulting from systemic drugs: is there strife between SDRIFE and allergic contact dermatitis syndrome? Contact Dermatitis 2004;51:297–310.

15 Bircher AJ, Scherer K: Delayed cutaneous manifestations of drug hypersensitivity. Med Clin North Am 2010;94:711–725.

16 Pirmohamed M: HIV and drug hypersensitivity; in Pichler W (ed): Drug Hypersensitivity. Basel, Karger, 2007, pp 84–94.

17 Litt JZ: Litt's Drug Eruptions & Reactions Manual, ed 16. London, Informa Healthcare, 2010.

18 Tohyama M, Hashimoto K, Yasukawa M, Kimura H, Horikawa T, Nakajima K, Urano Y, Matsumoto K, Iijima M, Shear N: Association of human herpesvirus 6 reactivation with the flaring and severity of drug-induced hypersensitivity syndrome. Br J Dermatol 2007;157:934–940.

19 Del Mar Campos-Fernández M, Ponce-de-León-Rosales S, Archer-Dubon C, Orozco-Topete R: Incidence and risk factors for cutaneous adverse drug reactions in an intensive care unit. Rev Invest Clin 2005;57:770–774.

20 Sparsa A, Boulinguez S, Le Brun V, Roux C, Bonnetblanc J, Bedane C: Acquired ichthyosis with pravastatin. J Eur Acad Dermatol Venereol 2007;21: 549–550.

21 Proksch E: Lipidsenker-induzierte Nebenwirkungen an der Haut. Hautarzt 1995;46:76–80.
22 Bork K: Pruritus precipitated by hydroxyethyl starch: a review. Br J Dermatol 2005;152:3–12.
23 Drago F, Broccolo F, Rebora A: Pityriasis rosea: an update with a critical appraisal of its possible herpesviral etiology. J Am Acad Dermatol 2009;61: 303–318.
24 Prantsidis A, Rigopoulos D, Papatheodorou G, Menounos P, Gregoriou S, Alexiou-Mousatou I, Katsambas A: Detection of human herpesvirus 8 in the skin of patients with pityriasis rosea. Acta Derm Venereol 2009;89:604–606.
25 Rongioletti F, Fiorucci C, Parodi A: Psoriasis induced or aggravated by drugs. J Rheumatol 2009; 83:59–61.
26 Ramdial PK, Naidoo DK: Drug-induced cutaneous pathology. J Clin Pathol 2009;62:493–504.
27 Mourão A, Rustin M, Isenberg D: Exacerbation of psoriatic skin lesions in patients with psoriatic arthritis receiving anti-tumour necrosis factor-alpha therapy: description of 3 cases and review of the literature. Clin Exp Rheumatol 2010;28:408–410.
28 Laquer V, Saedi N, Dann F, Kelly K: Sorafenib-associated psoriasiform skin changes (letter). Cutis 2010;85:301–302.
29 Park J-J, Choi YD, Lee J-B, Kim S-J, Lee S-C, Won YH, Yun SJ: Psoriasiform drug eruption induced by anti-tuberculosis medication: potential role of plasmacytoid dendritic cells. Acta Derm Venereol 2010; 90:305–306.
30 Ellgehausen P, Elsner P, Burg G: Drug-induced lichen planus. Clin Dermatol 1998;16:325–332.
31 Musumeci ML, Lacarrubba F, Micali G: Onset of lichen planus during treatment with etanercept. Am J Clin Dermatol 2010;11:55–56.
32 Van Renterghem D, De Vries EA: Pseudo-lymphoma and anticonvulsant hypersensitivity syndrome during the use of anti-epileptic agents. Tijdschr Geneesk 1997;53:399–403.
33 Bocquet H, Bagot M, Roujeau JC: Drug-induced pseudolymphoma and drug hypersensitivity syndrome (drug rash with eosinophilia and systemic symptoms: DRESS). Semin Cutan Med Surg 1996; 15:250–257.
34 Regula CG, Hennessy J, Clarke LE, Adams DR, Ioffreda MD, Graber EM, Helm KF: Interstitial granulomatous drug reaction to anakinra. J Am Acad Dermatol 2008;59:S25–S27.
35 Vila A, Puig L, Fernández-Figueras M, Laiz A, Vidal D, Alomar A: Adverse cutaneous reactions to anakinra in patients with rheumatoid arthritis: clinicopathological study of five patients. Br J Dermatol 2005;153:417–423.
36 Oh S, Schramme A, Stark A, Tilgen W, Gutwein P, Reichrath J: Overexpression of ADAM 10 and ADAM 12 in lesional psoriatic skin. Br J Dermatol 2008;158:1371–1373.
37 Cohen P: Sweet's syndrome – a comprehensive review of an acute febrile neutrophilic dermatosis. Orphanet J Rare Dis 2007;2:34.
38 Thompson DF, Montarella KE: Drug-induced Sweet's syndrome. Ann Pharmacother 2007;41:801–811.
39 van Rooijen MM, Brand CU, Ballmer-Weber BK, Yawalkar N, Hunziker TK: Medikamentös induziertes papulopurpurisches Gloves-and-Socks-Syndrom. Hautarzt 1999;50:280–283.
40 Bircher AJ: The lymphocyte transformation test in drug hypersensitivity. A useful diagnostic tool? in Nicolas JF (ed): Allergie aux médicaments: Tests immuno-biologiques. Montrouge, John Libbey Eurotext, 2006, pp 41–45.
41 Aberer W, Bircher A, Romano A, Blanca M, Campi P, Fernandez J, Brockow K, Pichler WJ, Demoly P: Drug provocation testing in the diagnosis of drug hypersensitivity reactions: general considerations. Allergy 2003;58:854–863.
42 Cernadas JR, Brockow K, Romano A, Aberer W, Torres MJ, Bircher A, Campi P, Sanz ML, Castells M, Demoly P, Pichler WJ, for the European Network of Drug Allergy and the EAACI interest group on drug hypersensitivity: General considerations on rapid desensitization for drug hypersensitivity – a consensus statement. Allergy 2010;65:1357–1366.
43 Scherer K, Bircher AJ: Danger signs in drug hypersensitivity. Med Clin North Am 2010;94:681–689.
44 Bircher AJ: Symptoms and danger signs in acute drug hypersensitivity. Toxicology 2005;209:201–207.
45 Pichler WJ: Drug hypersensitivity reactions: Classification and relationship to T-cell activation; in Pichler WJ (ed): Drug Hypersensitivity. Basel, Karger, 2007, pp 168–189.

Prof. Andreas J. Bircher
Allergy Unit, Department of Dermatology, University Hospital Basel
Petersgraben 4
CH–4031 Basel (Switzerland)
Tel. +41 61 265 43 59, E-Mail andreas.bircher@unibas.ch

French LE (ed): Adverse Cutaneous Drug Eruptions.
Chem Immunol Allergy. Basel, Karger, 2012, vol 97, pp 98–105

Drug-Induced Angioedema

Marianne Lerch

Allergy/Dermatology Unit, Department of Internal Medicine, Kantonsspital, Winterthur, Switzerland

Abstract

Angioedema (AE) is the end result of deep dermal, subcutaneous and/or submucosal swelling, and represents a major criterion in the definition of anaphylaxis. Drug-induced AE, like other cutaneous drug reactions, is most frequently elicited by betalactam antibiotics and nonsteroidal anti-inflammatory drugs. However, differences exist in their underlying pathophysiology (IgE mediated vs. pseudoallergic). Blockers of the renin-angiotensin-aldosterone system are the most common class of medications associated with isolated AE and are most probably related to elevated bradykinin levels. Typically, ACE inhibitor-associated AE can occur up to several years after initiating treatment, and may sporadically recur even after discontinuation. A comprehensive investigation of AE must include analysis of complement factors, tryptase levels as well as specific allergy tests. Furthermore, other possible causative agents ought to be excluded. Every patient with drug-induced AE must receive an allergy pass as well as emergency medication including epinephrine. In some cases, inhibitors of the bradykinin system may be considered for treatment.

Essentials in a Nutshell

- Drug-induced angioedema (AE) may be complicated by life-threatening anaphylaxis
- Drug-induced AE is most frequently elicited by betalactam antibiotics, nonsteroidal anti-inflammatory drugs (NSAIDs) as well as blockers of the renin-angiotensin-aldosterone system (ACE inhibitors – ACEIs, angiotensin II receptor blockers – ARBs, and direct renin inhibitors)

Introduction

Certain forms of AE were originally described more than 150 years ago. AE is defined as deep dermal, subcutaneous and/or submucosal swelling, whereas urticaria usually represents a more transient superficial swelling due to plasma leakage. C1 esterase

Table 1. Clinical findings in different forms of AE

	Form				
	HAE	AAE	RAE	A/PAE	IAE
Symptoms					
Abdominal symptoms	++	+	–/+	–/+	–
Urticaria	–	–	–	–/+	++

RAE = ACEI-, ARB- or renin inhibitor-induced AE; A/PAE = allergic/pseudoallergic AE; IAE = idiopathic AE.

inhibitor deficiency/dysfunction is characterized by recurrent AE without wheals that often also affects the bowel.

Regarding adverse drug reactions, exanthematous eruptions and urticaria represent the two most common forms of cutaneous clinical phenotypes. Drug-induced AE is associated with urticaria in 50% of cases and may be complicated by life-threatening anaphylaxis. The major drugs implicated in AE are betalactams, NSAIDs and ACEIs. Although the combination of urticaria and/or AE with systemic symptoms like hypotension is typical for IgE-mediated anaphylaxis and severe pseudoallergic reactions, delayed-type allergic reactions can manifest as urticarial lesions with a variable degree of AE as well. Also, facial edema is a cardinal symptom in a distinct T cell-mediated hypersensitivity syndrome called DRESS (drug reaction with eosinophilia and systemic symptoms) e.g. to carbamazepine as well as in contact dermatitis, e.g. to paraphenylenediamine (permanent black hair dye).

In the following chapter, different types of AE are briefly described, and an overview of AE-eliciting drugs will be provided. In this part, ACEI-induced AE including clinical presentation, underlying mechanisms, as well as treatment alternatives will be focused on. Finally, diagnostic procedures together with therapeutic measures for patients with drug-induced AE are summarized.

Types of Angioedema

In contrast to acute urticaria/AE, chronic forms of urticaria/AE last more than 6 weeks by definition, and are intermittent or persistent.

AE can be categorized into several forms [1, 2]: hereditary (HAE), acquired (AAE), idiopathic forms of AE, those associated with allergic/pseudoallergic reactions (i.e. venom hypersensitivity, latex allergy, some adverse drug reactions, food allergy, and (para)infectious reactions) and finally renin-angiotensin-aldosterone system blocker-induced AE (table 1).

HAE as well as AAE constitute C1 inhibitor deficiencies (low concentration or dysfunction). Whereas in HAE C1 inhibitor function is abnormal in combination

Table 2. Different groups of drug-induced AE according to pathomechanism (nonconclusive overview)

Specific	Nonspecific	
IgE mediated	intolerance	kinin-dependent
Penicillins, cephalosporins	NSAIDs	ACEIs ARBs
Iodinated contrast media	Iodinated contrast media	
Neuromuscular blocking agents	Neuromuscular blocking agents	
Pyrazolones	Pyrazolones	
Quinolones	Quinolones	

with a low or a normal C1 inhibitor concentration (HAE type I and HAE type II, respectively) and normal C1q, in HAE type III no complement C4 or C1 inhibitor abnormalities are found. AAE is associated with lymphoproliferative diseases/paraneoplastic syndromes or characterized by autoreactive IgG antibodies to C1 inhibitor.

AAE and HAE as well as other forms of AE are difficult to distinguish on clinical symptoms alone. However, in AAE a family history is absent. Also, onset of symptoms is much later. AAE patients have low levels (or activity) of C1 inhibitor, C4 and C1q [1, 3].

Patients with HAE do not have associated urticaria, but abdominal symptoms are common and at least 50% of them might have laryngeal swelling at some point [1]. Common triggers can include oral contraceptives, antiandrogenic treatment with cyproterone, hormonal replacement therapy, and ACEIs as well as other factors like trauma or infection. In addition to purified C1 inhibitor concentrate, more recently, icatibant, a bradykinin receptor antagonist, and ecallantide, a kallikrein inhibitor are available for the treatment of acute episodes of HAE [1, 4]. Furthermore, there is good evidence that icatibant and ecallantide might be effective in AAE as well [3]. In the future, the use of recombinant human C1 inhibitor (rhC1-INH) might reduce the risk of infection and the costs of C1 inhibitor therapy [2].

The true incidence of idiopathic urticaria/AE is not known. Idiopathic AE is a diagnosis of exclusion after thorough evaluation. Episodic (Gleich syndrome) and non-episodic AE with eosinophilia as well as the very rare capillary leak syndrome (Clarkson) are considered to be separate forms of idiopathic AE [1].

Drug-Induced Angioedema

Drug-induced AE can be differentiated into three main categories defined by the underlying eliciting mechanism (table 2).

Firstly, immediate hypersensitivity reactions to betalactam antibiotics constitute the most frequent allergic reactions which are IgE mediated [5]. Generally, penicillin allergies are the best-investigated hypersensitivity reactions as to the underlying immunological mechanism [6]. Other drugs that elicit AE by an IgE-mediated allergic mechanism are listed in table 2.

Secondly, adverse reactions to NSAIDs represent another important group with regard to drug-induced AE. However, this is classically via a non-allergic inhibition of cyclooxygenase and as a result major alterations in arachidonic acid metabolism such as cysteinyl leukotriene overproduction. Aspirin and other NSAIDs can also induce or aggravate clinical symptoms in the 20–40% of patients with chronic idiopathic urticaria/AE overlap. Another distinct clinical entity in this context is aspirin-induced asthma (AIA) which can also only be diagnosed with aspirin provocation challenges.

Although NSAIDs are common elicitors of non-allergic intolerance reactions, they may also be responsible for immediate or delayed allergic reactions, e.g. to pyrazolones, in a small subset of patients [7].

Non-immune-mediated hypersensitivity reactions or so-called pseudoallergic reactions are as frequent as true IgE-mediated reactions. However, higher drug doses than for true IgE-mediated reactions might be required. Also, it seems that these reactions tend to arise less rapidly (often after more than 15 min). Mast cell degranulation seems to play a role at least in some of these reactions. Pseudoallergic reactions can be elicited by many drugs like iodinated contrast media and plasma expanders [8]. However, recent data from a European multicenter study suggest that at least 50% of hypersensitivity reactions to contrast media are caused by an underlying immunological mechanism [9]. Detailed analysis of contrast media-specific T cells leads to better understanding of the molecular basis of contrast media hypersensitivity and may help identify for example contrast media that do not cross-react providing useful clinical alternatives [10, 11]. Unlike IgE-mediated immediate type reactions, delayed drug-induced cutaneous reactions can be subclassified based on clinical and immunological features [12].

Thirdly, the most frequently eliciting drugs of AE apart from NSAIDs and betalactams are ACEIs.

ACEIs are now widely prescribed for the treatment of hypertension as well as for providing cardiovascular and renal protection in patients with heart failure, chronic kidney disease, and at high risk of cardiovascular events [13]. Approximately 40 million people worldwide are currently receiving ACEIs. The most common adverse effects observed in patients treated with ACEIs are dry nonproductive cough occurring in 15–30% of patients and AE [14].

The reported incidence of ACEI-induced AE varies between 0.1 and 1%. Prevalence of ACEI-induced AE is higher in black than in white patients. Unlike in other cases of drug-induced AE, adverse reactions to ACEIs are frequently missed as they may develop long after the drug has been started. Also it may occur inconsistently while the drug is continued [15], and minor sporadic episodes of AE may even recur after discontinuation of the ACEI [16]. Life-threatening edema of the upper airways is present in up to 40%, and can be resistant to treatment or even fatal [14].

The underlying mechanism of ACEI-associated AE is the ACE inhibition itself, which as well as preventing the conversion of angiotensin I to angiotensin II also reduces the catabolism of bradykinin, a potent vasoactive peptide (vasodilator) [17].

Therefore, aside from conventional treatment with corticosteroids and epinephrine, the bradykinin inhibitor icatibant could be promising for the treatment of ACEI-associated AE [13, 18].

However, the most important measure to be taken is discontinuation of the eliciting drug.

In this context, the question arises as to how safe the replacement of ACEIs by ARBs is. ARBs were introduced in 1995 and have a pharmacological and metabolic profile similar to ACEIs [19, 20]. In the literature, several articles indicate a risk of development of any subsequent AE when taking an ARB of approximately 2–17% [14, 21]. Pathophysiologically, this might be due to the suggested participation of kinins in the effects of ARBs via activation of the angiotensin 2 receptor [22].

Thus, for practical purposes, ARBs should not be considered an ideal alternative for ACEI treatment. However, rare entities like calcium channel blocker-associated small bowel AE may have an impact on therapeutic decision-making in hypertensive patients as well [23].

The first oral direct renin inhibitor aliskiren received Food and Drug Administration approval for the treatment of hypertension in 2007 [24]. A more complete renin-angiotensin system inhibition than with existing agents is produced by its novel mechanism of action, namely inhibition of renin's catalytic activity. Thus, direct renin inhibitors may afford greater protection from hypertensive complications. As direct renin inhibition should not alter local or circulating bradykinin, aliskiren was thought to be an alternative in patients with ACEI and ARB-induced AE [25]. However, a recent pharmacovigilance analysis showed AE and renal dysfunction to be potential adverse events associated with exposure to aliskiren [26]. Therefore, treatment with renin inhibitors should be considered with caution in patients with ACEI- or ARB-induced AE.

Diagnostics and Treatment

In patients with AE of unknown etiology, a recommended diagnostic algorithm is summarized below.

Firstly, a thorough patient history is indispensable, particularly in determining frequency of occurrence, known allergies, comorbidities, medications and possible triggering cofactors such as physical exercise, alcohol, NSAID intake and infections. Secondly, a general predisposition for recurrent anaphylaxis due to systemic mastocytosis and a genuine predisposition to AE due to complement deficiency, respectively, have to be excluded. Finally, a previously unknown food hypersensitivity should be ruled out.

After physical examination, routine laboratory tests (blood cell count, immuno-electrophoresis, erythrocyte sedimentation rate, C-reactive protein, hepatic enzymes, renal function) are recommended. To exclude possible eliciting factors like infections and autoimmune disorders, further specific examinations have to be considered according to the patient history. Those would include stool analysis and serology for parasites and helminths, pharyngeal and urine cultures, sinus and dental radiography, determination of thyroid function and antithyroid antibodies as well as selected rheumatological parameters like antinuclear autoantibodies.

In cases of suspected drug-induced AE, specific allergy tests must be sequentially performed, including skin prick then intradermal tests, as well as in vitro determination of specific IgEs (if commercially available), basophil activation test (BAT), and lymphocyte transformation tests if available. Eventually, provocation testing may be considered in non-life threatening reactions to determine a tolerated alternative medication (table 3), e.g. provocation testing with COX 2-inhibitors (coxibs) in patients with AE to non-selective NSAIDs.

As emphasized earlier, the most important measure to be taken in drug-induced reactions is discontinuation of the eliciting drug. Also, all patients must be supplied with an allergy pass as well as emergency medication including epinephrine for self-administration after appropriate instruction on its use. A summary of therapeutic measures can be found in table 4.

Conclusions

Drug-induced AE can be elicited by three different pathophysiological mechanisms, namely IgE-mediated immediate hypersensitivity, pseudoallergic reactions e.g. due to inhibition of cyclooxygenase, and bradykinin-related reactions.

Interestingly, similar drugs like NSAIDs or contrast media may elicit adverse reactions by different pathways.

The specific allergic and the non-immune-mediated pseudoallergic reactions differ from ACEI-/ARB-induced AE with regard to the clinical picture. ACEI-associated AE might be missed as symptoms can occur several years after initiating therapy.

As continued ACEI treatment tends to worsen AE and because of the potentially life-threatening character of drug-induced AE in general, the eliciting medication must be promptly stopped and replaced by adequate alternative substances. Patients must also be provided with, and educated in the use of emergency medication including epinephrine when applicable.

In the future, the bradykinin inhibitor icatibant could be promising for the additional treatment of ACEI-associated AE. In this context, further studies are warranted to identify patients at risk of renin inhibitor-associated AE.

Table 3. Algorithm for the diagnosis of drug-induced AE

Physical examination
Emergency treatment
4–6 weeks

Standard workup	Specific evaluation
Complete blood cell count (eosinophilia?)	Skin test according to EAACI, except severe anaphylactic reactions
CRP	Determination of specific IgE: penicillins, anesthetics, etc.
Liver/kidney parameters	BAT, lymphocyte transformation test
Tryptase	Consider provocation test
Complement status: C1 inhibitor concentration/ function, C4, C1q	Allergy pass

Table 4. Current options for treatment of AE

	HAE	AAE	RAE*	A/PAE*	IAE
C1 inhibitor concentrate	X	X			
Fresh frozen plasma	X	X			
Epinephrine, corticosteroids		(X)	X	X	X
Anti-histamines (leukotriene antagonists)				X	X
Icatibant	X	X	X		
Ecallantide	X	X			
Immunotherapy, tolerance induction				X	

* Drug-induced AE.

References

1 Banerji A, Sheffer AL: The spectrum of chronic angioedema. Allergy Asthma Proc 2009;30:11–16.

2 Bas M, Adams V, Suvorava T, Niehues T, Hoffmann TK, Kojda G: Nonallergic angioedema: role of bradykinin. Allergy 2007;62:842–856.

3 Cicardi M, Zanichelli A: Acquired angioedema. Allergy Asthma Clin Immunol 2010;6:14.

4 Garnock-Jones KP: Ecallantide: in acute hereditary angioedema. Drugs 2010;70:1423–1431.

5 Antunez C, Martin E, Cornejo-Garcia JA, Blanca-Lopez N, Pena R, Mayorga C, Torres MJ, Blanca M: Immediate hypersensitivity reactions to penicillins and other betalactams. Curr Pharm Des 2006;12: 3327–3333.

6 Blanca M, Romano A, Torres MJ, Demoly P, DeWeck A: Continued need of appropriate betalactam-derived skin test reagents for the management of allergy to betalactams. Clin Exp Allergy 2007;37: 166–173.

7 Szczeklik A, Nizankowska-Mogilnicka E, Sanak M: Hypersensitivity to aspirin and other NSAIDs: mechanisms, clinical presentation and management; in Pichler WJ (ed): Drug Hypersensitivity. Basel, Karger, 2007, pp 340–349.

8 Pichler WJ: Drug hypersensitivity reactions: classification and relationship to T-cell activation; in Pichler WJ (ed): Drug Hypersensitivity. Basel, Karger, 2007, pp 168–189.

9 Brockow K, Romano A, Aberer W, Bircher AJ, Barbaud A, Bonadonna P, Faria E, Kanny G, Lerch M, Pichler WJ, Ring J, Rodrigues Cernadas J, Tomaz E, Demoly P, Christiansen C, European Network of Drug Allergy and the EAACI interest group on drug hypersensitivity: Skin testing in patients with hypersensitivity reactions to iodinated contrast media – a European multicenter study. Allergy 2009;64:234–241.

10 Lerch M, Keller M, Britschgi M, Kanny G, Tache V, Schmid DA, Beeler A, Gerber BO, Luethi M, Bircher AJ, Christiansen C, Pichler WJ: Cross-reactivity patterns of T cells specific for iodinated contrast media. J Allergy Clin Immunol 2007;119:1529–1536.

11 Keller M, Lerch M, Britschgi M, Tache V, Gerber BO, Luethi M, Lochmatter P, Kanny G, Bircher AJ, Christiansen C, Pichler WJ: Processing-dependent and -independent pathways for recognition of iodinated contrast media by specific human T cells. Clin Exp Allergy 2010;40:257–268.

12 Lerch M, Pichler WJ: The immunological and clinical spectrum of delayed drug-induced exanthems. Curr Opin Allergy Clin Immunol 2004;4:411–419.

13 Weber MA, Messerli FH: Angiotensin-converting enzyme inhibitors and angioedema: estimating the risk. Hypertension 2008;51:1465–1467.

14 Sanchez-Borges M, Gonzalez-Aveledo LA: Angiotensin-converting enzyme inhibitors and angioedema. Allergy Asthma Immunol Res 2010;2: 195–198.

15 Cicardi M, Zingale LC, Bergamaschini L, Agostoni A: Angioedema associated with angiotensin-converting enzyme inhibitor use. Arch Intern Med 2004; 164:910–913.

16 Zingale LC, Beltrami L, Zanichelli A, Maggioni L, Pappalardo E, Cicardi B, Cicardi M: Angioedema without urticaria: a large clinical survey. CMAJ 2006;175:1065–1070.

17 Kaplan AP, Joseph K, Silverberg M: Pathways for bradykinin formation and inflammatory disease. J Allergy Clin Immunol 2002;109:195–209.

18 Bas M, Greve J, Stelter K, Bier H, Stark T, Hoffmann TK, Kojda G: Therapeutic efficacy of icatibant in angioedema induced by angiotensin-converting enzyme inhibitors: a case series. Ann Emerg Med 2010;56:278–282.

19 Lerch M, Teuscher AU, Beissner P, Schneider M, Shaw SG, Weidmann P: Effects of angiotensin II-receptor blockade with losartan on insulin sensitivity, lipid profile, and endothelin in normotensive offspring of hypertensive parents. J Cardiovasc Pharmacol 1998;31:576–580.

20 Lerch M, Weidmann P, Ho MP, Gerber P, Eckenberger P, Kaemmereit A, Teuscher AU: Metabolic effects of temocapril in hypertensive patients with diabetes mellitus type 2. J Cardiovasc Pharmacol 1999;33:527–533.

21 Haymore BR, Yoon J, Mikita CP, Klote MM, DeZee KJ: Risk of angioedema with angiotensin receptor blockers in patients with prior angioedema associated with angiotensin-converting enzyme inhibitors: a meta-analysis. Ann Allergy Asthma Immunol 2008;101:495–499.

22 Yayama K, Okamoto H: Angiotensin II-induced vasodilation via type 2 receptor: role of bradykinin and nitric oxide. Int Immunopharmacol 2008;8: 312–318.

23 Turcu AF, White JA, Kulaga ME, Skluth M, Gruss CB: Calcium channel blocker-associated small bowel angioedema. J Clin Gastroenterol 2009;43: 338–341.

24 Shafiq MM, Menon DV, Victor RG: Oral direct renin inhibition: premise, promise, and potential limitations of a new class of antihypertensive drug. Am J Med 2008;121:265–271.

25 Anzaldua DA, Schmitz PG: Aliskiren as an alternative in a patient with life-threatening ACE inhibitor-induced angioedema. Am J Kidney Dis 2008;51: 532–533.

26 Ali AK: Pharmacovigilance analysis of adverse event reports for aliskiren hemifumarate, a first-in-class direct renin inhibitor. Ther Clin Risk Manag 2011;7: 337–344.

Dr. Marianne Lerch
Allergy/Dermatology Unit, Department of Internal Medicine, Kantonsspital
Brauerstrasse 15
CH–8401 Winterthur (Switzerland)
Tel. +41 52 266 55 18, E-Mail marianne.lerch@ksw.ch

French LE (ed): Adverse Cutaneous Drug Eruptions.
Chem Immunol Allergy. Basel, Karger, 2012, vol 97, pp 106–121

Fixed Drug Eruption: The Dark Side of Activation of Intraepidermal CD8+ T Cells Uniquely Specialized to Mediate Protective Immunity

Tetsuo Shiohara · Yoshiko Mizukawa

Department of Dermatology, Kyorin University School of Medicine, Tokyo, Japan

Abstract

Fixed drug eruption (FDE) is generally regarded as representing the mild end of drug-induced dermatitis, but the clinical importance of recognizing this disease as an abortive, localized variant of toxic epidermal necrolysis has received increasing attention in recent years. FDE often presents with a wide spectrum of clinical manifestations indistinguishable from those of other skin diseases, such as erythema multiforme, Stevens-Johnson syndrome /toxic epidermal necrolysis, cellulitis, paronychia, lichen planus, and parapsoriasis en plaques. These unusual forms of FDE are likely to be overlooked unless the possibility of a drug etiology is routinely considered in the differential diagnosis of any patient with these diseases. Clinical awareness and recognition of these unique forms are essential for avoiding a misdiagnosis. Intraepidermal CD8+ T cells resident in the FDE lesions that have the capacity to rapidly produce large amounts of IFN-γ are likely to have a key role in mediating localized epidermal injury, while they may represent a T cell subset uniquely specialized to mediate protective immunity against various pathogens.

Essentials in a Nutshell

- Fixed drug eruption (FDE) is a relatively common dermatitis
- Classic FDE is characterized by a solitary or small number of well-circumscribed, round and/or oval erythematous macules and plaques with dusky centers on the skin and/or mucous membrane which tend to recur at exactly the same site with each administration of the causative drug ('recall' or 'isotopic' phenomenon)
- FDE typically resolves after discontinuation of the causative drug, leaving hyperpigmentation at the site of lesions

- A nonpigmenting, multiple variant of FDE that closely resembles toxic epidermal necrolysis (TEN)/Stevens-Johnson syndrome (SJS) clinically is a diagnostic challenge, is often associated with systemic symptoms, and should be considered as a severe adverse cutaneous drug eruption
- Although the most frequently implicated medications are antibacterial agents and nonsteroidal anti-inflammatory drugs, the causative drugs differ from country to country
- FDE is mediated by skin-resident CD8+ T cells of the effector memory phenotype with the capacity to specifically recognize drug antigen

Introduction

FDE is a relatively common dermatitis, affecting individuals from childhood to adulthood of all ethnic backgrounds throughout the world, although susceptibility appears to be shaped by genetic influences [1]. Although the most frequently implicated medications are antibacterial agents and nonsteroidal anti-inflammatory drugs [2], the causative drugs differ from country to country and follow the local patterns of drug usage; thus, the number of cases of FDE caused by a particular drug is largely influenced by the amount of that drug taken nationwide, either on prescription or after purchase over the counter, in addition to its intrinsic ability to cause an FDE [3]. The traditional view of the pathogenesis is that localized cutaneous inflammation observed in FDE is mediated by T cells migrating from the circulation, with the capacity to specifically recognize drug antigen, like other drug eruptions. In the late 1990s, we demonstrated that FDE cases were associated with intraepidermal T cells originally resident in the lesional epidermis [4–7], validating the concept that FDE is mediated by such skin-resident T cells with overly aggressive activity of the effector memory phenotype which, on the other hand, preserve protective functions against pathogens [2, 4–7].

In recent years, attention has also been focused on the clinical and histological resemblance of the nonpigmenting, multiple variant to TEN, the most severe drug eruption. Although FDE is generally regarded as representing the mild end of drug-induced dermatitis, the clinical importance of recognizing this disease as an abortive, localized variant of TEN has received increasing attention over the last 5 years [8]. In addition, because a recall phenomenon or isotopic response can be typically seen in FDE lesions [9], this disease may also serve as an important clue in understanding the pathomechanism of a recall phenomenon [10]. Because the clinical spectrum of FDE is highly variable, contrary to the widely held belief, in this review we would also like to expand on the clinical and histopathologic spectrum of FDE by describing patients with unusual clinical features. The wide spectrum of clinical manifestations may highlight the complex role of skin-resident T cells in various cellular mechanisms.

Thus, we review these and other recent studies and their implications for our understanding of FDE.

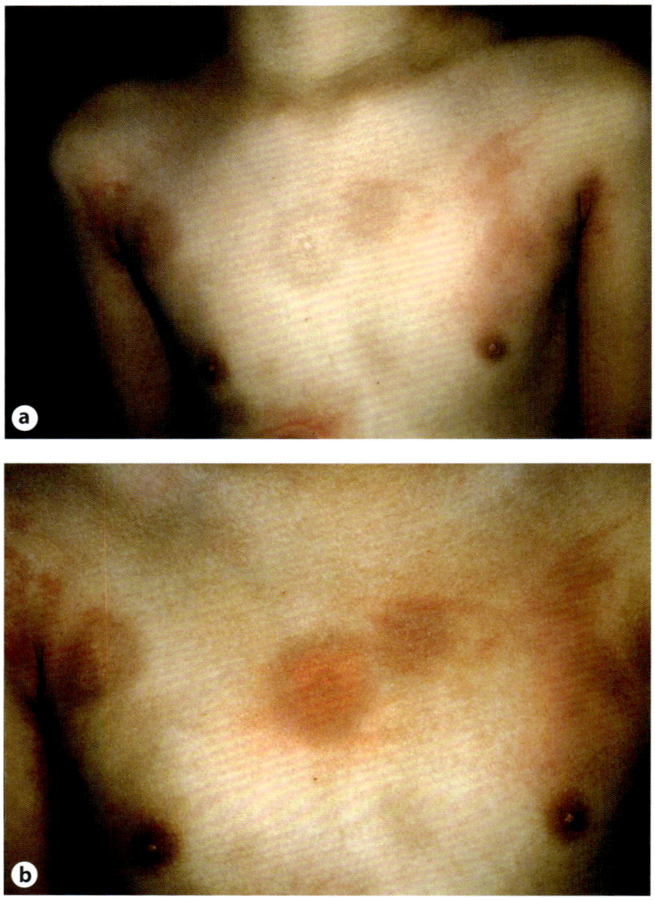

Fig. 1. a Typical multiple FDE lesions. Several round to oval, dusky red macules and plaques on the trunk 20 min after clinical challenge with the causative drug. **b** One h after clinical challenge, erythematous macules and plaques developed on most of the previously involved areas.

Clinical Manifestations of Fixed Drug Eruption

Clinical manifestations of FDE are not as straightforward as textbooks sometimes indicate and, as a result, FDE is undoubtedly underdiagnosed. The classic FDE lesions are characterized by a solitary or small number of well-circumscribed, round and/or oval erythematous macules and plaques with dusky centers on the skin (fig. 1) and/or mucous membrane; these lesions usually start abruptly at exactly the same site with each administration of the causative drug. The appearance of these lesions is often preceded and/or accompanied by sensation of itching or burning. These lesions typically resolve after discontinuation of the causative drug, leaving hyperpigmentation at the site of lesions. Therefore, the diagnosis of FDE is thought to be easy for many dermatologists even after clinical resolution, when these lesions are single or more round or oval demarcated hyperpigmented lesions. The individual lesions are 1–4 cm in diameter and rarely exceed 10 cm. The lesions usually appear within 30 min to 8 h after drug intake: mean length of time from drug intake to the onset of symptoms is approximately 2 h [11]. These FDE lesions become more numerous and more severe unless the causative drug is withdrawn. New FDE lesions often occur at the site of previously traumatized or inflamed skin such as insect bites, burn, and venepuncture sites [12]. Although FDE lesions occur anywhere on the skin or mucous or genital membranes, the most commonly affected locations are the lip, palms, soles, glans penis, and groin areas. Some FDE lesions evolve into bullous and generalized eruptions mimicking SJS and TEN. After discontinuation of the causative drug, these FDE lesions spontaneously resolve over several days, a finding that cannot be observed in severe drug eruptions such as SJS and TEN, in which lesions continue to increase in size and number several days after withdrawal of the causative drug.

Although systemic manifestations are usually absent in cases with typical FDE lesions, multiple lesions are often associated with systemic manifestations including malaise, high fever, nausea, and arthralgia [2, 5, 8, 13]. Because blister formation often occurs at an advanced stage in these patients, it is difficult to distinguish between TEN/SJS and such a multiple variant of FDE, particularly when the bullous lesions become more widespread in association with systemic manifestations and do not leave typical hyperpigmentation. In 1987, Shelley and Shelley coined the term nonpigmenting FDE (NPFDE) to refer to this variant [14]. Because the clinical features of such a nonpigmenting, multiple variant closely resemble those of TEN/SJS, this variant is frequently misdiagnosed as TEN/SJS unless dermatologists take special care to recognize the presence of this entity: this variant will be described later. The shade of the hyperpigmentation tends to become darker with each succeeding exacerbation. This tendency is more prominent in dark-skinned patients, such as Asians, while in light-skinned patients, such as Caucasians, the color of such lesions remains purplish gray to slate gray even after numerous episodes [15], making it difficult to identify the lesion as being 'fixed'. For this reason, FDE in light-skinned patients is easily misdiagnosed with erythema multiforme (EM) and inflammatory skin diseases.

Most FDE lesions occur with orally administered rather than injected drugs: the most common causative drugs are pseudoephedrine, trimethoprim, tetracycline, barbiturates, sulfonamide, mefenamic acid, acetylsalicylic acid, phenolphthalein, ibuprofen, and oxyphenbutazone. Over-the-counter drugs containing several medications often cause FDE. In some patients, FDE lesions can occur after sexual intercourse or kissing with their partners taking the offending drugs [16]: the lesions on the penis and the lip that were probably caused by contact with drugs seemingly present in the vaginal fluid and the oral cavity, respectively.

Although the incidence of FDE is generally thought to be decreasing, particularly in the Western world with a much lower usage of medications causing the FDE, the unusual form of FDE described later is likely to be increasing probably due to unawareness of the unusual presentation. Following each exacerbation, some FDE lesions fail to recur despite administration of the causative drug, which is known as the refractory period [7]. The duration of this period is variable, lasting from a few weeks to several months. Guin et al. [17] reported that the FDE lesions appeared to wander because some of the previously involved sites did not flare with each exposure while others flared: this peculiar eruption would be caused by a prolonged refractory period and the tendency to become completely refractory in some lesions, but not in others. Because of this period, in some patients there may be a delay of several weeks between drug intake and the development of FDE lesions.

FDE lesions can be reproduced upon administration of related drug/agents with chemical structures similar to the inducing offending drug, which is referred to as cross-reactivity. In some patients, however, drug/agents with totally different chemical structures can activate the FDE lesions at exactly the same sites as did the inducing offending drug, a phenomenon known as polysensitivity [18]. Polysensitivity is much more common than is actually reported and may have been overlooked in the past because of the relatively low recognition of this phenomenon.

In some patients, the FDE lesions can only be reproduced when multiple drugs are administered in combination but not separately [19]. Whatever the precise mechanism of action of the combination in causing the FDE lesions, combined stimulation by multiple drugs with unique immunomodulatory properties may be needed for precipitating exacerbations.

There have been many reports describing patients with typical FDE lesions but who had no significant history of drug intake preceding the eruption. Some of such cases of recurrent exacerbations of the FDE lesions without significant history of drug intake might be attributable to several nonspecific exogenous factors. Indeed, nonmedical factors, such as food, dermographism, and ultraviolet irradiation, have been reported to precipitate exacerbations of FDE lesions [20–24]. The FDE lesions precipitated by the ingestion of a particular food can be termed fixed food eruption [20–22], although it is unclear whether the triggering agents that originally induced the lesions were indeed drugs in these cases.

Despite the continued administration of the causative drug, the spontaneous resolution of FDE lesions has been known to occur in some patients, indicating that these patients would be spontaneously desensitized to the causative drug. Indeed, Kelso and Keating [25] reported successful desensitization for treatment of FDE to allopurinol.

Unusual Forms of Fixed Drug Eruption

FDE shows varying clinical and histologic expressions: very unusual forms including NPFDE have been reported. NPFDE is such a variant often associated with systemic manifestations, such as malaise, high fever, nausea, and arthralgia and represents the most extensive form of FDE. According to the original description by Shelley and Shelley [14], multiple, large, erythematous, well-circumscribed plaques are symmetrically located in the axillae, groins, pubis, flanks, and intergluteal fold (fig. 2). Although a classic form of pigmented FDE (PFDE) is generally recognized as representing the mild end of drug-induced reactions, generalized bullous NPFDE may

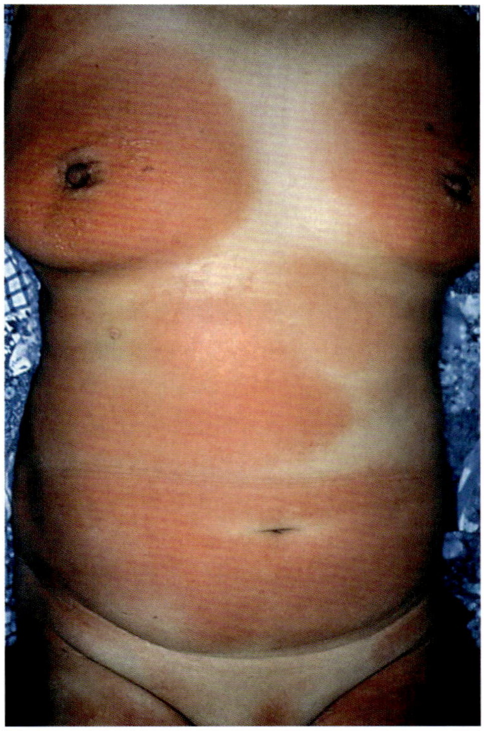

Fig. 2. Typical NPFDE lesions. Large, round to oval, erythematous plaques can be seen on the trunk. These lesions cleared without leaving pigmentary changes.

represent the severe end of FDE: it remains to be determined, however, whether this variant is a severe form of FDE or an abortive variant of the TEN spectrum [8]. In generalized bullous NPFDE, bullous lesions often continue to increase in number and may evolve into TEN/SJS-like lesions unless the causative drug is withdrawn. In this regard, some authors have argued that TEN/SJS may be a severe form of bullous FDE. At least, it should be recognized that, in many cases, TEN/SJS is defined empirically by its typical clinical and pathologic features without the confirmation of the causative agents, because of its clinical severity. The differential diagnosis of NPFDE includes bullous pemphigoid when large bullae appear on the involved areas.

NPFDE has been reported to develop in patients after general anesthesia [26]: because this reaction after the anesthesia is not generally recognized and it develops several hours after the anesthesia, it is difficult to note the link between drug administration and the appearance of a peculiar and rare type of the eruption. During the anesthesia, a variety of drugs able to be incriminated as the causative drug of FDE, such as codeine, morphine, opium, and barbiturates, are used. In this case, when anesthesia was induced with menthohexital sodium instead of thiopental, the patient had no reaction, suggesting a link between thiopental and appearance of the NPFDE lesions.

A peculiar linear pattern of FDE lesions have been also reported, although it is unclear whether the patient had preceding herpes zoster before onset of FDE [27]. Because the linear erythema occurred along the dermatomes suggesting a zoster sine herpete episode, this linear type of FDE may be caused by immune responses to herpes zoster previously unrecognized although triggered by the drug.

An unusual cellulitis-like FDE due to topotecan has also been reported [28]: an erythematous and edematous plaque with undermined borders mimicking cellulitis was elicited by the subsequent administration of the offending drug at the same sites, confirming the diagnosis of FDE. These findings suggest that FDE lesions can be reproduced at exactly the same sites of previously damaged skin by various exogenous stimuli, such as varicella-zoster virus [27] and previous cellulitis [28], or paronychia [29]. In these cases, not only the site but also the shape of the original disease can be reproduced in the FDE lesions. In this regard, we proposed the concept of trauma-localized FDE [10]: FDE lesions initially appeared at exactly the same sites of a previous trauma, such as burn scars and insect bites, and at venipuncture sites. This concept is helpful for our understanding of the mechanism of FDE and other inflammatory skin diseases such as lichen planus, which often appear in their particular areas of prediction, a finding known as 'recall phenomenon' [30, 31].

Another unique type of FDE shows multiple, chronic, superficial lesions persisting unchanged for several months [32]. The clinical picture nearly resembled parapsoriasis en plaques. In view of the fact that FDE has generally been regarded as an acutely inflamed skin disease, this chronic type of FDE is exceptional and may be easily overlooked. The diagnosis of the chronic type of FDE was made on the basis of prompt resolution upon withdrawal of the causative drug and the reproducibility of the eruption by administration of the drug: because in this case the patient took acetaminophen many times daily, this may have contributed to the chronic nature of the condition. In contrast, the classic 'acute' type of FDE would be induced by intermittently administered drug: on the other hand, the continued administration of the causative drug may result in desensitization to the drug.

Because FDE lesions of unusual forms as described above can be easily overlooked without a detailed history of drug intake and careful examination of the lesions, such cases may be at greater risk for repeated episodes of exacerbations by drug intake. Thus, the possible sequence of progressive exacerbation on repeated administration of the causative drug can mimic a variety of idiopathic skin diseases including EM, parapsoriasis, and mycosis fungoides [33]. The diagnosis of FDE is likely to be missed unless the possibility of a drug etiology is routinely considered in the differential diagnosis of patients with these diseases. The consequences of not diagnosing FDE or misdiagnosing these diseases could be devastating, because most of the improvement is seen over the first week after withdrawal of the causative drug: however, unless a search is made to identify a relevant causative drug, and exposure to the drug is avoided, repeated administration of the causative drug would result in progressive and irreversible disease. Keeping these considerations in mind, the spectrum of FDE has recently been expanded to include cases with such unusual clinical presentations. Clinical awareness and recognition of these unique features are essential for avoiding misdiagnosis.

Histology of Fixed Drug Eruption

The histologic picture of FDE is the prototype of a lichenoid tissue reaction [2, 5, 34] with melanin incontinence: the major changes are hydropic degeneration of basal keratinocytes associated with lymphocytic invasion of the epidermis involving mainly the interfollicular epidermis. These changes are typically observed in the FDE lesions on day 1 to 2 after administration of the causative drug, at which time most biopsy specimens are obtained. In interpreting these findings in FDE lesions at a given time, however, one must appreciate the fact that biopsy specimens obtained for diagnostic purposes represent a single time point in the evolving FDE lesions. The dynamics of evolving FDE lesions have unfortunately not been adequately investigated in the past. We therefore obtained biopsy specimens from virtually the same site after rechallenging patients with the causative drug, to follow the orchestrated series of events resulting in epidermal injury from the beginning [5, 8, 13]. The results showed remarkable differences depending on the time after rechallenging and the site biopsied.

Before rechallenge, a small number of lymphocytes were aligned along the epidermal side of the dermoepidermal junction and minimal perivascular lymphocytic infiltrates were detected: the epidermis appeared normal except for the presence of lymphocytes. At 2–3 h after rechallenge, when irritation and slight erythema appeared in the previously involved sites, lymphoid cells originally adhering to the basal layer moved upward to the lower half of the epidermis, while preserving the epidermal architectures. Neither hydropic degeneration of the basal layer nor an extensive exocytosis of lymphoid cells in the epidermis was seen at this time. Typical changes in FDE lesions consisting of hydropic degeneration of the basal layer and the extensive exocytosis of lymphoid cells were seen at 24–48 h. The extent of epidermal damage seen at the peak in FDE lesions is highly variable depending on the lesion examined, ranging from confluent epidermal necrosis resembling TEN to spongiotic epidermis. Thus, confluent epidermal necrosis, said to be specific for TEN but not in FDE, can be occasionally seen in FDE lesions and is largely a function of the site of lesions biopsied. Melanophages were abundantly detected in the upper dermis of classic PFDE lesions at any stage of lesions. In contrast, a few if any melanophages were present in NPFDE lesions, consistent with the lack of hyperpigmentation. Severe epidermal damage, however, can be also detected in some NPFDE lesions, not consistent with the original description by Shelley and Shelley [14], who proposed that the drug-induced immune responses in NPFDE are primarily directed against the dermis and spare the epidermis. Nevertheless, our finding can be reconciled with the severe nature of the clinical presentations of the NPFDE.

Although inflammatory cellular infiltrates observed at the peak of FDE lesions are predominantly composed of lymphoid cells, a mixed cellular infiltrate made up predominantly of neutrophils, nuclear dust, eosinophils and lymphohistiocytic cells can be also seen in some FDE lesions. FDE with the histopathological findings of a neutrophilic dermatosis has also been reported. Agnew and Liver [35] described this variant as neutrophilic FDE, because this case is clinically and histologically distinct from previously reported cases of FDE in that the basal epidermis is intact without lichenoid disruption and there is a marked perivascular and interstitial inflammatory infiltrate with a predominance of intact neutrophils. Despite their proposal, however, the presence of this variant has not been widely recognized. In our FDE case series, a mixed inflammatory infiltrate predominantly composed of neutrophils can only occasionally be seen. This neutrophil-rich infiltrate is often found when biopsy specimens are obtained from FDE lesions on the flexural areas, as in the case reported by Agnew and Liver [35]. Thus, this may have been a function of the site of lesions and would be expected in FDE lesions developing on the flexural areas.

Diagnosis of Fixed Drug Eruption

The diagnosis of classic PFDE is generally thought to be easy for many dermatologists even after clinical resolution, based on the history of episodes after drug intake and a single or multiple round or oval, demarcated hyperpigmented lesions. However, because the clinical spectrum is quite varied as described above, the diagnosis of FDE is not as straightforward as textbooks sometimes suggest. Indeed, FDE often presents with a wide spectrum of clinical manifestations indistinguishable from those of other skin diseases, such as EM [15], SJS/TEN, cellulitis [28], paronychia [29], neutrophilic dermatosis [35], lichen planus, and parapsoriasis en plaques [32]. In these cases, the time course of appearance of the FDE lesions in relation to any drug must be examined carefully, before attributing the lesions to a particular medication. Because blister formation often occurs at an advanced stage of FDE reactions in association with systemic symptoms such as fever, physicians often encounter a great deal of difficulty in distinguishing between the multiple, bullous variant of FDE and TEN, particularly when the bullous lesions become more widespread with systemic manifestations. Because this variant does not leave typical hyperpigmentation after clinical resolution as typically seen in NPFDE, this variant can be easily misdiagnosed as TEN or bullous pemphigoid. Bullous pemphigoid can be ruled out by negative immunofluorescence for subepidermal IgG and/or C3 in the biopsied lesions. Careful history taking into account drug intake and a prior history of recurrent lesions at the same sites are essential for the precise diagnosis of FDE, but patients often ignore medications they have been taking routinely for years, such as Chinese herbal medicines, and nonmedical agents such as food.

The diagnosis of FDE is made more complex by the recent recognition that exacerbations precisely similar to those caused by the inducing drug can be triggered at the same sites not only by drugs with totally different chemical structures, but also by other nonspecific exogenous factors such as ultraviolet irradiation. Moreover, we have learned to expect FDE lesions to initially occur at previously inflamed or traumatized skin sites, such as sites of burn scars and insect bites [12, 15]. In view of the fact that a 'recall' or 'isotopic' phenomenon is typically seen in FDE lesions and that the 'isotopic' phenomenon has also been well documented in EM, some cases with EM showing an 'isotopic' phenomenon may actually be a NPFDE variant. When the bullous lesions become rapidly widespread associated with high fever in the multiple, bullous variant, they need to be distinguished from TEN. The difference can be found in the clinical course after withdrawal of the causative drug: the bullous lesions in TEN progressively extend to involve the entire body despite drug withdrawal, while bullous FDE often resolves rapidly without the requirement for steroid administration.

Oral rechallenge and topical provocation tests are usually performed to identify the drug responsible for the FDE. Because no systemic symptoms can usually be induced by oral challenge tests, oral challenge tests with a single therapeutic dose of the suspected drug or one tenth of the therapeutic dose can be done with relative safety. Patch tests at the site of a previous lesion yield a positive response in up to 43% of cases [36]. However, false negative results have been reported and have been attributed to the reactivity of drugs with limited penetration properties. Although patch tests are usually performed with the pure original drug on the upper back in patients with other drug eruptions, this may give misleadingly negative results in FDE. There are several reasons for these negative results. First, patients are frequently not sensitized to the original drug but to its physiologic metabolites. Since these metabolites are usually neither known nor available for patch tests, the patch tests using the original drug may give false negative results. Second, when patch tests are performed with the original drug diluted at <1% in petrolatum and/or in water, this may also give false negative results. Thus, patch tests should be performed with the drug mixed in petrolatum to 10% or diluted in water. Although positive patch test reactions can be more easily obtained when the drug diluted at >50% is used, this should not be done: the stronger delayed reactions would occur on days 3–7, indicating patch test sensitization. Third, patch tests should be performed at the previously involved sites in FDE, because patch tests on the upper back usually yield false negative results. Patch tests are particularly useful to determine the causative drugs when multiple drugs are suspected. Thus, a positive patch test reaction confined to the previously involved areas is generally regarded as strong evidence that the FDE lesions are caused by the tested drug, although it must be kept in mind that a negative test does not necessarily exclude it. Some investigators suggest that patch tests would also be useful as a screening test when multiple drugs are suspected. Patch tests with multiple drugs, however, are not advised because of increased risk of a potential patch-test sensitization. The risk is also considered to be doubled when the drug diluted at >20% is used.

The lymphocyte transformation test has been successfully used for defining the culprit drug in maculopapular drug eruptions, acute generalized exanthematous pustulosis and drug-induced hypersensitivity syndrome [37, 38], but is rarely positive in FDE [26, 27]. Positive lymphocyte transformation test reactions are rarely obtained in patients with FDE, except for those with generalized FDE, such as NPFDE. Given the above, oral challenge remains the most reliable method for establishing the causative drug in FDE.

Clinically Relevant Issues of Disease Pathogenesis

Although extensive data exist on crosstalk between the intestinal epithelium and epithelial-resident lymphocytes under basal conditions and in chronic disease [39], this relation in human epidermis has not been studied to the same degree. In this regard, we previously demonstrated that CD8+ T cells with cytotoxic potential persist between basal keratinocytes as a stable subset in the lesions over a prolonged period of time after clinical resolution [40–42]. Given the presence of these T cells before the onset of clinical symptoms, it is evident that important immunological mechanisms take place for before patients consult a physician. While the T cell compartment in mouse epidermis is exclusively composed of γδ+ T cells with invariant T cell receptors (TCRs) designated as dendritic epidermal T cells [43], major resident T cells in human epidermis express TCR-αβ [4, 40]. Although skin-resident T cells in mice are crucial for tumor immunosurveillance [44] and skin homeostasis [40, 45, 46], little is known about the physiological role of human skin-resident T cells.

Our earlier studies reported that a phenotypically homogenous population of cells that express as TCR-αβ, CD3, CD8, CD45RA, CD103, CLA and CD11b but not CD27 and CD56 were preferentially detectable in FDE lesions before the onset of the disease, but rarely in the uninvolved epidermis of FDE patients and healthy individuals [4, 5, 40, 41]. This phenotype of T cells most closely resembles that of effector memory T cells [47–49], although some differences are present: these intraepidermal CD4+ T cells constitutively express markers common to the skin-homing memory T cells such as CLA and CD103, while effector memory T cells do not. Interestingly, such accumulations of T cells with an effector memory phenotype has been reported to be found at sites of repeated pathogen entry, such as the lung [50], suggesting that these T cells may confer protective immunity, like their murine counterpart. Consistent with this suggestion, T cells with an effector memory phenotype preferentially migrate into the sites of infection, such as mucosal sites and persist for long periods of time following infection [48, 49]. However, we demonstrated that intraepidermal CD8+ T cells resident in FDE lesions are critical in the initiation of cytotoxic immune responses against surrounding keratinocytes, the opposite of what would be expected if the role of T cells with an effector memory phenotype resident in the epithelium were simply a protective response to pathogens. If the intraepidermal CD8+ T cell population with an effector memory phenotype resident in the FDE lesions is a general mediator of this type of localized tissue injury, how can the detrimental effects of these T cells on epidermal tissues be reconciled with effects such as the mediation of protection in epithelial tissues?

These findings are not easily reconciled, unless one assumes that these intraepidermal T cells would be expected to play a previously unrecognized role in protection against pathogens under quiescent nonpathological conditions, but could nevertheless mediate localized epidermal damage through collaboration with cells of the acquired immune system such as CD4+ T cells. In support of this notion, Gebhardt

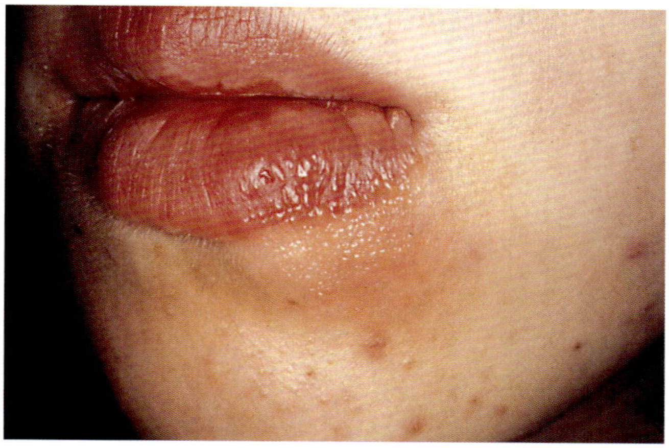

Fig. 3. A typical FDE lesion developed at exactly the same sites as the patient's previous herpes simplex lesions.

et al. [51] provided evidence to indicate that a unique memory T cell subset with the phenotype common to our intraepidermal CD8+ T cells remains resident in the skin after acute infection with herpes simplex virus (HSV) and provides enhanced local immunity during infection with HSV. Virus-specific CD8+ T cells have also been shown to accumulate near sensory nerve endings in genital skin during subclinical HSV-2 reactivation [52]. According to our scenario, CD8+ T cells with such an effector memory phenotype and skin-homing potential can initially be called to seed to the skin upon infection with HSV or other nonspecific stimuli, persist in these peripheral tissues for long periods of time following infection, and are noted for immediate expression of effector function, which mediate pathogen clearance. As shown in our previous studies [5, 41], such intraepidermal T cells can produce large amounts of cytokines, such as IFN-γ, in response to antigen without proliferative responses, a finding consistently observed in T cells with the effector memory phenotype [53]. The lack of an antigen-induced proliferative response by the intraepidermal CD8+ T cells in human skin despite the retention of a strong effector cytokine response within the lesional epidermis is consistent with these T cells having a protective role in mediating effector responses. Consistent with this scenario, the intraepidermal CD8+ T cells are not constitutively cytolytic, but, once activated via the CD3/TCR complex, display a strong cytolytic activity against NK-sensitive or NK-resistant tumor cells and cultured keratinocytes [41]. Support for this scenario also comes from our observations that the vast majority of patients with FDE are asymptomatic HSV-seropositive individuals without a known history of recognized herpetic lesions [54], and that FDE lesions often develop at the sites where herpes simplex repeatedly recurs, after complete resolution of HSV lesions. Furthermore, in some patients, HSV lesions appear to evolve into newly developed FDE lesions (fig. 3). Recent studies have also raised the possibility that the sustained functional T cell responses by HSV may provide protection not only against HSV but also bacterial infections [55, 56]. Thus, the T cell populations resident in peripheral tissues, which face repeated infection by microbial

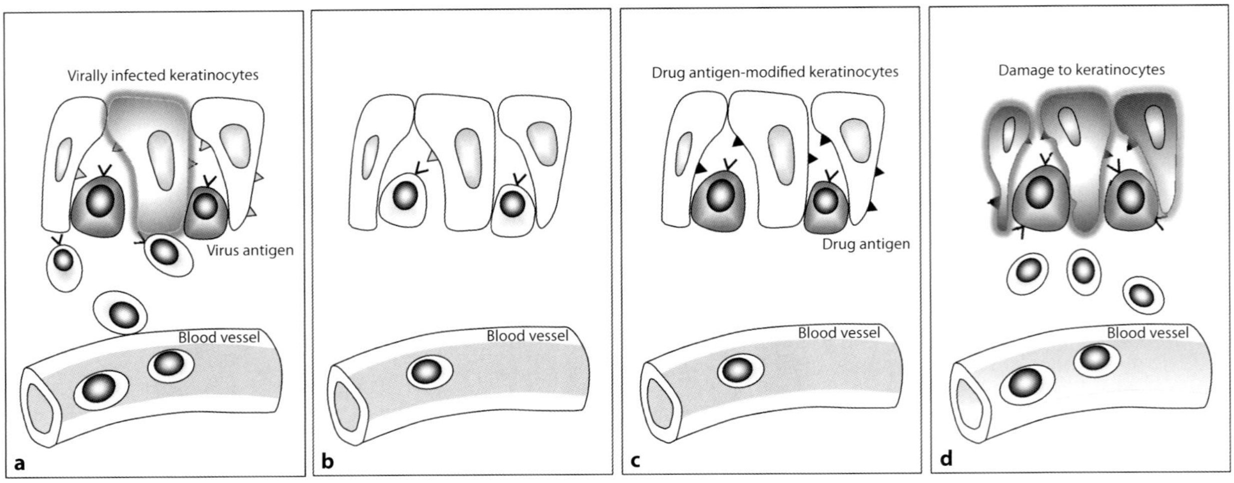

Fig. 4. Hypothetical model from the effector site of the antiviral immune responses to FDE lesions. **a** Migration of antiviral CD8+ T cells with the effector memory phenotype. **b** Retention of these intraepidermal T cells in the epidermis for protection against virus infection. **c** Acquisition of cross-reactivity to drug antigens on these intraepidermal T cells. **d** Recruitment of CD4+ T cells, including regulatory T cells, into the lesions.

pathogens, such as intraepidermal T cells, could play a key role in mediating T cell-dependent protective immunity against the pathogens.

If the intraepidermal CD8+ T cells are indeed mediators for protection against HSV and other microbial pathogens, what is the explanation for their activation by drug antigen? In this regard, there is now sufficient evidence to indicate that a large proportion of antigen-specific self-HLA restricted T cells are also directed toward infectious agents, particularly herpesviruses [57–59]. According to these studies, these cross-reactive T cells can recognize self- and nonself HLA molecules while maintaining a strong antiviral immune response by recruiting non-cross-reactive TCRs to control the virus [58, 60, 61]. In view of our observations that FDE lesions often appear at the sites of recent HSV and herpes zoster lesions (including zoster sine herpete), together with the recent data on the cross-reactivity of T cells with the effector memory phenotype, it is reasonable to speculate that virus-specific CD8+ T cells, once drug antigen is cross-recognized, can be activated to kill surrounding keratinocytes, resulting in localized epidermal injury (fig. 4). When the harmful consequences of such accidental activation of intraepidermal T cells by drug antigen become dominant, FDE would ensue.

Conclusion

It has long been speculated but not clearly shown that viruses are involved in the development of allergic diseases, such as FDE. The hypothesis that FDE lesions can be induced by a virus-driven process is attractive. FDE that reliably mimics in part features of severe drug eruptions often associated with viral infections would represent a useful disease model in helping us understand the mechanisms of how allergic diseases can be induced by the virus-driven process. Unraveling the complex dual roles of intraepidermal CD8+ T cells with the effector memory phenotype resident in the FDE lesions should also provide valuable insight toward the development of therapies to prevent excessive immunopathology, while maintaining efficient antiviral immune responses.

Acknowledgement

This work was supported in part by grants from the Ministry of Education, Culture, Sports, Science and Technology (to T.S.) and the Health and Labour Sciences Research Grants (Research on Intractable Diseases) from the Ministry of Health, Labour and Welfare of Japan (to T.S.).

References

1 Ozkaya-Bayazit E, Akar U: Fixed drug eruption induced by trimethoprim-sulfamethoxazole: evidence for a link to HLA-A30 B13 Cw6 haplotype. J Am Acad Dermatol 2001;45:712–717.
2 Shiohara T: Fixed drug eruption: pathogenesis and diagnostic tests. Curr Opin Allergy Clin Immunol 2009;9:316–321.
3 Savin JA: Current causes of fixed drug eruption in the UK. Br J Dermatol 2001;145:667–670.
4 Shiohara T, Moriya N: Epidermal T cells: their functional role and disease relevance for dermatologists. J Invest Dermatol 1997;109:271–275.
5 Mizukawa Y, Yamazaki Y, Terraki Y, Hayakawa J, Hayakawa K, Nuriya H, Kohara M, Shiohara T: Direct evidence for interferon-gamma production by effector-memory-type intraepidermal T cells residing at an effector site of immunopathology in fixed drug eruption. Am J Pathol 2002;161: 1337–1347.
6 Shiohara T, Mizukawa Y, Teraki Y: Pathophysiology of fixed drug eruption: the role of skin-resident T cells. Curr Opin Allergy Clin Immunol 2002;2: 317–323.
7 Shiohara T, Mizukawa Y: Fixed drug eruption: a disease mediated by self-inflicted responses of intraepidermal T cells. Eur J Dermatol 2007;17:201–208.
8 Mizukawa Y, Shiohara T: Nonpigmenting fixed drug eruption as a possible abortive variant of toxic epidermal necrolysis: immunohistochemical and serum cytokine analyses. Clin Exp Dermatol 2010; 35:493–497.
9 Ruocco V, Ruocco E, Ghersetich I, Bianchi B, Lotti T: Isotopic response after herpesvirus infection: an update. J Am Acad Dermatol 2002;46:90–94.
10 Shiohara T, Mizukawa Y: Recall phenomenon: some skin-resident cells remember previous insults. Dermatol 2003;207:127–129.
11 Korkij W, Soltani K: Fixed drug eruption. Arch Dermatol 1984;120:520–524.
12 Mizukawa Y, Shiohara T: Trauma-localized fixed drug eruption: involvement of burn scars, insect bites and venipuncture sites. Dermatology 2002;205: 159–161.
13 Mizukawa Y, Yamazaki Y, Shiohara T: In vivo dynamics of intraepidermal CD8+ T cells and CD4+ T cells during the evolution of fixed drug eruption. Br J Dermatol 2008;158:1230–1238.
14 Shelley WB, Shelley ED: Nonpigmenting fixed drug eruption as a distinctive reaction pattern: examples caused by sensitivity to pseudoephedrine hydrochloride and tetrahydrozoline. J Am Acad Dermatol 1987;17:403–407.
15 Shiohara T, Mizukawa Y: Fixed drug eruption: easily overlooked but needing new respect. Dermatology 2002;51:469–472.
16 Gruber F, Stasic A, Lenkovic M, Brajac I: Postcoital fixed drug eruption in a man sensitive to trimethoprim-sulphamethoxazole. Clin Exp Dermatol 1997;22:144–145.
17 Guin JD, Haynie LS, Jackson D, Baker GF: Wandering fixed drug eruption: a mucocutaneous reaction to acetaminophen. J Am Acad Dermatol 1987;17: 399–402.

18 Shiohara T, Kokaji T: Polysensitivity in fixed drug eruption. J Am Acad Dermatol 1997;37:1017–1018.
19 Verbov J: Fixed drug eruption due to a drug combination but not to its constituents. Dermatologica 1985;171:60–61.
20 Keiso JM: Fixed food eruption. J Am Acad Dermatol 1996;35:638–639.
21 Yanguas I, Oleaga JM, González-Güemes M, Goday JJ, Soloeta R: Fixed food eruption caused by lentils. J Am Acad Dermatol 1998;38:640–641.
22 Volz T, Berner D, Weigert C, Röcken M, Biedermann T: Fixed food eruption caused by asparagus. J Allergy Clin Immunol 2005;116:1390–1392.
23 Pellicano R, Camassa F, Lomuto M: Localized dermographism at the site of a fixed drug eruption. Br J Dermatol 1995;132:156–158.
24 del Rio E, Guimaraens D, Aguilar A, Conde-Salazar L, Sánchez Yus E: Fixed exanthema induced by ultraviolet radiation. Dermatology 1996;193:54–55.
25 Kelso JM, Keating RM: Successful desensitization for treatment of a fixed drug eruption to allopurinol. J Allergy Clin Immunol 1996;97:1171–1172.
26 Desmeules H: Nonpigmenting fixed drug eruption after anesthesia. Anesth Analg 1990;70:216–217.
27 Sigal-Nahum M, Konqui A, Gaulier A, Sigal S: Linear fixed drug eruption. Br J Dermatol 1988;118: 849–851.
28 Senturk N, Yanik F, Yildiz L, Aydin F, Canturk T, Turanli AY: Topotecan-induced celluitis-like fixed drug eruption. J Eur Acad Dermatol Venereol 2002; 16:414–416.
29 Baran R, Perrin C: Fixed-drug eruption presenting as an acute paronychia. Br J Dermatol 1991;125: 592–595.
30 Flax SH, Uhle P: Photo recall-like phenomenon following the use of cefazolin and gentamicin sulfate. Cutis 1990;46:59–61.
31 Goldfeder KL, Levin JM, Katz KA, Clarke LE, Loren AW, James WD: Ultraviolet recall reaction after total body irradiation, etoposide, and methotrexate therapy. J Am Acad Dermatol 2007;56:494–499.
32 Guin JD, Baker GF: Chronic fixed drug eruption caused by acetaminophen. Cutis 1988;4:106–108.
33 Rijlaarsdam U, Scheffer E, Meijer CJ, Kruyswijk MR, Willemze R: Mycosis fungoides-like lesions associated with phenytoin and carbamazepine therapy. J Am Acad Dermatol 1991;24:216–220.
34 Shiohara T, Mizukawa Y: The immunological basis of lichenoid tissue reaction. Autoimmune Rev 2005; 4:236–241.
35 Agnew KI, Liver GF: Neutrophilic fixed drug eruption. Australas J Dermatol 2001;42:200–202.
36 Barbaud A, Gonçalo M, Bruynzeel D, Bircher A: Guidelines for performing skin tests with drugs in the investigation of cutaneous adverse drug reactions. Contact Dermatitis 2001;45:321–328.
37 Pichler WJ, Tilch J: The lymphocyte transformation test in the diagnosis of drug hypersensitivity. Allergy 2004;59:809–820.
38 Takahashi R, Kano Y, Yamazaki Y, Kimishima M, Mizukawa Y, Shiohara T: Defective regulatory T cells in patients with severe drug eruption: timing of the dysfunction is associated with the pathological phenotype and outcome. J Immunol 2009;182: 8071–8079.
39 Chen Y, Chou K, Fuchs E, Havran WL, Boismenu R: Protection of the intestinal mucosa by intraepithelial γδ T cells. Proc Natl Acad Sci USA 2002;99: 14338–14343.
40 Shiohara T, Mizulawa Y, Teraki Y, Fukuda T: Gamma-delta T cells with emphasis on their functional role in the epidermis. Chem Immunol 2001; 79:66–86.
41 Komatsu T, Moriya N, Shiohara T: T cell receptor (TCR) repertoire and function of human epidermal T cells: restricted TCR Vα-Vβ genes are utilized by T cells residing in the lesional epidermis in fixed drug eruption. Clin Exp Immunol 1996;104:343–350.
42 Shiohara T, Mizukawa Y, Teraki Y: Pathophysiology of fixed drug eruption: the role of skin-resident T cells. Curr Opin Allergy Clin Immunol 2002;2: 317–323.
43 Havran WL, Chien YH, Allison JP: Recognition of self antigens by skin-derived T cells with invariant γδ antigen receptors. Science 1991;252:1430–1432.
44 Girardi M, Oppenheim DE, Steele CR, Lewis JM, Glusac E, Filler R, Hobby P, Sutton B, Tigelaar RE, Hayday AC: Regulation of cutaneous malignancy by γδ T cells. Science 2001;294:605–609.
45 Shiohara T, Moriya N, Hayakawa J, Itohara S, Ishikawa H: Resistance to cutaneous graft-vs.-host disease is not induced in T cell receptor δ gene-mutant mice. J Exp Med 1996;183:1483–1489.
46 Sharp LL, Jameson JM, Cauvi G, Havran WL: Dendritic epidermal T cells regulate skin homeostasis through local production of insulin-like growth factor 1. Nat Immunol 2005;6:73–79.
47 Sallusto F, Lenig D, Förster R, Lipp M, Lanzavecchia A: Two subsets of memory T lymphocytes with distinct homing potentials and effector functions. Nature 1999;401:708–712.
48 Masopust D, Vezys V, Marzo AL, Lefrançois L: Preferential localization of effector memory cells in nonlymphoid tissue. Science 2001;291:2413–2417.
49 Sallusto F, Mackay CR, Lanzavecchia A: The role of chemokine receptors in primary, effector, and memory immune responses. Annu Rev Immunol 2000;18:593–620.

50 Ely KH, Roberts AD, Woodland DL: Cutting edge: effector memory CD8+ T cells in the lung airways retain the potential to mediate recall responses. J Immunol 2003;171:3338–3342.
51 Gebhardt T, Wakim LM, Eidsmo L, Reading PC, Heath WR, Carbone FR: Memory T cells in non-lymphoid tissue that provide enhanced local immunity during infection with herpes simplex virus. Nat Immunol 2009;10:524–530.
52 Zhu J, Koelle DM, Cao J, Vazquez J, Huang ML, Hladik F, Wald A, Corey L: Virus-specific CD8+ T cells accumulate near sensory nerve endings in genital skin during subclinical HSV-2 reactivation. J Exp Med 2007;204:595–603.
53 van Panhuys N, Perret R, Prout M, Ronchese F, Le Gros G: Effector lymphoid tissue and its crucial role in protective immunity. Trends Immunol 2005;26:242–247.
54 Shiohara T, Mizukawa Y, Takahashi R, Kano Y: Pathomechanisms of lichen planus. Autoimmunity elicited by cross-reactive T cells; in Nickoloff BJ, Nesle FO (eds): Dermatologica Immunity. Curr Dir Autoimmun. Basel, Karger, 2008, pp 206–226.
55 Barton ES, White DW, Cathelyn JS, Brett-McClellan KA, Engle M, Diamond MS, Miller VL, Virgin HW 4th: Herpesvirus latency confers symbiotic protection from bacterial infection. Nature 2007;447:326–329.
56 Hansen SG,Vieville C, Whizin N, Coyne-Johnson L, Siess DC, Drummond DD, Legasse AW, Axthelm MK, Oswald K, Trubey CM, Piatak M Jr, Lifson JD, Nelson JA, Jarvis MA, Picker LJ: Effector memory T cell responses are associated with protection of rhesus monkeys from mucosal simian immunodeficiency virus challenge. Nat Med 2009;15:293–299.
57 Burrows SR, Khanna R, Burrows JM, Moss DJ: An alloresponse in humans is dominated by cytotoxic T lymphocytes (CTL) cross-reactive with a single Epstein-Barr virus CTL epitope: implications for graft-versus-host disease. J Exp Med 1994;179:1155–1161.
58 Burrows SR, Silins SL, Moss DJ, Khanna R, Misko IS, Argaet VP: T cell receptor repertoire for a viral epitope in humans is diversified by tolerance to a background major histocompatibility complex antigen. J Exp Med 1995;182:1703–1715.
59 Burrows SR, Silins SL, Khanna R, Burrows JM, Rischmueller M, McCluskey J, Moss DJ: Cross-reactive memory T cells for Epstein-Barr virus augment the alloresponse to common human leukocyte antigens: degenerate recognition of major histocompatibility complex-bound peptide by T cells and its role in alloreactivity. Eur J Immunol 1997;27:1726–1736.
60 Archbold JK, Macdonald WA, Gras S, Ely LK, Miles JJ, Bell MJ, Brennan RM, Beddoe T, Wilce MC, Clements CS, Purcell AW, McCluskey J, Burrows SR, Rossjohn J: Natural micropolymorphism in human leukocyte antigens provides a basis for genetic control of antigen recognition. J Exp Med 2009;206:209–219.
61 Archbold JK, Ely LK, Kjer-Nielsen L, Burrows SR, Rossjohn J, McCluskey J, Macdonald WA: T cell allorecognition and MHC restriction – a case of Jekyll and Hyde? Mol Immunol 2008;45:583–598.

Dr. Tetsuo Shiohara
Department of Dermatology, Kyorin University School of Medicine
6-20-2 Shinkawa, Mitaka
Tokyo 181-8611 (Japan)
Tel. +81 422 47 5511, E-Mail tpshio@ks.kyorin-u.ac.jp

French LE (ed): Adverse Cutaneous Drug Eruptions.
Chem Immunol Allergy. Basel, Karger, 2012, vol 97, pp 122–138

Drug-Induced Hypersensitivity Syndrome: Recent Advances in the Diagnosis, Pathogenesis and Management

Tetsuo Shiohara · Yoko Kano · Ryo Takahashi · Tadashi Ishida · Yoshiko Mizukawa

Department of Dermatology, Kyorin University School of Medicine, Tokyo, Japan

Abstract

Drug-induced hypersensitivity syndrome (DIHS), also referred to as drug reaction with eosinophilia with systemic symptoms, is a life-threatening multiorgan system reaction caused by a limited number of drugs such as anticonvulsants. This syndrome is characterized by fever, rash, lymphadenopathy, hepatitis, and leukocytosis with eosinophilia. DIHS has several unique features that include the delayed onset, paradoxical deterioration of clinical symptoms after withdrawal of the causative drug and unexplained cross-reactivity to multiple drugs with different structures. Because of these features and a lack of awareness of this syndrome, DIHS is undoubtedly underdiagnosed in many countries despite its worldwide distribution. The clinical variability in the presentation and course of clinical symptoms of DIHS could now be interpreted as an indication that several herpesviruses reactivate in a sequential manner independently in the different organs. Dramatic expansions of functional regulatory T (Treg) cells observed in the acute stage would serve to induce such sequential reactivations of herpesviruses while a gradual loss of Treg function occurring after resolution of DIHS could increase the risk of subsequently developing autoimmune disease. Although systemic corticosteroids are the mainstay of treatment, it remains to be determined whether this treatment is beneficial from a viewpoint of disease outcome and sequelae.

Essentials in a Nutshell

- Drug-induced hypersensitivity syndrome (DIHS) is also referred to as drug reaction with eosinophilia with systemic symptoms (DRESS)
- DIHS is a rare, but probably underdiagnosed adverse drug eruption with an estimated incidence of 10 per million person-years
- DIHS is a severe life-threatening multi-organ system reaction caused by a limited number of drugs the most frequent of which are anticonvulsants

- DIHS is characterized by fever, rash, lymphadenopathy, hepatitis, and leukocytosis with eosinophilia
- The pathogenesis involves the reactivation of herpesviruses (HHV-6, HHV-7, Epstein-Barr virus – EBV, cytomegalovirus – CMV), an oligoclonal expansion of activated memory CD8+ T cells that can specifically recognize herpesvirus antigens, and an expansion of Treg cells

Introduction

Severe drug eruptions encompass several distinct clinical entities, the most serious being toxic epidermal necrolysis (TEN). TEN and DIHS represent the opposite ends of a spectrum of severe drug eruptions: the two diseases differ in clinical presentation as well as histological findings, prognosis and pathomechanisms, although the same drugs can often cause these diseases. Although the incidence of DIHS was considered to be less than that of TEN and Stevens-Johnson syndrome (SJS), whose incidence ranges from 0.4 to 1.2 and 1.2 to 6 per million person-years, respectively [1], its incidence continues to increase worldwide probably due to better recognition of this syndrome by doctors or improved population-based surveillance.

The first description of this syndrome is generally credited to Meritt and Putnam, who in 1938 described the toxic symptoms caused by therapy with phenytoin and noted that the symptoms could be divided into two cutaneous reactions: the first one being a mild morbilliform eruption that healed when phenytoin was withdrawn without relapses, and the other being a severe exfoliative dermatitis with fever and eosinophilia [2]. By the time Chaiken et al. [3] described the systemic implications of the second, the link with lymphadenopathy and multivisceral involvement such as hepatitis was established. Since then, there had been many case reports describing similar symptoms induced by relatively long-term therapy with various anticonvulsants, under several different names including phenytoin hypersensitivity syndrome, based on names referring to the causative drug. Bocquet et al. [4] proposed the term 'drug reaction with eosinophilia and systemic symptoms (DRESS)' for this disorder to distinguish it from other severe drug eruptions. This syndrome was independently recognized as a new and distinct disorder in the late 1990s by us [5] and Hashimoto's group [6]: our reports describing an intimate relationship between the development of this disorder and reactivation of HHV-6 rekindled interest in the disorder in Japan [5, 6]. The clinical features, as the syndrome in its florid form is currently recognized, were outlined in 2006 by a Japanese consensus group by the aid of a nationwide survey in Japan [7–9]. Although there has been much debate about the criteria and considerable confusion about the name of this syndrome [7, 8, 10, 11], the clinical and histological findings reported under the name of DRESS are not significantly different from those reported under the name of DIHS. This review examines the laboratory and key clinical aspects of DIHS. Particular focus is given to the role of herpesviruses in view of its recent inclusion in the diagnostic criteria for DIHS. Since this syndrome was last reviewed in 2007 [12], considerably more data have become available on both the immune responses involved and the long-term sequelae of the disease.

Epidemiology

DIHS is now diagnosed earlier in its clinical course than it was in the past thanks to the diagnostic criteria. According to the previous study reported by Gennis et al. [13], the incidence of DIHS is estimated to be between 1 in 1,000 and 1 in 10,000 exposures to phenytoin. However, the frequency of DIHS could be increasing, because milder forms of the disease are being recognized. The most recent and careful population-based studies in Japan report an incidence of 10 per million person-years. In Japan and EU, the incidence increases steadily with advancing age. Incidence rose sharply from 5 per million during the time between 1991 and 2000 to 10 per million between 2001 and 2009. Although DIHS has been believed to have no age and sex predilection, women are about 1.3 times more likely to be affected than are men [Kaudaun, unpubl. data] as demonstrated in patients with SJS and TEN. Our series of this syndrome showed no increased incidence of a personal or family history of atopy and drug eruptions. About half of the patients have had a flu-like illness within the previous 4 weeks, suggesting viral infections as possible triggers for this syndrome.

Clinical Findings

The disease usually starts abruptly with cutaneous lesions or fever. In some cases, there may be a prodrome with upper airway infection. The cutaneous lesions are erythematous papules and patchy erythematous macules, which may be pruritic and can become confluent. The individual lesions are often with hemorrhage and symmetrically distributed on the face, trunk and extremities. Fever usually precedes the rash by 1–2 days and temperature ranges from 38 to 40°C with spikes that may generate concern regarding an underlying infection. The most characteristic cutaneous lesions during the eariest phase of the disease are periorbital and facial edema with pinhead-sized pustules [14], simulating acute generalized exanthematous pustulosis (AGEP). Usually, patients develop these clinical symptoms more than 3 weeks after starting therapy with a limited number of drugs, as shown in table 1. A dramatic deterioration of clinical symptoms often occurs 3–4 days after withdrawal of the causative drug (fig. 1), making the diagnosis of drug eruptions most difficult. The palms and soles are usually spared, but can occasionally show a few lesions. When the causative drug continues to be given after this syndrome has developed, the eruptions often generalize into severe exfoliative dermatitis or erythroderma. Blisters are occasionally present but mainly limited to the wrists and probably related to dermal edema. Follicular

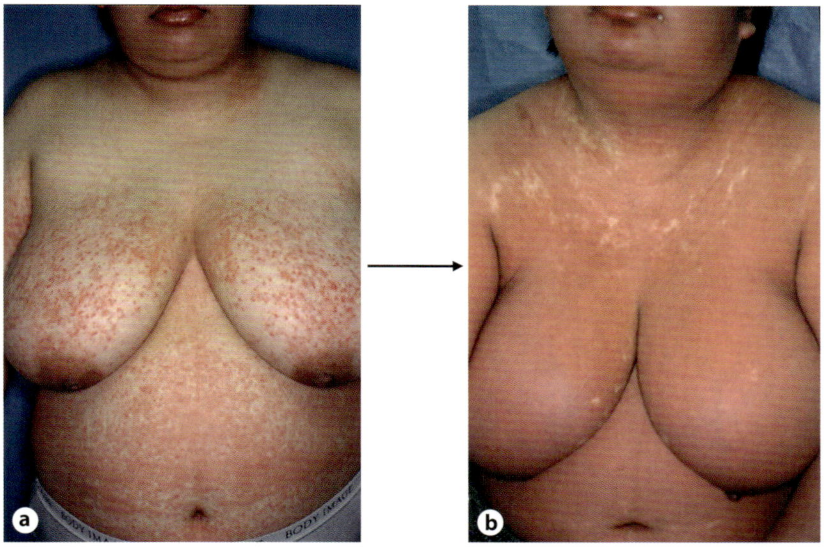

Fig. 1. The patient's clinical symptoms on the initial presentation (**a**) and 4 days after her initial presentation (**b**). A dramatic deterioration of the clinical symptoms is observed in association with an increase in body temperature despite withdrawal of the causative drug.

Table 1. Diagnostic criteria for DIHS established by a Japanese consensus group [7]

1	Maculopapular rash developing >3 weeks after starting with a limited number of drugs
2	Prolonged clinical symptoms after discontinuation of the causative drug
3	Fever (>38°C)
4	Liver abnormalities (ALT >100 U/l)[1]
5	Leukocyte abnormalities (at least one present)
	a Leukocytosis ($>11 \times 10^9$/l)
	b Atypical lymphocytosis (>5%)
	c Eosinophilia ($>1.5 \times 10^9$/l)
6	Lymphadenopathy
7	HHV-6 reactivation

The diagnosis is confirmed by the presence of the seven criteria above (typical DIHS) or of five of the seven (atypical DIHS).
[1] This can be replaced by other organ involvement, such as renal involvement.

accentuation of the erythematous papules is a characteristic finding of DIHS [15]. Mucosal surfaces show a few lesions, particularly lips and oral mucous membranes, more frequently than generally thought, although much less severe and hemorrhagic than SJS/TEN.

Tender lymphadenopathy can be found in >70% of patients early in the course of the illness, predominantly affecting the cervical, axillary, or inguinal nodes. Bilateral swelling of the salivary glands with severe xerostomia can be frequently seen early in the course, suggesting that mumps virus may be reactivated before onset of this syndrome. Some patients may often complain of oral dryness which makes swallowing of dry food difficult.

Two or more internal organs are involved in many patients with DIHS. Most frequently involved organs are liver (70%) [12, 16–18], kidney (11%) [8, 12, 17, 18], and lung [18]. If hepatitis is present, it is usually anicteric [8]. Hepatomegaly accompanied by splenomegaly is a common finding. Which organs are prefentially involved is likely to be determined in part by the drug used: hepatitis is often observed in phenytoin-, minocycline-, or dapsone-induced DIHS [8, 17, 18], and kidney involvement is frequently seen in allopurinol-induced DIHS [12, 18]. Thus, various organ involvement emerges after an undefined period of critical illness of days to weeks: resolution of symptoms in one organ may be often followed by a stepwise development of other organ failures, despite withdrawal of the causative drugs. Such clinical variability in the presentation and course of clinical symptoms allows for a delay in diagnosis which may arouse suspicion of infection in doctors of first contact who may not have seen patients with DIHS. As a result, unnecessary empirical antibiotic therapy which could increase the risk of developing additional drug rashes may be started. Indeed, patients with DIHS often show unexplained cross-reactivity to multiple drugs with different structures, including those used after onset of symptoms. In some patients, to make matters worse, the fever often persists even for weeks despite discontinuation of the causative drug.

Overlap with Other Severe Drug Eruptions

Clinical and histologic observations support the view that DIHS and SJS/TEN are opposite clinical poles of a continuous spectrum of severe drug eruptions: a particular, predilection for mucosal surfaces is typically seen in SJS/TEN, but not in DIHS. More than 30% of patients with DIHS, however, also possess mucous membrane lesions, although less than those in SJS/TEN. Thus, there is considerable overlap in the clinical manifestations of both conditions. Indeed, some of our patients with DIHS had concurrent or sequential development of SJS-like mucosal and cutaneous lesions. Most of them initially presented with clinical features typical of DIHS but went on to develop SJS-like mucosal and cutaneous lesions: these patients initially present with both clinical and immunologic findings, including HHV-6 reactivation, consistent with a diagnosis of DIHS, but whose subsequent clinical pattern has evolved to become more typical of SJS/TEN. As we have recently demonstrated [19], both conditions are mediated by activated effector T (Teff) cells that can recognize drug antigen, but expansions of functional regulatory T cells are only observed in the setting of DIHS: this expansion has a proven causal relationship with the clinical symptoms and viral reactivations observed in DIHS. Thus, although the skin lesions of both clinical entities were thought to rarely change from one clinical type to the other, it is important to understand that the conversion from DIHS to SJS/TEN is not the rare event: in many cases, SJS/TEN is usually preceded by DIHS. In these cases, occurrence of SJS-like lesions is delayed for a week after onset of clinical symptoms consistent with DIHS: this delay may be diagnostic of identifying the patients with DIHS evolving into SJS/TEN, because patients with widely distributed purpuric erythematous macules rapidly progressing into blisters and erosions over a period of a few days are likely to have SJS/TEN not associated with DIHS. Because these cases indicate that specific factors determining the expression of a particular disease phenotype may vary with time, detailed kinetic information on these patients would be helpful in determining disease expression.

Facial erythema and edema with pinhead-sized pustules as one of the relatively early symptoms of DIHS are often indistinguishable from those observed in AGEP. Clinicians who are less familiar with the clinical symptoms of DIHS and AGEP may experience the difficulties in assigning a specific diagnosis to patients presenting with facial erythema and edema associated with pustules. There is, however, considerable evidence that the two are distinct conditions with divergent clinical features. Nevertheless, the pattern of erythematous lesions in AGEP, initially with distribution around the flexural areas, is very different from DIHS where lesions usually occur on the face and upper trunk. The marked difference between the two can be also found in their disease course after withdrawal of the causative drug: spontaneous resolution of the pustules occurs in less than 15 days with characteristic desquamation [20], while DIHS usually runs a chronic unremitting course. Clearly, the clinical phenotype of severe drug eruptions varies with time and definitive diagnostic categorization is not always possible at the initial presentation.

Laboratory Findings

The peripheral blood usually shows marked leukocytosis with atypical lymphocytosis or eosinophilia of various degree. In some patients, leucopenia or lymphopenia may be seen, especially at the early stage of the illness [8, 12, 21]: this occasionally precedes leukocytosis. While eosinophilia can be seen in 60–70% of the patients in our series [8, 12], other recent studies reported that transient eosinophilia (95%) was far more frequently present [Kardaun et al., submitted] than previously reported. Occasionally, the number of monocytes is also increased, although this is a relatively late event as compared with neutrophilia and lymphocytosis, both of which can often be seen in the early stage of the disease. The increase in either CD4+ T cells or CD8+ T cells can be seen in the early phase of the disease. According to our series of 12 patients (6 male and 6 female, age range 25–70 years) with DIHS diagnosed and managed at our institution, CD4+ T-cell numbers initially increased at the early stage in >90% of these patients [22]; this increase, however, was followed by a gradual decrease reaching normal values by 2 months after onset. In some patients, the increase in CD8+ T cell numbers was seen, although this difference was not reflected in clinical symptoms. A profound decrease in CD19+ B-cell numbers and CD56+ NK-cell numbers was observed at their initial presentation [23]. The subsequent decrease in CD4+ T cell numbers was usually coincident with improvements in clinical status. The degree of the increase in CD4+ T cell numbers best correlated with the severity of clinical symptoms, such as the extent of skin lesions and the magnitude of viral reactivations, as mentioned later.

A dramatic decrease in serum IgG, IgA, and IgM levels is typically observed at onset, and the lowest levels are usually detected a week after withdrawal of the causative drug [23]. Immediately 1–2 weeks after the nadir in their levels, the overshoot in their levels can be observed, and they eventually return to normal upon full recovery. Because these alterations in Ig levels during the course of the illness were never observed in patients with SJS/TEN and AGEP, this finding can only be diagnostic of DIHS when Ig levels are carefully measured at various points after onset. In some patients, this decrease may be only apparent when compared with those levels after full recovery, while those levels at onset may be within normal limits. Thus, it should be noted that Ig levels at a single time point are not sufficiently enough to conclude their decrease.

A marked increase in the serum alanine aminotransferase values can be seen in up to 70% of patients. In some patients, γ-glutamyl-transpeptidase, total bilirubin, and alkaline phosphatase increase to a variable degree. Such liver abnormalities often occur in association with the increase in circulating atypical lymphocytes, suggesting that activated lymphocytes may contribute to liver damage. Various forms of renal involvement have also been reported [24, 25], ranging from tubulointerstitial nephritis to granulomatous necrotizing angiitis. The mortality is likely to depend in part on the degree of renal involvement rather than hepatic involvement.

Although in earlier studies HHV-6 was thought to be the only virus that was reactivated in patients with DIHS [6], it has become clear that other herpesviruses, such as EBV, HHV-7, and CMV are also reactivated during the course of the disease [5, 26–28]. Our results of PCR analyses performed at various time points after onset showed that various herpesviruses sequentially reactivate during the course of DIHS in the order as demonstrated in graft-versus-host disease (GVHD) [27]: the cascade of reactivation events initiated by EBV or HHV-6 extends, with some delay, to HHV-7 as well, and eventually to CMV, as shown in figure 2. Our clinical observations demonstrated that reactivations of these herpesviruses can be detected coincident with the onset of various clinical symptoms, such as liver abnormalities in some patients while in other patients they occur without the evidence of overt clinical symptoms. In order to demonstrate full cascades of reactivation events during the course of DIHS, frequent sampling of blood at least on a weekly basis is needed, because the changes in viral loads are so rapid. Thus, the true peak of viral loads can easily be missed on a routine examination performed at a single time point on a routine basis.

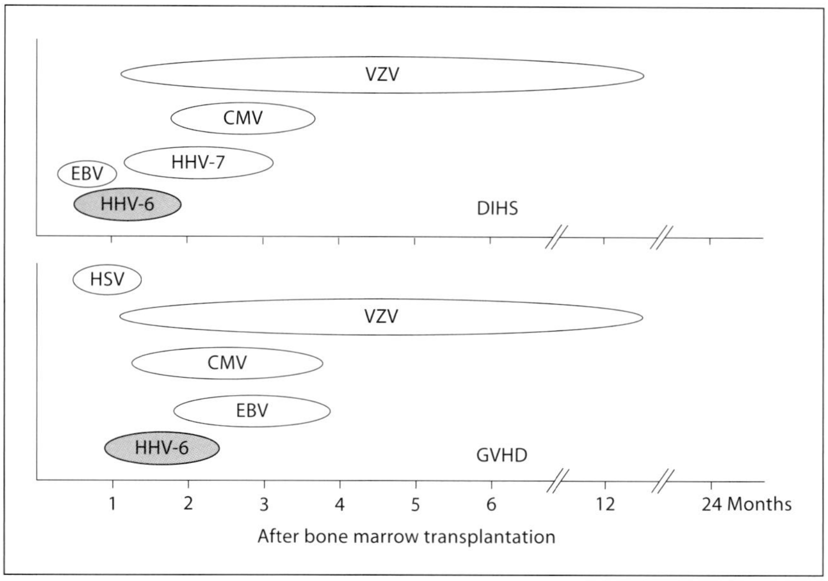

Fig. 2. The sequence of herpesvirus reactivation events observed in DIHS (upper) and GVHD (lower). Modified from our previous paper [12]. VZV = Varicella zoster virus.

Diagnosis of Drug-Induced Hypersensitivity Syndrome

The diagnosis of DIHS is usually not difficult for dermatologists who are familiar with clinical symptoms of DIHS, if a history of drug intake, particularly drugs listed in table 1, is sought in all patients presenting with fever, erythematous skin lesions predominating on the face and upper trunk, lymphoadenopathy, and other organ involvement. The diagnosis, however, can be challenging for physicians who have seen such patients before. There are a number of differential diagnostic considerations that may usually play a greater role in atypical or very early cases: they include EBV- or CMV-induced infectious mononucleosis (IM), measles, exfoliative erythroderma, a drug-induced erythrodermic condition, Kawasaki syndrome, Kikuchi-Fujimoto disease, and drug-induced pseudolymphomas. The clinical findings alone can be difficult to differentiate from IM: IM occurs most commonly in teenagers or young adults, and the eruption usually occurs 2–10 days after starting therapy with antibiotics which rarely cause DIHS, while DIHS typically occurs 3 weeks to 3 months after starting therapy with anticonvulsants in adults or elderly patients.

Although this syndrome had been recognized as a distinct disorder in the early 1960s, much of the confusion has resulted from the inconsistent and variable terminology and the lack of a specific and sensitive diagnostic test. In this regard, we and Hashimoto's group independently demonstrated that HHV-6 can be reactivated at a particular time point, 2–3 weeks after onset of rash in the vast majority of patients regardless of treatment [5, 6]. Since then, a strong association between HHV-6

Table 2. Drugs frequently causing DIHS/DRESS

• Carbamazepine	• Dapsone
• Phenytoin	• Salazosulfapyridine
• Phenobarbital	• Allopurinol
• Zonisamide	• Minocycline
• Mexiletine	• Abacavir[1]
• Lamotrigine	• Nevirapine[1]

[1] These drugs cause systemic hypersensitivity reactions with some peculiar symptoms [12].

reactivation and this syndrome has been supported by a large number of independent groups over the years in Japan. In 2006, we, a Japanese consensus group named the Japanese Research Committee on Severe Cutaneous Adverse Reaction established a set of criteria for diagnosis of this syndrome (table 2) and proposed the term 'DIHS' [7, 8]. DIHS is currently diagnosed by using the seven criteria in Japan: diagnosis of typical DIHS requires all seven criteria, although, in many cases, the criteria for DIHS are not all present on any given day. Our case series diagnosed by clinical and laboratory findings alone have shown that HHV-6 reactivation can be detected in the vast majority of patients who satisfy the other six criteria. The concept of 'atypical DIHS' can be used for patients with typical clinical presentations, in whom HHV-6 reactivation cannot be detected due to inappropriate timing of sampling or the lack of a specific test for detecting HHV-6 reactivation: the detection of HHV-6 reactivation can be evidenced by the significant rise in HHV-6 IgG titers or HHV-6 DNA levels.

Recently, an international consensus group named RegiSCAR has proposed a standardized scoring system for diagnosis [Kardaun et al., submitted], based on clinical and biological characteristics in 117 cases prospectively enrolled from 2005 to mid-2009. There is no fundamental difference in the clinical and laboratory findings except for HHV-6 reactivation between this system and our criteria, although the major concern is that, when this scoring system is used for diagnosis, the syndrome may be overdiagnosed or underdiagnosed due to the lack of a specific diagnostic test for HHV-6 reactivation. According to our experience, patients with clinical symptoms and laboratory findings consistent with those of DIHS but without the evidence of HHV-6 reactivation have shown to exhibit a tendency toward milder disease [7]. In our case series, patients who had more than two episodes of worsening after initial improvement, either treatment-related or -unrelated fluctuations, were more likely to run a chronic, unremitting course, probably due to repeated reactivations of various herpesviruses. The magnitude of HHV-6 reactivations as evidenced by the increase in HHV-6 DNA levels is thought to reflect the severity of inflammatory responses that occur in vivo in patients with DIHS. We recommend that HHV-6 testing be used to confirm a clinical diagnosis rather than simply as a screening tool.

The lymphocyte transformation test (LTT) [29] is a frequently used as a tool to confirm a clinical diagnosis of allergic drug reaction and determine the causative drug. We previously demonstrated that positive LTT reactions were obtained at the recovery stage but not the acute stage in DIHS, while in SJS/TEN and other types of drug eruptions, positive LTT reactions were only obtained when the test was performed at the acute stage [30]. Our analyses performed with the use of samples at various time points after onset showed that LTT reactions became positive from 5 weeks onward after onset in the majority of patients, regardless of whether patients were on therapy with prednisolone or not [30]. Because this finding was only observed in patients with DIHS, the LTT is a reliable method to define the causative drug in DIHS when the test is performed at the right timing. Ideally, this test should be done as soon as possible after presentation and should be repeated after 2 months. Negative LTT reactions at the acute stage could alternatively be interpreted as suggesting a diagnosis of DIHS.

Pathology

The histologic picture of DIHS is not diagnostic. The common pathological findings are superficial perivascular lymphocytic infiltrates and some extravasated erythrocytes and eosinophils. On rare occasions, DIHS may feature a lichenoid infiltrate with apoptotic keratinocytes, a finding frequently seen in other drug eruptions such as erythema multiforme type and SJS/TEN. Full-thickness epidermal necrosis and detachment can only be seen in patients with DIHS evolving into SJS/TEN. The pattern of inflammation in DIHS involves mixed infiltration composed of CD4+ and CD8+ T cells with hemorrhage. In our earlier study, high levels of HHV-6 genome and viral antigens were detected in infiltrating cells in the skin lesions taken at the early stage [5], despite the absence of HHV-6 DNA in the blood simultaneously obtained from the same patient. These results indicate that there exist other distinct, undefined compartments, such as skin, liver and lymph nodes, where herpesviruses can reactivate in sequential order independent of the blood. This may be reflected in differences in the nature of the localized immune process taking place in the target organs of DIHS.

Pathogenesis

Activated T cells seem to play an important role in DIHS, as suggested in other severe drug eruptions [19]. Previously, it was believed that DIHS merely represents an exaggerated, hyperinflammatory response with inflammation-induced viral reactivations and subsequent organ injury [9]. According to this theory, reactivations of herpesviruses specifically observed in patients with DIHS are a consequence, not a cause, of excessive activation of T cells. In this regard, we have suggested the existence of a more complex scenario: sequential reactivations of herpesviruses would occur far earlier than onset probably due to protracted use of anticonvulsants, thereby causing the generation and activation of virus-specific memory CD8+ T cells. However, recent studies including our own have somewhat revised this theory and found that antiviral T cells can directly influence the course of DIHS and regulatory T cells confer protective immunity in this setting. In view of the fact that the clinical symptoms of DIHS remain dormant for prolonged periods after starting therapy with the causative drug, there could exist some mechanisms, whereby antiviral CD8+ T cell responses can be silenced to limit possible immunopathology before onset. If this balance mechanism is eventually disturbed, a condition is set that leads to onset of the disease. According to this scenario, memory T cells specific for a viral peptide presented in the context of certain HLA-A or -B could play a central role in the pathogenesis of DIHS, and drug antigens could serve to induce accidental activation of those virus-specific T cells with cross-reactivity to drug antigens. Consistent with this scenario, Hung et al. [31] provided evidence for a genetic predisposition in DIHS showing a strong association (100%) between allopurinol-induced DRESS and HLA-B*5801. Prospective studies of 40 patients presenting with well-characterized DRESS by Picard et al. [32] provide ample support for our scenario. They demonstrated that EBV, HHV-6, or HHV-7 reactivation can be detected in 76% of patients with DRESS and that the cutaneous and visceral symptoms of DRESS are associated with an oligoclonal expansion of activated memory CD8+ T cells that can specifically recognize one of viral antigens derived from herpesviruses. Importantly, viral replication has been shown to be enhanced by the causative drug, but not an irrelevant drug that has not been involved in the occurrence of DRESS [32]. A likely interpretation of these findings, in consideration of our own data, is that the cutaneous and visceral symptoms of DIHS can be mediated by the activation and migration into the target organ of antiviral CD8+ T cells resulting from sequential reactivation of herpesviruses.

If antiviral T cells play a central role in tissue injury, it is logical to ask by which mechanism(s) these antiviral T cells can be silenced over a prolonged period of time before onset. The most promising new insight into the protective mechanism(s) comes from the work from our group investigating the role of regulatory T (Treg) cells in patients with DIHS [19]. We have recently investigated whether Treg cell frequency and function can influence the clinical manifestations and course of DIHS. In this study, patients with TEN were also analyzed in comparison with DIHS. Dramatic expansions of fully functional CD4+CD25+FoxP3+ Treg cells were specifically found in the acute stage of DIHS [19]; in contrast, in TEN their capacity to migrate into the skin and to suppress the activation of Teff cells was profoundly impaired during the acute stage, although they are present in normal frequency in the blood. These expanded Treg cells have been shown to inhibit drug-induced cytokine production by Teff cells in vitro, indicating that the expanded Treg cells could serve to inhibit activation of antiviral T cells for a prolonged period of time before onset of DIHS, and induce sequential reactivations of herpesviruses. Our further unpublished observations show that the causative drug can trigger the expansion of Treg cells from patients with DIHS. Our findings provide explanations for why the onset of DIHS is delayed in relation to the introduction of the causative drug, and why severe epidermal damage cannot be detected in the skin lesions of DIHS despite activation of Teff cells, why viral reactivations are induced, and why positive LTT reactions cannot be detected during the acute stage. In view of their ability to induce B cell death [33], a decrease in serum Ig levels and B cell number specifically observed during the acute stage would be explained by expansions of functional Treg cells.

Surprisingly, the Treg cells gradually lose their original suppressing function when contracted upon resolution of IDHS [19]. In contrast, a functional impairment of Treg cells during the acute stage of TEN was restored upon resolution. This progressive dysfunction of Treg cells specifically observed after resolution of DIHS could be due to their exhaustion as a consequence of repeated activation of Treg cells in response to excessive activation of Teff cells including antiviral T cells driven by a high viral load in patients.

Complications and Long-Term Sequelae

Our series of patients and a review of the English literature have suggested the following features of the natural history of DIHS. Less than 10% of patients die within 1 year after onset, and autoimmune disease or production of autoantibodies occur as a sequela of DIHS in 10% of surviving patients, regardless of whether they were treated with systemic corticosteroids. Because they appear for several months to years after the acute illness was resolved, it is difficult to find a link between preceding DIHS and the subsequent autoimmune diseases unless special attention is given to a history of a clinical illness compatible with DIHS. It should be recognized that they cannot necessarily occur immediately after resolution of DIHS but rather occur after a disease-free interval of several months to years and that there is the long prodromal period preceding clinical onset of autoimmune diseases [34]. These autoimmune diseases include type 1 diabetes mellitus [35–38], autoimmune thyroid disease [8, 12, 38], sclerodermoid GVHD-like lesions [39] and lupus erythematosus [34, 40]. In a patient who subsequently developed GVHD-like lesions, antinuclear antibody (ANA) was negative during the course of DIHS and became detectable (1:40), coincident with the development of alopecia: a dramatic increase in ANA (1:5,120) was eventually found 4 years after onset of DIHS, at her initial presentation to our Department because of sclerodermoid GVHD-like lesions, indicating that the disease process of DIHS may act as a trigger for the subsequent development of autoimmune disease [39]. Given the strong association between EBV infection and systemic lupus erythematosus (SLE) [41, 42], it is likely that EBV reactivations occurring during the episode of DIHS could profoundly influence the autoimmune sequelae of DIHS. Indeed, EBV reactivations were confirmed on two occasions, during the episode of DIHS and at the time of the presentation with clinical manifestations of SLE in our reported case [34, 40]. In addition to the role of EBV reactivations, a gradual loss of Treg function after resolution of DIHS [19] could increase the risk of subsequently developing autoimmune disease.

Management of Drug-Induced Hypersensitivity Syndrome

Early recognition of clinical symptoms compatible with DIHS is essential in improving patient outcomes. Because paradoxical deterioration of clinical symptoms and laboratory findings is often seen 3–4 days after withdrawal of the causative drug, a concern of an underlying infection may be generated; and, as a result, empirical treatment with antibiotics or nonsteroidal anti-inflammatory drugs may be initiated, which often confuse or worsen the clinical picture probably due to unexplained cross-reactivity to these drugs. The use of those drugs should be avoided, particularly during the acute phase.

Systemic corticosteroids is the mainstay of treatment, particularly in the earlier stages of the disease. Rapid resolution of rashes and fever occurs within several days after starting a moderate dose of systemic corticosteroids (prednisolone, 40–50 mg/day). Because marked deterioration of various clinical symptoms is frequently seen with abrupt discontinuation or rapid tapering of corticosteroids, corticosteroid dose should be reduced gradually even upon resolution of clinical manifestation: tapering corticosteroids more gradually over a prolonged period of time (usually 6–8 weeks) can help to limit the severe flare-ups. One should recognize that patients with DIHS are at greater risk of subsequently developing the wide spectrum of immune reconstitution syndrome (IRS) ranging from CMV disease to autoimmune disease [8, 12, 22, 34] (table 3), and the use of systemic corticosteroids represents an important factor that increases the risk of disease progression to full manifestations of IRS upon the withdrawal or reductions. Indeed, HHV-6 and CMV, but not EBV, viral loads were significantly higher in patients with DIHS receiving systemic corticosteroids compared with those without corticosteroid therapy [Ishida et al., submitted]. This finding indicates that the degree and duration of HHV-6 and CMV reactivations would be greatly influenced by the use of immunosuppressive drugs. Nevertheless, this effect of corticosteroids on viral reactivations is likely to be an unanticipated consequence of a tapering corticosteroid dose, because our frequent monitoring of viral loads in patient with DIHS revealed that the increase in CMV viral loads coincided with a tapering of corticosteroid dose [43]. Given the high risk of sequelae from CMV reactivation in patients with DIHS [43], the direct anti-CMV medications with a gradual reducing dose of corticosteroids may help to avoid disease progression to full manifestations of IRS [22].

The use of intravenous immunoglobulin (IVIG) has so far only been assessed in some patients; however, our trials of combining treatments, giving IVIG (0.1 g/kg per

Table 3. Reported clinical illness consistent with IRS in HIV-negative hosts [22]

Mycobacterium avium complex infection
Tuberculosis
Cryptococcosis[1]
Herpes simplex[1]
Herpes zoster[1]
Hepatitis C virus
Hepatitis B virus
CMV[1]
Kaposi sarcoma
Sarcoidosis
Graves' disease
Hashimoto thyroiditis[1]
DIHS

[1] Infectious and autoimmune diseases often observed during the course of DIHS or long after its resolution.

day for 3 days) together with systemic corticosteroids, have failed to show extra benefit compared with corticosteroids alone. Because patients with moderate disease can often recover from this syndrome by supportive care without the need of systemic corticosteroids within 3 weeks, the use of systemic corticosteroids is not necessarily recommended as a treatment option of DIHS. Particularly, a small dose (prednisolone, 10–20 mg/day) of systemic corticosteroids followed by small increments in dosage at short intervals should be avoided even for mild cases, because this may not be sufficient to ameliorate clinical symptoms and may result in unnecessarily protracted use of corticosteroids. Thus, although systemic corticosteroids have become accepted as the gold standard treatment for DIHS, it remains to be determined whether treatment with systemic corticosteroids is also beneficial from a viewpoint of disease outcome and sequleae. Nevertheless, the benefit is greatest during the first 2–3 weeks when treatment was given early. Likewise, there was also no significant improvement in patients treated with corticosteroids for other important outcomes including time to discharge, death and disability after 1 year. Our longitudinal PCR analyses of viral loads in patients with DIHS justify the frequent monitoring of viral reactivations to predict and improve the short-term or long-term outcome.

Conclusion

The development of an internationally standardized scoring system to clearly identify patients with DIHS will be critical in treating those who had suffered from preventable morbidity and mortality. Considerations for the development of therapies that can reduce the risk of long-term sequelae such as autoimmune disease would seem a reasonable path to pursue.

Acknowledgement

This work was supported in part by grants from the Ministry of Education, Culture, Sports, Science and Technology (to T.S.) and the Health and Labour Sciences Research Grants (Research on Intractable Diseases) from the Ministry of Health, Labour and Welfare of Japan (to T.S.).

References

1 Roujeau JC, Stern RS: Severe adverse cutaneous reactions to drugs. N Engl J Med 1994;331:1272–1285.
2 Merritt HH, Putnam TJ: Sodium diphenylhydantoinate in the treatment of convulsive disorders. JAMA 1938;111:1068–1073.
3 Chaiken BH, Goldberg BI, Segal JP: Dilantin hypersensitivity: report of a case of hepatitis with jaundice, pyrexia, and exfoliative dermatitis. N Engl J Med 1950;242:897–898.
4 Bocquet H, Bagot M, Roujeau JC: Drug-induced pseudolymphoma and drug hypersensitivity syndrome (Drug Rash with Eosinophilia and Systemic Symptoms: DRESS). Semin Cutan Med Surg 1996; 15:250–257.
5 Suzuki Y, Inagi R, Aono T, Yamanishi K, Shiohara T: Human herpesvirus 6 infection as a risk factor for the development of severe drug-induced hypersensitivity syndrome. Arch Dermatol 1998;134:1108–1112.
6 Tohyama H, Yahata Y, Yasukawa M, Inagi R, Urano Y, Yamanishi K, Hashimoto K: Severe hypersensitivity syndrome due to sulfasalazine associated with reactivation of human herpesvirus 6. Arch Dermatol 1998;134:1113–1117.
7 Shiohara T, Iijima M, Ikezawa Z, Hashimoto K: The diagnosis of a DRESS syndrome has been sufficiently established on the basis of typical clinical features and viral reactivations. Br J Dermatol 2007; 156:1083–1084.
8 Shiohara T, Inaoka M, Kano Y: Drug-induced hypersensitivity syndrome (DIHS): a reaction induced by a complex interplay among herpesviruses and antiviral and antidrug immune responses. Allergol Int 2006;55:1–8.
9 Hashimoto K, Yasukawa M, Tohyama M: Human herpesvirus 6 and drug allergy. Curr Opin Allergy Clin Immunol 2003;3:255–260.
10 Peynére H, Dereure O, Breton H, Demoly P, Cociglio M, Blayac JP, Hillaire-Buys D: Variability in the clinical pattern of cutaneous side-effects of drugs with systemic symptoms: does a DRESS syndrome really exist? Br J Dermatol 2006;155:422–428.
11 Kardaun SH, Sidoroff A, Valeyrie-Allanore L, Halevy S, Davidovici BB, Mockenhaupt M, Roujeau JC: Variability in the clinical pattern of cutaneous side-effects of drugs with systemic symptoms: does a DRESS syndrome really exist? Br J Dermatol 2007; 156:609–611.
12 Shiohara T, Takahashi R, Kano Y: Drug-induced hypersensitivity syndrome and viral reactivation; in Pichler WJ (ed): Drug Hypersensitivity. Basel, Karger, 2007, pp 251–266.
13 Gennis MA, Vemuri R, Burns EA, Hill JV, Miller MA, Spielberg SP: Familiar occurrence of hypersensitivity to phenytoin. Am J Med 1991;91:631–634.
14 Vittorio CC, Muglia JJ: Anticonvulsant hypersensitivity syndrome. Arch Intern Med 1995;155:2285–2290.
15 Stanley J, Fallon-Pellicci V: Phenytoin hypersensitivity reaction. Arch Dermatol 1978;114:1350–1353.
16 Hari Y, Frutig-Schnyder K, Humi M, Yawalkar N, Zanni MP, Schnyder B, Kappeler A, von Greyerz S, Braathen LR, Pichler WJ: T cell involvement in cutaneous drug eruptions. Clin Exp Allergy 2001;31: 1398–1408.
17 Kano Y, Shiohara T: The variable clinical picture of drug-induced hypersensitivity syndrome/drug rash with eosinophilia and systemic symptoms in relation to the eliciting drug. Immunol Allergy Clin North Am 2009;29:481–501.

18 Kano Y, Ishida T, Hirahara K, Shiohara T: Visceral involvements and long-term sequelae in drug-induced hypersensitivity syndrome. Med Clin North Am 2010;94:743–759.
19 Takahashi R, Kano Y, Yamazaki Y, Kimishima M, Mizukawa Y, Shiohara T: Defective regulatory T cells in patients with severe drug eruptions: timing of the dysfunction is associated with the pathological phenotype and outcome. J Immunol 2009;182: 8071–8079.
20 Sidoroff A, Dunant A, Viboud C, Halevy S, Bavinck JN, Naldi L, Mockenhaupt M, Fagot JP, Roujeau JC: Risk factors for acute generalized exanthematous pustulosis (AGEP)-results of a multinational case-control study (EuroSCAR). Br J Dermatol 2007; 157:989–996.
21 Horneff G, Lenard HG, Wahn V: Severe adverse reaction to carbamazepine: significance of humoral and cellular reactions to the drug. Neuropediatrics 1992;23:272–275.
22 Shiohara T, Kurata M, Mizukawa Y, Kano Y: Recognition of immune reconstitution syndrome necessary for better management of patients with severe drug eruptions and those under immunosuppressive therapy. Allergol Int 2010;59: 333–343.
23 Kano Y, Inaoka M, Shiohara T: Association between anticonvulsant hypersensitivity syndrome and human herpesvirus 6 reactivation and hypogammaglobulinemia. Arch Dermatol 2004;140: 183–188.
24 Hogg RJ, Sawyer M, Hecox K, Eigenbrodt E: Carbamazepine-induced acute tubulointestinal nephritis. J Pediatr 1981;83:830–832.
25 Imai H, Nakamoto Y, Hirokawa M, Akihama T, Miura A: Carbamazepin-induced granulomatous necrotizing angiitis with acute renal failure. Nephron 1989;51:405–408.
26 Descamps V, Mahe E, Houhou N, Abramowitz L, Rozenberg F, Ranger-Rogez S, Crickx B: Drug-induced hypersensitivity syndrome associated with Epstein-Barr virus infection. Br J Dermatol 2003; 148:1032–1034.
27 Kano Y, Hirahara K, Sakuma K, Shiohara T: Several herpesviruses can reactivate in a severe drug-induced multiorgan reaction in the same sequential order as in graft-versus-host disease. Br J Dermatol 2006;155:301–306.
28 Aihara M, Sugita Y, Takahashi S, Nagatani T, Arata S, Takeuchi K, Ikezawa Z: Anticonvulsant hypersensitivity syndrome associated with reactivation of cytomegalovirus. Br J Dermatol 2001;144:1231–1234.
29 Pichler WJ, Tilch J: The lymphocyte transformation test in the diagnosis of drug hypersensitivity. Allergy 2004;59:809–820.
30 Kano Y, Hirahara K, Mitsuyama T, Takahashi R, Shiohara T: Utility of the lymphocyte transformation test in the diagnosis of drug sensitivity: dependence on its timing and the type of drug eruption. Allergy 2007;62:1439–1444.
31 Hung SI, Chung WH, Liou LB, Chu CC, Lin M, Huang HP, Lin YL, Lan JL, Yang LC, Hong HS, Chen MJ, Lai PC, Wu MS, Chu CY, Wang KH, Chen CH, Fann CS, Wu JY, Chen YT: HLA-B*5801 allele as a genetic marker for severe cutaneous adverse reactions caused by allopurinol. Proc Natl Acad Sci USA 2005;102:4134–4139.
32 Picard D, Janela B, Descamps V, D'Incan M, Courville P, Jacquot S, Rogez S, Mardivirin L, Moins-Teisserenc H, Toubert A, Benichou J, Joly P, Musette P: Drug reaction with eosinophilia and systemic symptoms (DRESS): a multiorgan antiviral T cell response. Sci Transl Med 2010;2:46–62.
33 Zhao DM, Thomton AM, DiPaolo RJ, Shevach EM: Activated CD4+CD25+ T cells selectively kill B lymphocytes. Blood 2006;107:3925–3932.
34 Aota N, Shiohara T: Viral connection between drug rashes and autoimmune disease: how autoimmune responses are generated after resolution of drug rashes. Autoimmun Rev 2009;8:488–494.
35 Sommers LM, Schoene RB: Allopurinol hypersensitivity syndrome associated with pancreatic exocrine abnormalities and new-onset diabetes mellitus. Arch Intern Med 2002;162:1190–1192.
36 Seino Y, Yamauchi M, Hirai C, Okumura A, Kondo K, Yamamoto M, Okazaki Y: A case of fulminant type 1 diabetes associated with mexiletine hypersensitivity syndrome. Diabet Med 2004;21:1156–1157.
37 Chiou CC, Chung WH, Hung SI, Ynag LC, Hong HS: Fulminant type 1 diabetes mellitus caused by drug hypersensitivity syndrome with human herpesvirus 6 infection. J Am Acad Dermatol 2006;54: S14–S17.
38 Brown RJ, Rother KI, Artman H, Mercurio MG, Wang R, Looney RJ, Cowen EW: Minocycline-induced drug hypersensitivity syndrome followed by multiple autoimmune sequelae. Arch Dermatol 2009;145:63–66.
39 Kano Y, Sakuma K, Shiohara T: Sclerodermoid graft-versus-host disease-like lesions occurring after drug-induced hypersensitivity syndrome. Br J Dermatol 2007;156:1061–1063.

40 Aota N, Hirahara K, Kano Y, Fukuoka T, Yamada A, Shiohara T: Systemic lupus erythematosus presenting with Kikuchi-Fujimoto's disease as a long-term sequela of drug-induced hypersensitivity syndrome. A possible role of Epstein-Barr virus reactivaton. Dermatology 2009;218:275–277.
41 Kang I, Quan T, Nolasco H, Park SH, Hong MS, Crouch J, Pamer EG, Howe JG, Craft J: Defective control of latent Epstein-Barr virus infection in systemic lupus erythematosus. J Immunol 2004;172: 1287–1294.
42 Gross AJ, Hochberg D, Rand WM, Thorley-Lawson DA: EBV and systemic lupus erythematosus: a new perspective. J Immunol 2005;174:6599–6607.
43 Asano Y, Kagawa H, Kano Y, Shiohara T: Cytomegalovirus disease during severe drug eruptions: report of 2 cases and retrospective study of 18 patients with drug-induced hypersensitivity syndrome. Arch Dermatol 2009;145:1030–1036.

Dr. Tetsuo Shiohara
Department of Dermatology, Kyorin University School of Medicine
6-20-2 Shinkawa, Mitaka
Tokyo 181-8611 (Japan)
Tel. +81 422 47 5511, E-Mail tpshio@ks.kyorin-u.ac.jp

French LE (ed): Adverse Cutaneous Drug Eruptions.
Chem Immunol Allergy. Basel, Karger, 2012, vol 97, pp 139–148

Acute Generalized Exanthematous Pustulosis

Alexis Sidoroff

Department of Dermatology and Venereology, Medical University of Innsbruck, Innsbruck, Austria

Abstract

The key clinical features of acute generalized exanthematous pustulosis (AGEP) are the acute occurrence of numerous pinhead-sized nonfollicular sterile pustules on an edematous erythema accompanied by fever and leukocytosis. Histology shows mainly spongiform subcorneal and/or intraepidermal pustules, frequently a marked edema of the papillary dermis, neutrophils, and often eosinophils. AGEP is a reaction pattern mostly caused by drugs, the ones with the highest risk being antibacterial agents like ampicillin/amoxicillin, and quinolones, pristinamycin, anti-infective sulfonamides, the antimycotic drug terbinafine, (hydroxy)chloroquine, and diltiazem. In addition, a large number of other drugs as well as infections have been reported as triggers. AGEP is an acute and sometimes severe reaction. When the causative agent is withdrawn, it usually resolves quickly without specific treatment.

Essentials in a Nutshell

- Acute generalized exanthematous pustulosis (AGEP) is characterized by an acute occurrence of numerous nonfollicular pinhead-sized, sterile pustules. The underlying exanthema is most pronounced in large flexural areas.
- Drugs with an elevated risk of causing AGEP are ampicillin/amoxicillin, quinolones, pristinamycin, anti-infective sulfonamides, terbinafine, (hydroxy) chloroquine, and diltiazem
- The main therapeutic measure to be taken is to withdraw the causative agent
- In contrast to most other adverse drug eruptions patch testing can be very useful in revealing the culprit drug
- Although mortality in AGEP is much lower than in other severe cutaneous drug reactions (like SJS/TEN or DRESS), it has quite dramatic clinical features suggesting a very severe disease, and confusion with other SCARs may thus be

quite common. Nevertheless, in patients with poor general clinical condition, AGEP can be a life-threatening disease.

Introduction

The term 'pustulose exanthématique aiguë généralisée (PEAG)' was coined by Beylot et al. [1] in 1980, and found its way into the English literature as acute generalized exanthematous pustulosis or its acronym AGEP. It is increasingly accepted as a clinical reaction pattern – mainly caused by drugs – whose hallmark is the occurrence of a quite characteristic disseminated nonfollicular pustular rash. Despite this, the terminology found in the literature may be confusing. Already in 1968, Baker and Ryan [2] reported on 104 cases of pustular psoriasis in which 5 patients without previous history of psoriasis showed a very acute pustular eruption that resolved quickly, and in which drugs and/or infections had been suspected as trigger. They used the term exanthematic pustular psoriasis for this subgroup. In other publications, denominations like pustular drug rash [3] or toxic pustuloderma [4] were used for patients sharing similar clinical features, or they were interpreted as being affected by special variants of other pustular diseases. Further confusion may arise from the term 'pustulosis acuta generalisata' which is used to describe a poststreptococcal reaction totally unrelated to AGEP, affecting mainly children [5].

Epidemiology

Epidemiological data on AGEP are unreliable – not only because of the semantic confusion, but also because the episode in which pustules can be seen is often of very transient nature, or the pustules are not given special attention to, leading to more general diagnoses like drug rash or viral exanthema. Some vague estimates about the incidence of AGEP range between 1 and 5 cases per million inhabitants per year. All ages can be affected, but according to some publications, women seem to be affected more often than men [6], especially in association with acetaminophen (paracetamol), and pregnancy may also play a role [7]. The issue of genetic predisposition is yet to be clarified, but in a study by Bernard et al. [8] HLA B51, DR11 and DQ3 were found to be more frequent than in the average population.

Clinical Features

The hallmark of AGEP [9] is the usually rapid appearance of at least dozens, but often hundreds to thousands of small, pinhead-sized, sterile nonfollicular pustules arising on an often edematous diffuse erythema (fig. 1). Classical predilection sites for the

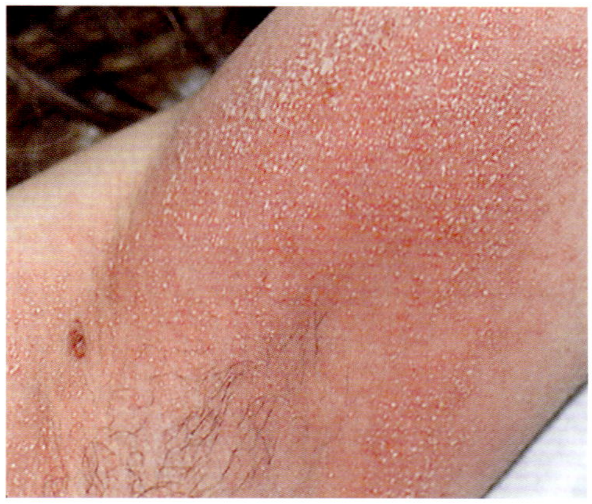

Fig. 1. AGEP with multiple pinhead-sized nonfollicular pustules on an edematous erythematous base.

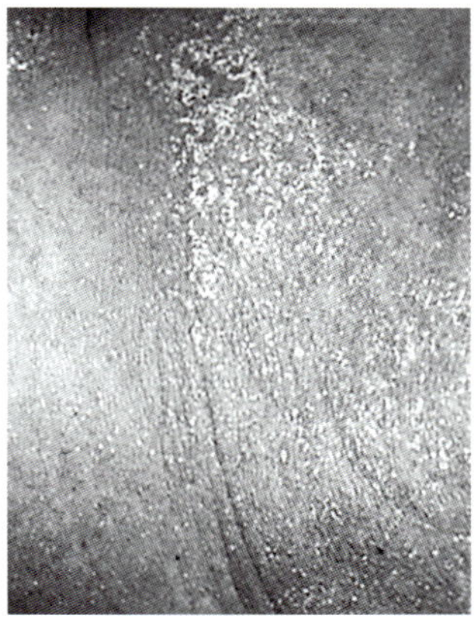

Fig. 2. Typical postpustular desquamation in AGEP.

skin lesions are the large body flexures (inguinal, axillar, and submammary areas), but cases with more irregularly distributed patches are not uncommon. An edematous erythema of the face is frequently present, blisters and vesicles, purpura (especially on the lower extremities), and Stevens-Johnson syndrome-like atypical targets can also be seen, but are not specific for AGEP. The cutaneous manifestations may be accompanied by itching or burning. Only exceptionally are mucous membranes (mostly lips and/or the oral cavity) affected (e.g. mild erosions of lips or in the oral cavity). The acute phase of the disease is often accompanied by fever above 38°C, leukocytosis (neutrophil counts above 7×10^9/l) and sometimes a mild eosinophilia [10]. Lymphadenopathy, a slightly reduced creatinine clearance, or a mild elevation of liver enzymes may be present, but internal organ involvement is rather exceptional in AGEP [11].

Skin lesions usually resolve rapidly (within a few days) after withdrawal of the causative agent. At this point, a characteristic collaret-shaped postpustular desquamation may still be a clue to the diagnosis (fig. 2). In general, AGEP heals without residual skin changes.

Histopathology

The histomorphological equivalents of the skin lesions found in AGEP are spongiform subcorneal and/or intraepidermal pustules frequently associated with a marked edema of the papillary dermis. Some single cell necrosis of keratinocytes may be present. The inflammatory infiltrate in the dermis tends to have a perivascular accentuation and mainly consists of neutrophils and often eosinophils [12]. Occasionally, erythrocyte extravasation can be observed. Histological features of a series of 102 cases have been recently described in detail by Halevy et al. [13].

A constant matter of debate remains the question whether AGEP can be distinguished from acute exanthematic pustular psoriasis. A couple of publications have addressed this issue. Although some clues might speak in favor of AGEP (presence of eosinophils in the pustules or dermis, necrotic keratinocytes, a mixed neutrophil-rich interstitial and mid-dermal infiltrate and the absence of tortuous, dilated blood vessels) [14, 15], in individual cases, AGEP might not be differentiated from acute exanthematic pustular psoriasis on histological grounds alone. The cell proliferation marker Ki67 is highly expressed in both entities [16].

Even if the clinical diagnosis of AGEP is quite straightforward in many cases, taking a biopsy is recommended. This should preferentially be done as soon as possible due to the transient nature of the reaction. Even if – as mentioned before – differentiation from acute pustular psoriasis may not be possible, histology is helpful in cases were the clinical presentation is not clear. Given the rapid evolution of the disease, the possibility of obtaining the result of emergency biopsies rapidly is of great advantage.

Differential Diagnoses

Generalized Acute Pustular Psoriasis (von Zumbusch Type)

The question whether AGEP is an entity of its own or a variant of acute generalized pustular psoriasis of the von Zumbusch type is a consequence of their sometimes very similar clinical appearance. Nevertheless, differentiation between the two diseases seems to be justified based on a number of specific features. Only a minority of patients with AGEP report on a history of psoriasis (personal or familiar) and/or show other morphological clues for psoriasis (e.g. nail changes, related arthritis). The major difference though seems to be the evolution of the rash over time: while AGEP resolves quickly (even without treatment), when the trigger is withdrawn, pustular psoriasis has a more prolonged course. Medications (mainly beta-blockers or lithium) might rarely be involved in triggering psoriatic flares. AGEP is mainly a drug reaction, and the associated drugs are not the same [17]. These facts have clear impact on treatment considerations and the patients' prognosis.

Stevens-Johnson Syndrome and Toxic Epidermal Necrolysis

When many pustules are standing close together, their confluence may form larger pustules. Due to their fragility, they result in erosions similar to those in Stevens-Johnson syndrome and toxic epidermal necrolysis (SJS/TEN), and a positive direct Nikolski's sign is mimicked. Thus the combination of a drug reaction and erosions might lead to a wrong diagnosis [18], especially when lesions resembling atypical targets are present. In addition, rare cases with clinical and histological features of both reaction types AGEP and SJS/TEN at the same time have been reported [19]. A more superficial epidermal detachment and the lack of mucous membrane erosions are more suggestive of AGEP, while full-thickness necrosis of the epidermis with a sparse inflammatory infiltrate in the histopathology speak in favor of TEN.

Drug Hypersensitivity Syndrome

Drug hypersensitivity syndrome, DRESS (an acronym for drug rash with eosinophilia and systemic symptoms) or DIHS (drug induced hypersensitivity syndrome) are just different denominations for intolerance reactions to drugs that are typically characterized by fever, eosinophilia, atypical lymphocytosis, lymphadenopathy, and severe internal organ involvement like hepatitis, nephritis, pneumonitis, myocarditis and more. Skin manifestations of DRESS are not specific, but may include edema of the face, a rather edematous rash and even papulovesicles or papulopustules, and – in rare cases – even numerous real pustules suggestive of AGEP. In general, patients suffering from DRESS are more severely ill, and the adverse cutaneous drug reaction lasts longer, sometimes beyond the point where the causative agent would be expected to be eliminated from the body. This might be due to viral reactivation (especially HHV6), which seems to be very common in DRESS, but is not a hallmark of AGEP.

Subcorneal Pustular Dermatosis (Sneddon-Wilkinson)

Another pustular dermatosis is Sneddon Wilkinson's disease, but here the nonfollicular pustules – that often have a circinate distribution – are larger, flaccid and typically show hypopyon formation. Onset is less acute than in AGEP, and the course of disease is more chronic.

Pustular Vasculitis

Leukocytoclastic vasculitis is characterized by palpable purpuric lesions, but bullous or pustular lesions may be present. Clinically, even special cases of vasculitis with many small pustules, mainly located on the dorsum of the hands and sometimes triggered by drugs should be easily distinguishable from AGEP. In cases of doubt, histology is helpful as it shows clear features of leukocytoclastic vasculitis [20, 21]. Confusion is mainly semantic, as the term pustulosis acuta generalisata [5, 22, 23] attributed to a poststreptococcal form of leukocytoclastic vasculitis sounds very similar to AGEP. Further confusion arises from the fact that another source of ambiguity might be related to the fact that some vasculitic changes are not uncommon in biopsies of AGEP lesions.

Candidiasis

Numerous pustules, especially in the big flexures can be caused by candida infection. This diagnosis can easily be confirmed by the detection of hyphae.

Others

There is an extensive list of dermatoses showing pustules in a variable degree. When pustules are predominantly follicular, differential diagnosis is rarely a problem. Examples are acne and acneiform pustules, localized pustular contact dermatitis, bacterial folliculitis, furunculosis, dermatophyte infections, impetigo, impetiginized eczema, varicella, pyoderma vegetans, Kaposi's varicelliform eruption, Sweet's syndrome, infantile chronic acropustulosis, or pustules in migratory necrolytic eruption of glucagonoma, bowel bypass syndrome, Behcet's disease or pemphigus foliaceus and other autoimmune bullous disorders (like IgA pemphigus which might have some histological resemblances). Also in cases with confluent pustules and erosions, differentiation from staphylococcal scalded skin syndrome can rarely represent a diagnostic challenge. Only in cases where pustules are few or have already ruptured and left large areas of desquamation, the differentiation from erythroderma or exfoliative dermatitis might be difficult.

Etiology and Pathogenesis

The vast majority of AGEP cases are drug induced, although viral infections, for example, can also be associated with the disease [25–30]. Literature provides a long list of single case reports and case series in which a large number of different drugs is documented as potential triggers. Giving all references would go beyond the scope of this textbook, but reports on the following anti-infective agents have been frequently reported: β-lactam antibiotics, macrolides, cephalosporins, quinolones, tetracyclines, other antibiotics (chloramphenicol, imipenem, gentamycin, isoniazid, metronidazole, trimethoprim-sulfamethoxazole, vancomycin), antimycotics (terbinafine, griseofulvin, itraconazole, nystatin, amphotericin B), other anti-infectives [(hydroxy-)chloroquine, diaphenylsulfone, nifuroxazide, pyrimethamine, protease inhibitors]. Other drugs that have been described as causative agents are (in alphabetical order): acetylsalicylic acid, allopurinol, allylisopropylacetylurea, amoxapine, azathioprine, buphenine, bufexamac, calcium channel blockers, carbamazepine, carbimazole, carbutamide, high-dose chemotherapy, chromium picolinate, cimetidine, clemastine, clobazam, clozapine, contrast media (nonionic), corticosteroids, dalteparin, dexamethasone, disulfiram, enalapril, eprazinone, epoetin-α, fenoterol, fluinidone, furosemide, gefitinib, icodextrin, imantinib, isotretinoin, kerorin, lansoprazole, morphine, nadoxolol, nifedipine, nimesulide, meladinine, mercury, olanzapine, paracetamol, piperazine ethionamate, pneumococcal vaccine, propafenone, prostaglandin E1, pseudoephedrine, quinidine sulbutiamine, ritodrine, sulfasalazine, thalidomide, as well as herbal medications (gingko biloba and other herbs used in traditional Chinese medicine), Rhus (lacquer), topical agents [2-chlorobenzylidene malononitrile (CS) gas, metronidazole, mephenesin], spider bites or PUVA. It has to be mentioned that this list is neither complete nor definite, as new reports are constantly being published. A synopsis of these reports and the result of systematic studies allow to give a better estimate on which drugs have a higher risk of inducing AGEP [17, 24]: strongly associated drugs seem to be antibacterial agents like ampicillin/amoxicillin, and quinolones, pristinamycin (a macrolide not widely marketed), anti-infective sulfonamides, the antimycotic drug terbinafine, (hydroxy)chloroquine, and diltiazem.

These results show that the spectrum of drugs that often act as trigger for AGEP clearly differ from the compounds that are the usual suspects for other skin reactions like SJS/TEN. Classical triggers for the latter, like allopurinol, antiepileptic drugs, or nevirapine do not seem to play a prominent role in AGEP, while terbinafine, diltiazem and pristinamycin are not of major importance in SJS/TEN. Only antibiotic agents are often associated with both types of reaction.

A number of cases in which infections are the suspected trigger for AGEP can be found in the literature [10] (e.g. parvovirus B19, mycoplasma, cytomegalovirus, coxsackie B4). In many cases, the infectious trigger is well documented, and the sole probable reason for the reaction – AGEP caused by infectious agents – seems to be an exception. In this context, one must be aware that confounding by indication (drug given for an underlying infection or already for the first symptoms of the reaction), makes causality assessment for drugs particularly difficult. Yet, present data suggest that infections – although possible – are not very common in triggering AGEP.

It is obvious that neutrophils play an important role in AGEP, and the role of drug-specific (CD4+) T cells that produce neutrophil-attracting factors like interleukin-8 and cytotoxic (CD8+) T cells has been extensively investigated [31–35]. Recently, it has been shown that T helper 17 cells and interleukin-22 are increased in AGEP patients [36]. Yet, a number of questions in the pathomechanism of AGEP remain to be answered. One of them arises from the observation that there seem to be two timing patterns for the reaction. One is similar to that of other drug rashes, i.e. the reaction occurs in a time frame between 1 and 2 weeks. But for a large number of cases (especially those triggered by antibiotics), the interval between first intake and cutaneous reaction can be as short as a few hours. This could be explained by prior sensitization and rechallenge to the specific drug, but in the majority of cases, evidence for such a prior exposure cannot be found [17]. Another field of interest for future research is the genetic predisposition that might lead patients to react in a neutrophilic direction.

Treatment

As AGEP is mainly caused by drugs, detection of the probable trigger(s) and its/their withdrawal is the main therapeutic step to be taken. The culprit agent though may not be obvious in cases where patients might have taken a large number of drugs. In addition, a thorough drug history is necessary to discriminate drugs that have been taken after the onset of the reaction. Usually, withdrawal of the causative agent leads to a resolution of active lesions within a few days. Postpustular desquamation may persist a little bit longer, but no new lesions should arise. It is a common practice to apply topical and systemic steroids. Although this is not an evidence-based approach, it is acceptable, as the drugs are given for a short time-period and do not bear the risk of significant side effects. If antipyretics are not part of the spectrum of suspected drugs, they can be given for symptomatic relief.

After the acute phase, causality assessment is still a very important procedure that needs to be done, as reexposure to the drug might lead to another episode of AGEP [37]. Patch testing with suspected triggers in AGEP leads more often to positive test results than in other drug rashes (like SJS/TEN), usually revealing many small sterile pustules at the site of testing [38, 39]. Rarely, systemic reactions can occur [40]. Positive patch testing is quite helpful to identify the culprit agent when two or more drugs are suspected to have caused the reaction. Negative patch tests do not however prove that a certain substance was not the cause for the reaction.

There have been reports on drug specific in vitro tests, but until now they cannot be regarded as standardized diagnostic tools. The mast cell degranulation test [41, 42], macrophage migration inhibition factor test, interferon-γ release test [43] and lymphocyte proliferation responses [44] have been published. For the latter, it could be demonstrated that it correlated with patch tests in 2 patients [45]. As with many drug intolerance reactions, a thorough drug history and understanding of the reaction remain the main pillars of determining the culprit drug, while in vivo and laboratory tests may be of confirmatory help.

References

1 Beylot C, Bioulac P, Doutre MS: Acute generalized exanthematic pustuloses four cases (in French). Ann Dermatol Venereol 1980;107:37–48.
2 Baker H, Ryan TJ: Generalized pustular psoriasis. A clinical and epidemiologssssical study of 104 cases. Br J Dermatol 1968;80:771–793.
3 Macmillan AL: Generalised pustular drug rash. Dermatologica 1973;146:285–291.
4 Staughton RC, Payne CM, Harper JI, McMichen H: Toxic pustuloderma – a new entity? J R Soc Med 1984;77(suppl 4):6–8.
5 Auer-Grumbach P, Pfaffenthaler E, Soyer HP: Pustulosis acuta generalisata is a post-streptococcal disease and is distinct from acute generalized exanthematous pustulosis. Br J Dermatol 1995;133: 135–139.
6 Tamir E, Wohl Y, Mashiah J, Brenner S: Acute generalized exanthematous pustulosis: a retrospective analysis showing a clear predilection for women. Skinmed 2006;5:186–188.
7 Brenner S, Wohl Y: Acute generalized exanthematous pustulosis in pregnancy: more common than previously estimated. Skinmed 2005;4:336.
8 Bernard P, Lizeaux-Parneix V, Miossec V, et al: HLA et prédisposition génétique dans les pustuloses exanthématiques (PEAG) et les exanthémes maculo-papuleux (EMP). Ann Dermatol Venerol 1995; 122:S38–S39.
9 Sidoroff A, Halevy S, Bavinck JN, Vaillant L, Roujeau JC: Acute generalized exanthematous pustulosis (AGEP) – a clinical reaction pattern. J Cutan Pathol 2001;28:113–119.
10 Roujeau JC, Bioulac-Sage P, Bourseau C, Guillaume JC, Bernard P, Lok C, Plantin P, Claudy A, Delavierre C, Vaillant L, et al: Acute generalized exanthematous pustulosis. Analysis of 63 cases. Arch Dermatol 1991;127:1333–1338.
11 Leclair MA, Maynard B, St-Pierre C: Acute generalized exanthematous pustulosis with severe organ dysfunction. CMAJ 2009;181:393–396.
12 Burrows NP, Russell Jones RR: Pustular drug eruptions: a histopathological spectrum. Histopathology 1993;22:569–573.
13 Halevy S, Kardaun SH, Davidovici B, Wechsler J: The spectrum of histopathological features in acute generalized exanthematous pustulosis: a study of 102 cases. Br J Dermatol 2010;163:1245–1252.
14 Beylot C, Doutre MS, Beylot-Barry M: Acute generalized exanthematous pustulosis. Semin Cutan Med Surg 1996;15:244–249.
15 Kardaun SH, Kuiper H, Fidler V, Jonkman MF: The histopathological spectrum of acute generalized exanthematous pustulosis (AGEP) and its differentiation from generalized pustular psoriasis. J Cutan Pathol 2010;37:1220–1229.
16 Chang SL, Hu S, Hung SI, Huang YL, Hsiao WC, Chung WH: A comparison of Ki-67 antigen presentation in acute generalized exanthematous pustulosis and pustular psoriasis. Arch Dermatol Res 2010; 302:525–529.
17 Sidoroff A, Dunant A, Viboud C, Halevy S, Bavinck JN, Naldi L, Mockenhaupt M, Fagot JP, Roujeau JC: Risk factors for acute generalized exanthematous pustulosis (AGEP)-results of a multinational case-control study (EuroSCAR). Br J Dermatol 2007;157: 989–996.
18 Cohen AD, Cagnano E, Halevy S: Acute generalized exanthematous pustulosis mimicking toxic epidermal necrolysis. Int J Dermatol 2001;40:458–461.
19 Meiss F, Helmbold P, Meykadeh N, Gaber G, Marsch W, Fischer M: Overlap of acute generalized exanthematous pustulosis and toxic epidermal necrolysis: response to antitumour necrosis factor-alpha antibody infliximab: report of three cases. J Eur Acad Dermatol Venereol 2007;21:717–719.
20 Rockl H: Leukocytoclastic vasculitis due to drug allergy presenting as generalized pustular exanthema (in German). Hautarzt 1981;32:467–470.
21 Strutton G, Weedon D, Robertson I: Pustular vasculitis of the hands. J Am Acad Dermatol 1995;32: 192–198.
22 Braun-Falco O, Luderschmidt C, Maciejewski W, Scherer R: Generalized acute pustulosis. An unusual presentation of leukocytoclastic vasculitis (in German). Hautarzt 1978;29:371–377.
23 Patrizi A, Savoia F, Giacomini F, Neri I, Ricci G: Diffuse acute pustular eruption after streptococcal infection – a new instance of pustulosis acuta generalisata. Pediatr Dermatol 2007;24:272–276.
24 Saissi EH, Beau-Salinas F, Jonville-Bera AP, Lorette G, Autret-Leca E: Drugs associated with acute generalized exanthematic pustulosis (in French). Ann Dermatol Venereol 2003;130:612–618.
25 Feio AB, Apetato M, Costa MM, Sa J, Alcantara J: Acute generalized exanthematous pustulosis due to Coxsackie B4 virus (in Portugese). Acta Med Port 1997;10:487–491.
26 Haro-Gabaldon V, Sanchez-Sanchez-Vizcaino J, Ruiz-Avila P, Gutierrez-Fernandez J, Linares J, Naranjo-Sintes R: Acute generalized exanthematous pustulosis with cytomegalovirus infection. Int J Dermatol 1996;35:735–737.

27 Rouchouse B, Bonnefoy M, Pallot B, Jacquelin L, Dimoux-Dime G, Claudy AL: Acute generalized exanthematous pustular dermatitis and viral infection. Dermatologica 1986;173:180–184.
28 Naides SJ, Piette W, Veach LA, Argenyi Z: Human parvovirus B19-induced vesiculopustular skin eruption. Am J Med 1988;84:968–972.
29 Manzano S, Guggisberg D, Hammann C, Laubscher B: Acute generalized exanthematous pustulosis: first case associated with a Chlamydia pneumoniae infection (in French). Arch Pediatr 2006;13: 1230–1232.
30 Ofuji S, Yamamoto O: Acute generalized exanthematous pustulosis associated with a human parvovirus B19 infection. J Dermatol 2007;34:121–123.
31 Britschgi M, Pichler WJ: Acute generalized exanthematous pustulosis, a clue to neutrophil-mediated inflammatory processes orchestrated by T cells. Curr Opin Allergy Clin Immunol 2002;2:325–331.
32 Britschgi M, Steiner UC, Schmid S, Depta JP, Senti G, Bircher A, Burkhart C, Yawalkar N, Pichler WJ: T-cell involvement in drug-induced acute generalized exanthematous pustulosis. J Clin Invest 2001; 107:1433–1441.
33 Britschgi M, von Greyerz S, Burkhart C, Pichler WJ: Molecular aspects of drug recognition by specific T cells. Curr Drug Targets 2003;4:1–11.
34 Pichler WJ: T cells in drug allergy. Curr Allergy Asthma Rep 2002;2:9–15.
35 Schmid S, Kuechler PC, Britschgi M, Steiner UC, Yawalkar N, Limat A, Baltensperger K, Braathen L, Pichler WJ: Acute generalized exanthematous pustulosis: role of cytotoxic T cells in pustule formation. Am J Pathol 2002;161:2079–2086.
36 Tokura Y, Mori T, Hino R: Psoriasis and other Th17-mediated skin diseases. J UOEH 2010;32:317–328.
37 Greco M, Plantin P: Acute generalized exanthematous pustulosis (AGEP) induced by terbinafine with involuntary positive reintroduction. Eur J Dermatol 2005;15:116.
38 Wolkenstein P, Chosidow O, Flechet ML, Robbiola O, Paul M, Dume L, Revuz J, Roujeau JC: Patch testing in severe cutaneous adverse drug reactions, including Stevens-Johnson syndrome and toxic epidermal necrolysis. Contact Dermatitis 1996;35: 234–236.
39 Barbaud A: Drug patch testing in systemic cutaneous drug allergy. Toxicology 2005;209:209–216.
40 Mashiah J, Brenner S: A systemic reaction to patch testing for the evaluation of acute generalized exanthematous pustulosis. Arch Dermatol 2003;139: 1181–1183.
41 Lazarov A, Livni E, Halevy S: Generalized pustular drug eruptions: confirmation by in vitro tests. J Eur Acad Dermatol Venereol 1998;10:36–41.
42 Pichler WJ, Yawalkar N, Britschgi M, Depta J, Strasser I, Schmid S, Kuechler P, Naisbitt D: Cellular and molecular pathophysiology of cutaneous drug reactions. Am J Clin Dermatol 2002;3:229–238.
43 Halevy S, Cohen A, Livni E: Acute generalized exanthematous pustulosis associated with polysensitivity to paracetamol and bromhexine: the diagnostic role of in vitro interferon-gamma release test. Clin Exp Dermatol 2000;25:652–654.
44 Beltraminelli HS, Lerch M, Arnold A, Bircher AJ, Haeusermann P: Acute generalized exanthematous pustulosis induced by the antifungal terbinafine: case report and review of the literature. Br J Dermatol 2005;152:780–783.
45 Girardi M, Duncan KO, Tigelaar RE, Imaeda S, Watsky KL, McNiff JM: Cross-comparison of patch test and lymphocyte proliferation responses in patients with a history of acute generalized exanthematous pustulosis. Am J Dermatopathol 2005;27: 343–346.

Ao. Univ.-Prof. Dr. Alexis Sidoroff
Department of Dermatology and Venereology, Medical University of Innsbruck
Anichstrasse 35
AT–6020 Innsbruck (Austria)
Tel. +43 512 504 22971, E-Mail alexis.sidoroff@i-med.ac.at

French LE (ed): Adverse Cutaneous Drug Eruptions.
Chem Immunol Allergy. Basel, Karger, 2012, vol 97, pp 149–166

Stevens-Johnson Syndrome and Toxic Epidermal Necrolysis

Thomas Harr · Lars E. French

Department of Dermatology, University Hospital Zurich, Zurich, Switzerland

Abstract

Toxic epidermal necrolysis (TEN) and Stevens-Johnson syndrome (SJS) are rare but severe adverse cutaneous drug reactions that are to be considered medical emergencies. The average reported mortality rate for SJS is 1–5%, and up to 25–35% for TEN. TEN and SJS are characterized by more or less extensive painful erythematous and erosive lesions of the skin, conjunctiva and mucous membranes resulting from massive apoptosis of epithelial cells, and are considered to be two ends of a spectrum of severe epidermolytic adverse cutaneous drug reactions, differing only by their extent of skin detachment. Drugs including allopurinol, antibiotics, anticonvulsants and NSAIDs of the oxicam type are the main cause of SJS/TEN in most cases. Recent evidence supports a genetic susceptibility to SJS and TEN as exemplified by the strong association observed in Han Chinese between the human leukocyte antigen HLA-B*1502, and SJS induced by carbamazepine. Diagnosis relies mainly on clinical signs together with the histological analysis of a skin biopsy showing typical full-thickness epidermal necrolysis due to extensive keratinocyte apoptosis. Differential diagnoses include autoimmune bullous dermatoses, acute generalized exanthematous pustulosis, disseminated fixed bullous drug eruption and staphyloccocal scalded skin syndrome. Due to the high risk of mortality, management of patients with SJS/TEN requires rapid diagnosis, evaluation of the prognosis using SCORTEN, rapid identification and interruption of the culprit drug, specialized supportive care ideally in an intensive care unit, and the consideration of immunomodulatory agents such as high-dose intravenous immunoglobulin.

Essentials in a Nutshell

- Stevens-Johnson syndrome (SJS) and toxic epidermal necrolysis (TEN) are severe adverse mucocutaneous drug eruptions with a mortality rate of 1–5% for SJS and 25–30% for TEN
- SJS and TEN are considered to be two ends of a spectrum of severe epidermolytic adverse cutaneous drug reactions with increasing severity ranging from SJS to TEN

- Allopurinol, antibiotics, anticonvulsants and NSAIDs of the oxicam-type are the main causes of SJS/TEN
- The pathogenesis involves a genetic susceptibility, an inappropriate allergic response to the culprit drug, and massive apoptosis of epithelial cells of the skin and mucous membranes
- Rapid diagnosis, identification of the culprit drug, and discontinuation of its intake can reduce mortality
- No specific therapy with a proven high evidence level exists
- High-dose intravenous immunoglobulin (IVIG) may have a benefit if given early at a total dose of 3 g/kg bodyweight

Introduction

SJS was first described in 1922 as an acute mucocutaneous syndrome in two young boys. The condition was characterized by severe purulent conjunctivitis, severe stomatitis with extensive mucosal necrosis, and purpuric macules. It became known as SJS and was recognized as a severe mucocutaneous disease with a prolonged course and potentially lethal outcome that is in most cases drug-induced, and should be distinguished from erythema multiforme majus. Recent clinical studies highlight the fact that erythema multiforme majus and SJS are clinically and etiologically distinct disorders that should be classified as such [1–4].

Toxic epidermal necrolysis was the name given in 1956 by a Scottish dermatologist Alan Lyell to a not previously described eruption resembling scalding of the skin which he observed in 4 patients [4]. It was only as more patients with TEN were reported in the years following Lyell's original publication, that it became clear that TEN was drug induced, and that selected drugs such as sulfonamides, pyrazolones, barbiturates, and antiepileptics were frequent triggers of TEN. Increasingly to date, SJS and TEN are considered to be two ends of a spectrum of severe epidermolytic adverse cutaneous drug reactions, differing only by their extent of skin detachment.

Epidemiology

SJS and TEN are rare diseases in absolute numbers with an incidence of approximately 1.9 cases per million inhabitants per year [5, 6]. Certain infectious diseases may affect the incidence of TEN as is the case for HIV, in which the annual incidence is approximately 1,000-fold higher than in the general population, with approximately 1 case of TEN per thousand per year in the HIV-positive population [7].

Regional differences in drug prescription, the genetic background of patients (HLA, metabolizing enzymes), the coexistence of cancer, and concomitant radiotherapy have also been reported to impact on the incidence of SJS and TEN [8, 9].

To a lesser extent than drugs, certain infections have in rare instances been reported as the sole identifiable cause of SJS/TEN. *Mycoplasma pneumoniae* infections have been documented to cause SJS and TEN without initial exposure to drugs [10–12], and herpes simplex virus was reported in several cases of SJS, especially in children [13]. Despite the above, there are still cases of SJS/TEN without any obvious identifiable cause.

Clinical Features

Acute Phase

Initial symptoms of TEN and SJS are unspecific and include symptoms such as fever, stinging eyes and discomfort upon swallowing. Typically, these symptoms precede cutaneous manifestations by hours to days. Usually the first and predominantly involved sites of cutaneous involvement are the presternal region and the face, but also the palms and soles. Involvement of the buccal, genital and/or ocular mucosa, characterized by erythema and erosions, occurs in more than 90% of patients, and in some cases the respiratory and gastrointestinal tracts are also affected [14, 15]. Ocular involvement is frequent, and can range from acute conjunctivitis to conjunctival membrane or pseudomembrane formation or corneal erosion, and, in severe cases, to cicatrizing lesions, symblepharon, fornix foreshortening, and corneal ulceration [16, 17]. The severity of acute ocular manifestation is not however predictive of late complications [18]. The morphology of early skin lesions includes erythematous and livid macules, which may or may not be slightly infiltrated, and have a tendency to rapid coalescence and evolve to the formation of tense bullae (table 1; fig. 1a). The above-mentioned skin signs associated with mucosal involvement are clear danger signs and warrant rapid diagnostic confirmation with immediate cryosections of a skin biopsy. Histological examination including direct immunofluorescence analysis of the skin biopsy is also important in order to rule out differential diagnoses such as autoimmune blistering diseases, bullous fixed drug eruption, acute generalized exanthematic pustulosis, and staphyloccocal scalded skin syndrome.

In a second phase, large areas of epidermal detachment develop (fig. 1). In the absence of epidermal detachment, more detailed skin examination should be performed by exerting tangential mechanical pressure on several erythematous zones (Nikolsky sign). The Nikolsky sign is positive if mechanical pressure induces epidermal detachment, but is not specific for TEN or SJS, as it can also be positive in, for example, autoimmune bullous skin diseases.

The extent of skin involvement is a major prognostic factor. It should be emphasized that only necrotic skin, which is already detached (e.g. blisters, erosions) or detachable skin (Nikolsky positive) should be included in the evaluation of the extent of skin involvement. Bastuji-Garin et al. [1] proposed classifying patients into three

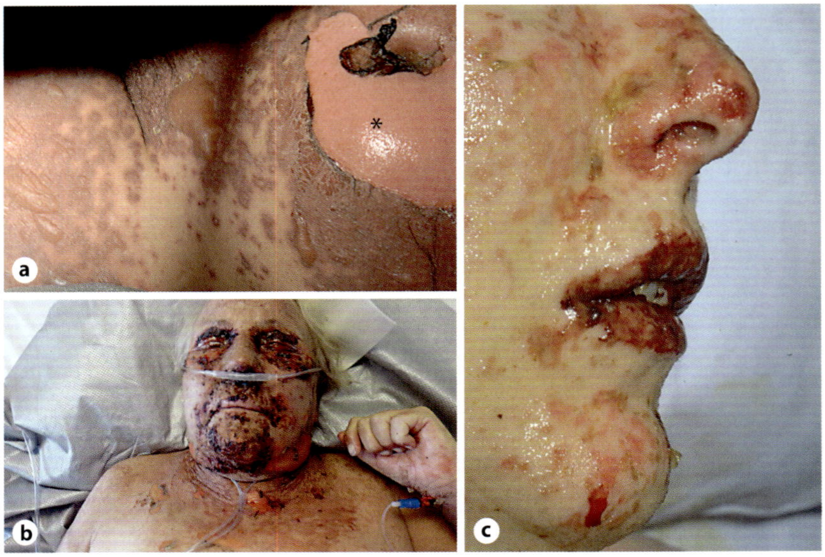

Fig. 1. **a** Dusky red confluent macular lesions associated with tense bullae and large areas of dermoepidermal detachment or denuded skin (asterisk). **b** Typical distribution of skin and mucous membrane lesions in SJS and/or TEN with predominance of confluent erythema and skin detachment initially in the prethoracic region and face, associated with buccal and ocular erythema, hemorrhagic crusts and mucous membrane detachment. **c** Overt mucous membrane involvement (lips) and moderate skin detachment with crusts in a case of SJS.

Table 1. Clinical features that distinguish SJS, SJS/TEN overlap, and TEN

Clinical entity	SJS	SJS/TEN overlap	TEN
Primary lesions	Dusky red lesions Flat atypical targets	Dusky red lesions Flat atypical targets	Poorly delineated erythematous plaques Epidermal detachment Dusky red lesions Flat atypical targets
Distribution	Isolated lesions Confluence (+) on face and trunk	Isolated lesions Confluence (++) on face and trunk	Isolated lesions (rare) Confluence (+++) on face, trunk, and elsewhere
Mucosal involvement	Yes	Yes	Yes
Systemic symptoms	Usually	Always	Always
Detachment (% body surface area)	<10	10–30	>30

Adapted from Bachot et al. [54].

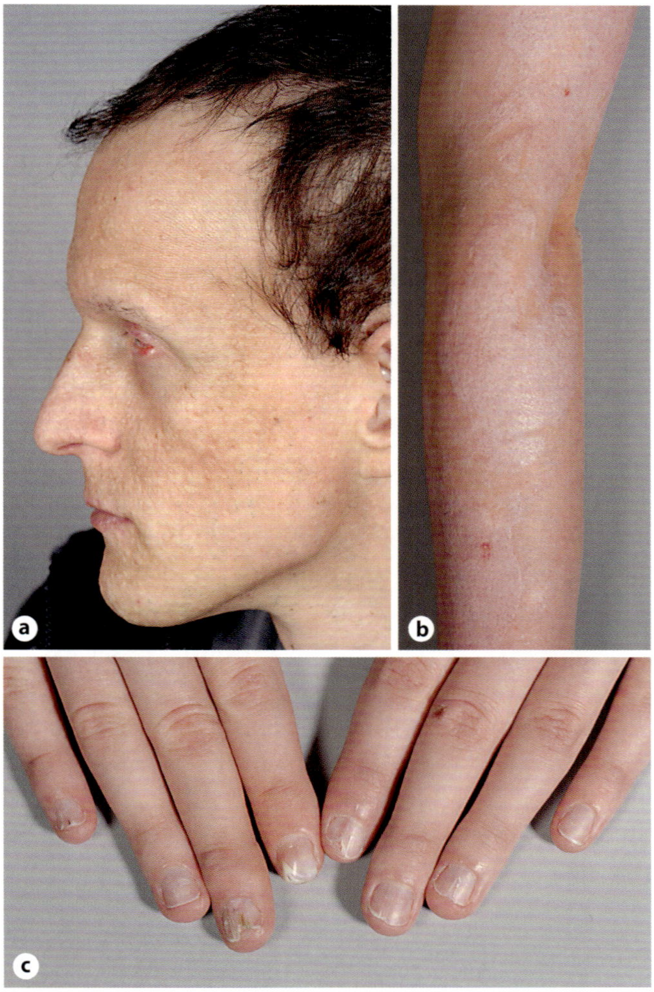

Fig. 2. Sequelae are common features of late-phase SJS and/or TEN. Hyper- and hypopigmentation of the skin on the face (**a**) and arm (**b**) associated with superficial scarring (**a**, **b**), ocular complications such as keratoconjunctivitis (**a**), and nail dystrophies (**c**).

groups according to the degree of skin detachment: 1–10% defined as SJS, 11–30% defined as SJS-TEN overlap, and greater than 30% defined as TEN (table 1).

Late Phase and Sequelae

Sequelae are common features of late-phase TEN, and include hyper- and hypopigmentation of the skin (62.5% of cases), nail dystrophies (37.5% of cases), and ocular complications (50% of cases) [18, 19] (fig. 2). Long-term complications of mucosal involvement occur in 73% of patients, and involve mainly the oral and esophageal mucosa, and to a lesser extent lung and genital mucosa [20]. Xerostomia or keratoconjunctivitis or both resembling Sjögren-like syndrome have also been reported [21, 22].

Etiology and Pathogenesis

Genetic Susceptibility

Great progress has recently been made in elucidating the genetic underpinnings of SJS/TEN, and it is becoming clear that a genetic predisposition is a major pathogenic factor in this disease. A unique and strong association between HLA (HLA-B*1502) and carbamazepine drug hypersensitivity in the form of SJS was discovered for Han Chinese [23]. This association has been confirmed in Hong Kong Han Chinese and in a Thai population [24, 25], but not in Japanese or Europeans [26–29]. In Europeans developing a hypersensitivity reaction to carbamazepine, including SJS/TEN and DRESS (drug rash with eosinophilia and systemic symptoms), recent data have shown that there is a significant association with another distinct HLA allele, namely HLA-A*3101 [30]. A second strong association between HLA genotype and SJS/TEN has been reported for allopurinol. Indeed, 100% of Han Chinese patients with a severe adverse drug reaction to allopurinol were HLA-B*5801 positive [31]. Subsequently, a strong association between SJS/TEN and HLA-B*5801 was also demonstrated in Japanese [27], Thai [25], and also to a lesser extent (55% of cases) in patients of European origin [29].

Of extreme interest and relevance with respect to the predictive value of the above-described genetic markers, is the fact – as recently revealed by a prospective study in Taiwan – that carbamazepine-induced SJS/TEN can indeed be prevented by using HLA-B*1502 genotype screening to prospectively identify subjects at genetic risk for the condition [32].

Pathomechanism of Stevens-Johnson Syndrome and Toxic Epidermal Necrolysis

The pathogenesis of SJS/TEN is not fully understood but is believed to be immune mediated, as rechallenging an individual with the same drug can result in rapid recurrence of SJS/TEN [33, 34]. The histopathology of SJS/TEN lesions shows that keratinocyte apoptosis followed by necrosis is the pathogenic basis of the widespread epidermal detachment observed in SJS/TEN. The clinical, histopathological and immunological findings in SJS/TEN support the currently prevalent concept that SJS and TEN are specific drug hypersensitivity reactions in which cytotoxic T lymphocytes (CTL) play a role in the initiation phase. Indeed, in the early phase of disease, blister fluid contains mainly cytotoxic CD8+T lymphocytes [35, 36], suggesting that a major histocompatibility class I restricted drug presentation leads to clonal expansion of CD8+ CTLs, and the subsequent – to date only incompletely understood – immune reaction that causes SJS/TEN. These CD8+ T cells express common cutaneous leukocyte antigen and are negative for CD45RA and CD28. Nassif et al. [37] were able to demonstrate that blister T cells from patients exert drug-specific cytototoxic activity against both autologous B-lymphocyte cell lines and keratinocytes, and furthermore demonstrated that this cell-mediated cytotoxicity was mediated by granzyme B. The discrepancy between the paucity of the infiltration of immune cells (including CTLs) in the skin of patients with SJS/TEN and the overwhelming keratinocyte apoptosis has however led to the search for cytotoxic proteins and/or cytokines that may amplify the extent of keratinocyte apoptosis that CTLs alone could induce upon cell-cell contact. To date, the strongest evidence suggests a key contribution of the cytotoxic molecules FasL and granulysin as molecules responsible for the disseminated keratinocyte apoptosis in SJS/TEN [38, 39]. However, it is still not fully understood what causes the upregulation of FasL/Fas on keratinocytes or granulysin in immune cells, and how the immune system, including T cells found in blister fluid at the onset of disease may regulate this.

The role of soluble FasL (sFasL) in SJS/TEN remains controversial. It appears clear now that increased levels of sFasL can be found in the serum of patients with SJS/TEN, and levels of sFasL are consistently elevated when analysis is performed preceding skin detachment [40]. sFasL as opposed to membrane-bound FasL is, however, very poorly cytolytic, and it is therefore unlikely to be a cause of keratinocyte apoptosis in TEN [41]. Nevertheless, one study showed that sera of SJS/TEN were able to induce abundant keratinocyte apoptosis, and furthermore that peripheral blood monuclear cells of patients stimulated by the causative drug excreted high levels of sFasL [42]. But it should be noted that sera can contain small membrane vesicles with membrane-bound FasL that can account for the observed activity.

In conclusion, and based on our knowledge to date, CD8 T cells as well as the cytolytic molecules FasL and granulysin are key players in the pathogenesis of SJS/TEN. How a culprit drug in a given patient who will develop SJS/TEN regulates the function of these key players is the subject of ongoing research.

Drugs

In absolute case numbers, allopurinol is currently the most common cause of SJS/TEN in Europe and Israel [43], and mostly in patients receiving daily doses of at least 200 mg.

In a case-control study performed in Europe between 1989 and 1993, the following drugs were found to be at increased risk of inducing SJS/TEN when used over a short period of time: trimethoprim-sulfamethoxazole and other sulfonamide antibiotics, aminopenicillins, cephalosporins, quinolones and chlormezanone [7]. Among drugs usually taken for longer periods of time and associated with SJS/TEN, including carbamazepine, phenytoin, phenobarbital, valproic acid, nonsteroidal anti-inflammatory drugs of the oxicam type, allopurinol and corticosteroids, the highest risk of induction of SJS/TEN was observed during the first 2 months of treatment with a sharp drop in incidence thereafter [7]. Although these drugs have a high relative risk compared to other drugs, the actual risk remained low with 5 cases or less per million users per week. A similar population studied more recently (1997–2001) with special attention for newly marketed drugs identified nevirapine, lamotrigine, and sertraline, as drugs with a significantly increased risk of inducing SJS/TEN [44]. Older drugs identified as having a high risk of inducing SJS/TEN were sulfamethoxazole/trimethoprim, sulfonamides (sulfasalazine, sulfadiazine, sulfadoxine, sulfafurazole), allopurinol, carbamazepine, phenytoin, phenobarbital, and NSAIDs of the oxicam type (meloxicam, piroxicam, tenoxicam). However, the incidence of SJS/TEN under treatment with valproic acid is confounded by the concomitant use of other drugs, such as lamotrigine [5].

Diagnosis and Diagnostic Methods

The diagnosis of SJS and TEN is clinical, confirmed by histological features. Typical clinical signs have been previously described and initially include areas of erythematous and livid macules on the skin on which a positive Nikolsky sign can be induced by mechanical pressure on the skin. To distinguish SJS, SJS-TEN and TEN the surface area of the detachment is the main discriminating factor (table 1). Histological workup of immediate cryosections or conventional formalin-fixed sections of the skin revealing widespread necrotic epidermis involving all layers confirms the diagnosis. In order to rule out autoimmune blistering diseases, direct immune fluorescence staining should be performed.

Differential Diagnosis

Major differential diagnosis of SJS/TEN are autoimmune blistering diseases, including linear IgA dermatosis and paraneoplastic pemphigus but also pemphigus vulgaris and bullous pemphigoid, acute generalized exanthematous pustulosis, disseminated fixed bullous drug eruption and staphyloccocal scalded skin syndrome.

Management and Therapy

Treatment in Acute Stage

Management in the acute stage involves sequentially evaluating the severity and prognosis of disease, rapid identification and withdrawal of the culprit drug(s), rapidly initiating best supportive care in an appropriate setting, and eventual specific drug therapy as described in detail below.

Table 2. SCORTEN severity of illness score

Clinical-biologic parameter	Individual score	SCORTEN	Predicted mortality, %
Age >40 years	Yes = 1, No = 0	0–1	3.2
Malignancy	Yes = 1, No = 0	2	12.1
Tachycardia (>120/min)	Yes = 1, No = 0		
Epidermal detachment >10%	Yes = 1, No = 0	3	35.3
Serum urea >10 mmol/l	Yes = 1, No = 0	4	58.3
Serum glucose >14 mmol/l	Yes = 1, No = 0		
Bicarbonate <20 mmol/l	Yes = 1, No = 0	≥5	90

Evaluation of Severity and Prognosis

As soon as the diagnosis of SJS or TEN has been established, the severity and prognosis of the disease should be determined so as to define the appropriate medical setting for further management. The validated SCORTEN disease severity scoring system can be used for this (see table 2). Patients with a SCORTEN score of 3 or above should be managed in an intensive care unit if possible.

Rapid Withdrawal of Culprit Drug(s)

Research has shown that the earlier the causative drug is withdrawn, the better the prognosis, and that patients exposed to causative drugs with long half-lives have an increased risk of dying [45]. In order to identify the culprit drug(s), it is important to consider the chronology of administration of the drug and the reported ability of the drug to induce SJS/TEN using sources such as Pubmed/Medline or the Litt's drug eruption reference manual [46].

Best Supportive Care

Best supportive care is an essential part of the therapeutic approach to SJS and TEN [47]. A multicenter study conducted in the USA [48], and including 15 regional burn centers with 199 admitted patients, showed that survival rate – independent of the severity of disease (APACHE score and TBSA = total body surface area) – was significantly higher in patients who were transferred to a burn unit within 7 days after disease onset compared to patients admitted after 7 days (29.8 vs. 51.4%; $p < 0.05$). This positive association of early referral and survival has been confirmed in other studies [20, 49].

A critical element of supportive care is the management of fluid and electrolyte requirements. Intravenous fluid should be given to maintain urine output of 50–80 ml per h with 0.5% NaCl supplemented with 20 mEq of KCl. Appropriate early

Table 3. Published studies/reports documenting effect of IVIG use in TEN (with 10 or more reported patients/study)

	Viard [39]	Trent [62]	Prins [59]	Campione [58]	Al-Mutairi [56]	Shortt [60]	Tan [61]
Study design	Prosp N/Cont	Retro N/Cont	Retro N/Cont	Prosp N/Cont	Prosp N/Cont	Retro N/Cont	Retro N/Cont
Patients	10	24	48	10	12	16	12
Detachment, %	39	44	45	49	58	65	–
Total dose IVIG, g/kg	3	4	3	2	2.5	2.8	2
Predicted mortality (SCORTEN/APACHE*), %	–	33	–	35%	–	38*	–
Actual mortality, %	0	4	12	10	0	25	8

and aggressive replacement therapy is required in case of hypernatremia, hypokalemia or hypophosphatemia, which occur quite frequently. Wounds should be treated conservatively, without skin debridement which is often performed in burn units, as blistered skin acts as a natural biological dressing which likely favors reepithelialization. Nonadhesive wound dressings are used where required, and topical sulfa-containing medications should be avoided.

Specific Therapy

To date, a specific therapy for SJS/TEN that has shown efficacy in controlled clinical trials does not exist. Several treatment modalities given in addition to supportive care are reported in the literature and are listed below.

– Systemic steroids were the standard treatment until the early 1990s, although no benefit has been proven in controlled or case-controlled studies [50]. A recent retrospective monocenter study suggests that a short course pulse of high-dose corticosteroids (dexamethasone) may be of benefit [51].

– Thalidomide, a medication with known anti-TNF-α and immunomodulatory activity has been evaluated for the treatment of TEN in a double-blind, randomized, placebo-controlled study, and higher mortality was observed in the thalidomide-treated group suggesting that thalidomide is detrimental in TEN [52, 53].

– High-dose IVIG. As a consequence of the discovery of the anti-Fas potential of pooled human IVIG in vitro [39], IVIG have been tested for the treatment of TEN, and their effect reported in different noncontrolled studies. To date, numerous case reports and 15 noncontrolled clinical studies containing 10 or more patients have analyzed the therapeutic effect of IVIG in TEN (table 3). All except one study [54], confirm the known excellent tolerability and a low toxic potential of IVIG when used with appropriate precaution in patients with potential risk factors (renal insufficiency, cardiac insufficiency, IgA deficiency, thromboembolic risk) [55]. Taken together,

Stella [64]	Yang [93]	Molgó [94]	Rajaratnam [63]	Chen [95]	Bachot [54]	Brown [57]	Schneck [50]
Retro Cont	Retro N/Cont	Retro N/Cont	Retro N/Cont	Retro N/Cont	Prosp N/Cont	Retro N/Cont	Retro Cont
23	20	15	14	24	34	24	75
–	–	–	44	30.2	19	49	–
–	2 (+steroids)	2.3	3.3	2.7 (+steroids)	2	1.6	1.9 (0.7–2.3)
35.8	17.5	–	36	22	24	28.6	25
26	15	20	21	12.5	32	41.7	34

although each study has its potential biases and the 15 studies are not directly comparable, 12 of the 15 studies suggest that there may be a benefit of high-dose IVIG on the mortality associated with TEN [39, 50, 54, 56–64]. Analysis of published studies (table 3) suggests that total IVIG doses of 3 g/kg bodyweight or more may be of greater benefit than lower doses [65]. Given the favorable side effect profile of IVIG and the data existing to date, in the authors' opinion early administration of high-dose immunoglobulin (3 g/kg total dose given over 3–4 days) should be considered alongside supportive care for the treatment of TEN, given the absence of other validated specific therapeutic alternatives.

– Cyclosporin (CsA). CsA, a calcineurin inhibitor, is an efficient drug in transplantation and autoimmune diseases. Arevalo et al. [66] have performed a study as a case series with two treatment arms: CsA alone versus cyclophosphamide (CPP) in combination with corticosteroids. Patients treated with CsA had significantly shorter time to complete reepithelialization, and fewer patients with multi-organ failure and death were observed. A small case series with 3 TEN patients treated initially with high doses of intravenous dexamethasone followed by CsA showed a stop in disease progression within 72 h [67]. Other single case reports also reported a positive effect of the use of CsA in TEN [68, 69]. Recently, Valeyrie-Allanore et al. [70] conducted an open, phase II trial to determine the safety and possible benefit of CsA. Twenty-nine patients were included in the trial (10 SJS, 12 SJS-TEN overlap and 7 TEN), and 26 completed the treatment with CsA administered orally (3 mg/kg/day for 10 days) and tapered over a month. The prognostic score predicted 2.75 deaths and none occurred ($p = 0.1$), suggesting that, although not statistically significant, CsA may be useful for the treatment of TEN.

– TNF antagonists. A new therapeutic approach targeting the proinflammatory cytokine TNF-α has been proposed by Hunger et al. [71]. They treated one patient with a single dose of the chimeric anti-TNF-α antibody (infliximab 5 mg/kg) and reported that disease progression stopped within 24 h followed by a complete reepithelialization within 5 days. Meiss et al. [72] report 3 cases with an overlap of acute generalized exanthematous pustulosis and TEN and treatment response to infliximab. Administration of the soluble TNF-α receptor etanercept 25 mg on days 4 and 8 after onset of TEN in a single case resulted in cessation of epidermal detachment within 24 h but subsequent death of the patient. The published data are currently insufficient to draw a conclusion on the therapeutic potential of TNF antagonists in TEN.

– Plasmapheresis/plasma exchange (PE). PE has also been tried in SJS/TEN, but the current data do not allow a conclusion to be drawn as to the potential of this approach due to the small number of patients treated, the frequent confounding factors including different or combined treatments, and other potential biases [73–76].

– Cyclophosphamide (CCP). CPP has been studied in small case series, either in combination with other treatments such as CsA [66], in conjunction with high-dose corticosteroids [77], or alone [78]. Although a beneficial effect of CPP is suggested by the authors of these small trials, larger studies are needed to clarify these preliminary results with a special attention to potential side effects.

Treatment of Sequelae

Due to the frequent combined involvement of the skin, eyes and mucous membranes, follow-up and treatment of sequelae should be interdisciplinary. Special attention should be given to the prevention of ocular complications. Early referral to an ophthalmologist is mandatory for assessment of the extent of eye involvement and prompt treatment with topical steroids. Visual outcome is reported to be significantly better in patients who receive specific ophthalmological treatment during the first week of disease [17]. Some of the ocular complications have an inflammatory background and have to be treated occasionally with ophthalmic steroids and/or extensive lubrication of the eye [79] in order to prevent progression leading ultimately to the need for corneal transplantation. The benefit of local antibiotic treatment (ointments) is not clear [18]. Hypopharyngeal stenosis combined with dysphagia and esophageal strictures are long-term complications which are difficult to treat [80, 81] and may require laryngectomy.

Allergological Testing

A detailed drug history is very important when striving to identify the culprit drug in SJS/TEN. In some cases, several drugs are possible candidates, and allergological testing can be of help in identifying the most likely candidate. In principle, the severity of SJS and TEN excludes rechallenge and intradermal testing with the culprit drugs, although two case reports describe intradermal testing without triggering of a second episode of TEN [82, 83]. Induction of SJS/TEN has, however, been documented following local eye treatment [84, 85].

Patch testing is an investigational option, but not a routine diagnostic option at the moment. Low sensitivity is a problem with patch testing in SJS/TEN, as only two of 22 tested patients in a study had a relevant positive patch test [86].

Currently, the focus of allergological testing is more on ex vivo/in vitro tests. The lymphocyte transformation test, which measures the proliferation of T cells to a drug in vitro, has shown a sensitivity of 60–70% for patients allergic to β-lactam antibiotics [87]. Unfortunately, the sensitivity of the lymphocyte transformation test is still very low in SJS/TEN even if performed within one week after onset of the disease [88].

Another recently reported approach looks for upregulation of CD69 on T-lymphocytes 2 days after lymphocyte stimulation in vitro as a sign of drug hypersensitivity [89]. Novel in vitro methods to help identify culprit drug in SJS/TEN are needed [90].

Prognosis

SJS and TEN are severe and life-threatening. The average reported mortality rate of SJS is 1–5%, and of TEN is 25–35%; it can be even higher in elderly patients and those with a large surface area of epidermal detachment [47]. In order to standardize the evaluation of risk and prognosis in patients with SJS/TEN, different scoring systems have been proposed. The SCORTEN is now the most widely used scoring system; it evaluates the following parameters: age, malignancy, tachycardia, initial body surface area of epidermal detachment, serum urea, serum glucose, and bicarbonate (table 2) [91]. Yun et al. [92] recently reported that lactate dehydrogenase may be an additional useful parameter in the evaluation of disease severity.

References

1 Bastuji-Garin S, Rzany B, Stern RS, Shear NH, Naldi L, Roujeau JC: Clinical classification of cases of toxic epidermal necrolysis, Stevens-Johnson syndrome, and erythema multiforme. Arch Dermatol 1993;129:92–96.

2 Fiessinger N, Rendu R: Sur un syndrome charactérisé par l'inflammation simultanée de toutes les muqueuses externes coexistant avec une éruption vésiculeuse des quatre membres, non douloureuse et non recidivante. Paris Med 1917;25:54–58.

3 Stevens AM, Johnson FC: A new eruptive fever associated with stomatitis and ophtalmia; report of two cases in children. Am J Dis Child 1922;24:526–533.

4 Lyell A: Toxic epidermal necrolysis: an eruption resembling scalding of the skin. Br J Dermatol 1956; 68:355–361.

5 Rzany B, Correia O, Kelly JP, Naldi L, Auquier A, Stern R: Risk of Stevens-Johnson syndrome and toxic epidermal necrolysis during first weeks of antiepileptic therapy: a case-control study. Study Group of the International Case Control Study on Severe Cutaneous Adverse Reactions. Lancet 1999; 353:2190–2194.

6 La Grenade L, Lee L, Weaver J, Bonnel R, Karwoski C, Governale L, Brinker A: Comparison of reporting of Stevens-Johnson syndrome and toxic epidermal necrolysis in association with selective COX-2 inhibitors. Drug Saf 2005;28:917–924.

7 Roujeau JC, Kelly JP, Naldi L, Rzany B, Stern RS, Anderson T, Auquier A, Bastuji-Garin S, Correia O, Locati F, Mockenhaupt M, Paoletti C, Shapiro S, Shear N, Schöpf E, Kaufman DW: Medication use and the risk of Stevens-Johnson syndrome or toxic epidermal necrolysis. N Engl J Med 1995;333: 1600–1607.

8 Aguiar D, Pazo R, Duran I, Terrasa J, Arrivi A, Manzano H, Martin J, Rifa J: Toxic epidermal necrolysis in patients receiving anticonvulsants and cranial irradiation: a risk to consider. J Neurooncol 2004;66:345–350.

9 Aydin F, Cokluk C, Senturk N, Aydin K, Canturk MT, Turanli AY: Stevens-Johnson syndrome in two patients treated with cranial irradiation and phenytoin. J Eur Acad Dermatol Venereol 2006;20: 588–590.

10 Fournier S, Bastuji-Garin S, Mentec H, Revuz J, Roujeau JC: Toxic epidermal necrolysis associated with *Mycoplasma pneumoniae* infection. Eur J Clin Microbiol Infect Dis 1995;14:558–559.

11 Mulvey JM, Padowitz A, Lindley-Jones M, Nickels R: *Mycoplasma pneumoniae* associated with Stevens Johnson syndrome. Anaesth Intensive Care 2007;35: 414–417.

12 Schalock PC, Dinulos JG: *Mycoplasma pneumoniae*-induced Stevens-Johnson syndrome without skin lesions: fact or fiction? J Am Acad Dermatol 2005; 52:312–315.

13 Forman R, Koren G, Shear NH: Erythema multiforme, Stevens-Johnson syndrome and toxic epidermal necrolysis in children: a review of 10 years' experience. Drug Saf 2002;25:965–972.

14 Lebargy F, Wolkenstein P, Gisselbrecht M, Lange F, Fleury-Feith J, Delclaux C, Roupie E, Revuz J, Roujeau JC: Pulmonary complications in toxic epidermal necrolysis: a prospective clinical study. Intensive Care Med 1997;23:1237–1244.

15 Revuz J, Penso D, Roujeau JC, Guillaume JC, Payne CR, Wechsler J, Touraine R: Toxic epidermal necrolysis. Clinical findings and prognosis factors in 87 patients. Arch Dermatol 1987;123:1160–1165.

16 Chang YS, Huang FC, Tseng SH, Hsu CK, Ho CL, Sheu HM: Erythema multiforme, Stevens-Johnson syndrome, and toxic epidermal necrolysis: acute ocular manifestations, causes, and management. Cornea 2007;26:123–129.

17 Sotozono C, Ueta M, Koizumi N, Inatomi T, Shirakata Y, Ikezawa Z, Hashimoto K, Kinoshita S: Diagnosis and treatment of Stevens-Johnson syndrome and toxic epidermal necrolysis with ocular complications. Ophthalmology 2009;116:685–690.

18 Yip LW, Thong BY, Lim J, Tan AW, Wong HB, Handa S, Heng WJ: Ocular manifestations and complications of Stevens-Johnson syndrome and toxic epidermal necrolysis: an Asian series. Allergy 2007;62: 527–531.

19 Magina S, Lisboa C, Leal V, Palmares J, Mesquita-Guimaraes J: Dermatological and ophthalmological sequels in toxic epidermal necrolysis. Dermatology 2003;207:33–36.

20 Oplatek A, Brown K, Sen S, Halerz M, Supple K, Gamelli RL: Long-term follow-up of patients treated for toxic epidermal necrolysis. J Burn Care Res 2006;27:26–33.

21 Roujeau JC, Guillaume JC, Revuz J, Touraine R: Reporting adverse drug reactions. Lancet 1985;2: 1244–1247.

22 Saban J, Pais JR, Rodriguez JL, Boixeda D: Sjogren-like pluriglandular exocrine insufficiency after drug-induced toxic epidermal necrolysis. Postgrad Med J 1991;67:195–197.

23 Chung WH, Hung SI, Hong HS, Hsih MS, Yang LC, Ho HC, Wu JY, Chen YT: Medical genetics: a marker for Stevens-Johnson syndrome. Nature 2004;428: 486.

24 Man CB, Kwan P, Baum L, Yu E, Lau KM, Cheng AS, Ng MH: Association between HLA-B*1502 allele and antiepileptic drug-induced cutaneous reactions in Han Chinese. Epilepsia 2007;48:1015–1018.

25 Tassaneeyakul W, Tiamkao S, Jantararoungtong T, Chen P, Lin SY, Chen WH, Konyoung P, Khunarkornsiri U, Auvichayapat N, Pavakul K, Kulkantrakorn K, Choonhakarn C, Phonhiamhan S, Piyatrakul N, Aungaree T, Pongpakdee S, Yodnopaglaw P: Association between HLA-B*1502 and carbamazepine-induced severe cutaneous adverse drug reactions in a Thai population. Epilepsia 2010;51:926–930.

26 Alfirevic A, Jorgensen AL, Williamson PR, Chadwick DW, Park BK, Pirmohamed M: HLA-B locus in Caucasian patients with carbamazepine hypersensitivity. Pharmacogenomics 2006;7:813–818.

27 Kaniwa N, Saito Y, Aihara M, Matsunaga K, Tohkin M, Kurose K, Sawada J, Furuya H, Takahashi Y, Muramatsu M, Kinoshita S, Abe M, Ikeda H, Kashiwagi M, Song Y, Ueta M, Sotozono C, Ikezawa Z, Hasegawa R, JSAR research group: HLA-B locus in Japanese patients with anti-epileptics and allopurinol-related Stevens-Johnson syndrome and toxic epidermal necrolysis. Pharmacogenomics 2008; 9:1617–1622.

28 Lonjou C, Thomas L, Borot N, Ledger N, de Toma C, LeLouet H, Graf E, Schumacher M, Hovnanian A, Mockenhaupt M, Roujeau JC: A marker for Stevens-Johnson syndrome . . . : ethnicity matters. Pharmacogenomics J 2006;6:265–268.

29 Lonjou C, Borot N, Sekula P, Ledger N, Thomas L, Halevy S, Naldi L, Bouwes-Bavinck JN, Sidoroff A, de Toma C, Schumacher M, Roujeau JC, Hovnanian A, Mockenhaupt M, RegiSCAR study group: A European study of HLA-B in Stevens-Johnson syndrome and toxic epidermal necrolysis related to five high-risk drugs. Pharmacogenet Genomics 2008;18:99–107.

30 McCormack M, Alfirevic A, Bourgeois S, Farrell JJ, et al: HLA-A*3101 and carbamazepine-induced hypersensitivity reactions in Europeans. N Engl J Med 2011;364:1134–1143.

31 Hung SI, Chung WH, Liou LB, Chu CC, Lin M, Huang HP, Lin YL, Lan JL, Yang LC, Hong HS, Chen MJ, Lai PC, Wu MS, Chu CY, Wang KH, Chen CH, Fann CS, Wu JY, Chen YT: HLA-B*5801 allele as a genetic marker for severe cutaneous adverse reactions caused by allopurinol. Proc Natl Acad Sci USA 2005;102:4134–4139.

32 Chen P, Lin JJ, Lu CS, Ong CT, et al: Taiwan SJS Consortium: Carbamazepine-induced toxic effects and HLA-B*1502 screening in Taiwan. N Engl J Med 2011;364:1126–1133.

33 Halevi A, Ben-Amitai D, Garty BZ: Toxic epidermal necrolysis associated with acetaminophen ingestion. Ann Pharmacother 2000;34:32–34.

34 Schmidt D, Kluge W: Fatal toxic epidermal necrolysis following reexposure to phenytoin: a case report. Epilepsia 1983;24:440–443.

35 Correia O, Delgado L, Ramos JP, Resende C, Torrinha JA: Cutaneous T-cell recruitment in toxic epidermal necrolysis. Further evidence of CD8+ lymphocyte involvement. Arch Dermatol 1993;129: 466–468.

36 Le Cleach L, Delaire S, Boumsell L, Bagot M, Bourgault-Villada I, Bensussan A, Roujeau JC: Blister fluid T lymphocytes during toxic epidermal necrolysis are functional cytotoxic cells which express human natural killer (NK) inhibitory receptors. Clin Exp Immunol 2000;119:225–230.

37 Nassif A, Bensussan A, Boumsell L, Deniaud A, Moslehi H, Wolkenstein P, Bagot M, Roujeau JC: Toxic epidermal necrolysis: effector cells are drug-specific cytotoxic T cells. J Allergy Clin Immunol 2004;114:1209–1215.

38 Chung WH, Hung SI, Yang JY, Su SC, Huang SP, Wei CY, Chin SW, Chiou CC, Chu SC, Ho HC, Yang CH, Lu CF, Wu JY, Liao YD, Chen YT: Granulysin is a key mediator for disseminated keratinocyte death in Stevens-Johnson syndrome and toxic epidermal necrolysis. Nat Med 2008;14:1343–1350.

39 Viard I, Wehrli P, Bullani R, Schneider P, Holler N, Salomon D, Hunziker T, Saurat JH, Tschopp J, French LE: Inhibition of toxic epidermal necrolysis by blockade of CD95 with human intravenous immunoglobulin. Science 1998;282:490–493.

40 Murata J, Abe R, Shimizu H: Increased soluble Fas ligand levels in patients with Stevens-Johnson syndrome and toxic epidermal necrolysis preceding skin detachment. J Allergy Clin Immunol 2008;122: 992–1000.

41 Schneider P, Holler N, Bodmer JL, Hahne M, Frei K, Fontana A, Tschopp J: Conversion of membrane-bound Fas(CD95) ligand to its soluble form is associated with downregulation of its proapoptotic activity and loss of liver toxicity. J Exp Med 1998;187: 1205–1213.

42 Abe R, Shimizu T, Shibaki A, Nakamura H, Watanabe H, Shimizu H: Toxic epidermal necrolysis and Stevens-Johnson syndrome are induced by soluble Fas ligand. Am J Pathol 2003;162: 1515–1520.

43 Halevy S, Ghislain PD, Mockenhaupt M, Fagot JP, Bouwes Bavinck JN, Sidoroff A, Naldi L, Dunant A, Viboud C, Roujeau JC: Allopurinol is the most common cause of Stevens-Johnson syndrome and toxic epidermal necrolysis in Europe and Israel. J Am Acad Dermatol 2008;58:25–32.

44 Mockenhaupt M, Viboud C, Dunant A, Naldi L, Halevy S, Bouwes Bavinck JN, Sidoroff A, Schneck J, Roujeau JC, Flahault A: Stevens-Johnson syndrome and toxic epidermal necrolysis: assessment of medication risks with emphasis on recently marketed drugs. The EuroSCAR-study. J Invest Dermatol 2008;128:35–44.

45 Garcia-Doval I, LeCleach L, Bocquet H, Otero XL, Roujeau JC: Toxic epidermal necrolysis and Stevens-Johnson syndrome: does early withdrawal of causative drugs decrease the risk of death? Arch Dermatol 2000;136:323–327.

46 Litt JZ: Litt's Drug Eruptions and Reactions Manual, ed 16. London, Informa, 2010.

47 Roujeau JC, Stern RS: Severe adverse cutaneous reactions to drugs. N Engl J Med 1994;331: 1272–1285.

48 Palmieri TL, Greenhalgh DG, Saffle JR, Spence RJ, Peck MD, Jeng JC, Mozingo DW, Yowler CJ, Sheridan RL, Ahrenholz DH, Caruso DM, Foster KN, Kagan RJ, Voigt DW, Purdue GF, Hunt JL, Wolf S, Molitor F: A multicenter review of toxic epidermal necrolysis treated in U.S. burn centers at the end of the twentieth century. J Burn Care Rehabil 2002;23:87–96.

49 McGee T, Munster A: Toxic epidermal necrolysis syndrome: mortality rate reduced with early referral to regional burn center. Plast Reconstr Surg 1998; 102:1018–1022.

50 Schneck J, Fagot JP, Sekula P, Sassolas B, Roujeau JC, Mockenhaupt M: Effects of treatments on the mortality of Stevens-Johnson syndrome and toxic epidermal necrolysis: a retrospective study on patients included in the prospective EuroSCAR Study. J Am Acad Dermatol 2008;58:33–40.

51 Kardaun SH, Jonkman MF: Dexamethasone pulse therapy for Stevens-Johnson syndrome/toxic epidermal necrolysis. Acta Derm Venereol 2007;87: 144–148.

52 Wolkenstein P, Latarjet J, Roujeau JC, Duguet C, Boudeau S, Vaillant L, Maignan M, Schuhmacher MH, Milpied B, Pilorget A, Bocquet H, Brun-Buisson C, Revuz J: Randomised comparison of thalidomide versus placebo in toxic epidermal necrolysis. Lancet 1998;352:1586–1589.

53 Namazi MR: Increased mortality in toxic epidermal necrolysis with thalidomide: corroborating or exonerating the pathogenetic role of TNF-alpha? Br J Dermatol 2006;155:842–843.

54 Bachot N, Revuz J, Roujeau JC: Intravenous immunoglobulin treatment for Stevens-Johnson syndrome and toxic epidermal necrolysis: a prospective noncomparative study showing no benefit on mortality or progression. Arch Dermatol 2003;139: 33–36.

55 Prins C, Gelfand EW, French LE: Intravenous immunoglobulin: properties, mode of action and practical use in dermatology. Acta Derm Venereol 2007;87:206–218.

56 Al-Mutairi N, Arun J, Osama NE, Amr Z, Mazen AS, Ibtesam el A, Nazeha el B: Prospective, noncomparative open study from Kuwait of the role of intravenous immunoglobulin in the treatment of toxic epidermal necrolysis. Int J Dermatol 2004;43: 847–851.

57 Brown KM, Silver GM, Halerz M, Walaszek P, Sandroni A, Gamelli RL: Toxic epidermal necrolysis: does immunoglobulin make a difference? J Burn Care Rehabil 2004;25:81–88.

58 Campione E, Marulli GC, Carrozzo AM, Chimenti MS, Costanzo A, Bianchi L: High-dose intravenous immunoglobulin for severe drug reactions: efficacy in toxic epidermal necrolysis. Acta Derm Venereol 2003;83:430–432.

59 Prins C, Kerdel FA, Padilla RS, Hunziker T, Chimenti S, Viard I, Mauri DN, Flynn K, Trent J, Margolis DJ, Saurat JH, French LE, TEN-IVIG Study Group: Treatment of toxic epidermal necrolysis with high-dose intravenous immunoglobulins: multicenter retrospective analysis of 48 consecutive cases. Arch Dermatol 2003;139:26–32.

60 Shortt R, Gomez M, Mittman N, Cartotto R: Intravenous immunoglobulin does not improve outcome in toxic epidermal necrolysis. J Burn Care Rehabil 2004;25:246–255.

61 Tan AW, Thong BY, Yip LW, Chng HH, Ng SK: High-dose intravenous immunoglobulins in the treatment of toxic epidermal necrolysis: an Asian series. J Dermatol 2005;32:1–6.

62 Trent JT, Kirsner RS, Romanelli P, Kerdel FA: Analysis of intravenous immunoglobulin for the treatment of toxic epidermal necrolysis using SCORTEN: The University of Miami Experience. Arch Dermatol 2003;139:39–43.

63 Rajaratnam R, Mann C, Balasubramaniam P, Marsden JR, Taibjee SM, Shah F, Lim R, Papini R, Moiemen N, Lewis H: Toxic epidermal necrolysis: retrospective analysis of 21 consecutive cases managed at a tertiary centre. Clin Exp Dermatol 2010;35:853–862.

64 Stella M, Clemente A, Bollero D, Risso D, Dalmasso P: Toxic epidermal necrolysis (TEN) and Stevens-Johnson syndrome (SJS): experience with high-dose intravenous immunoglobulins and topical conservative approach. A retrospective analysis. Burns 2007;33:452–459.

65 Trent JT, Fangchao M, Kerdel F, Fie S, French LE, Romanelli P, Kirsner RS: Dose of intravenous immunoglobulin and patient survival in SJS and toxic epidermal necrolysis. Expert Rev Dermatol 2007;2:299–303.

66 Arevalo JM, Lorente JA, Gonzalez-Herrada C, Jimenez-Reyes J: Treatment of toxic epidermal necrolysis with cyclosporin A. J Trauma 2000;48: 473–478.

67 Rai R, Srinivas CR: Suprapharmacologic doses of intravenous dexamethasone followed by cyclosporine in the treatment of toxic epidermal necrolysis. Indian J Dermatol Venereol Leprol 2008; 74:263–265.

68 Hashim N, Bandara D, Tan E, Ilchyshyn A: Early cyclosporine treatment of incipient toxic epidermal necrolysis induced by concomitant use of lamotrigine and sodium valproate. Acta Derm Venereol 2004;84:90–91.

69 Robak E, Robak T, Gora-Tybor J, Chojnowski K, Strzelecka B, Waszczykowska E, Sysa-Jedrzejowska A: Toxic epidermal necrolysis in a patient with severe aplastic anemia treated with cyclosporin A and G-CSF. J Med 2001;32:31–39.

70 Valeyrie-Allanore L, Wolkenstein P, Brochard L, Ortonne N, Maitre B, Revuz J, Bagot M, Roujeau J: Open trial of ciclosporin treatment for Stevens-Johnson syndrome and toxic epidermal necrolysis. Br J Dermatol 2010;163:847–853.

71 Hunger RE, Hunziker T, Buettiker U, Braathen LR, Yawalkar N: Rapid resolution of toxic epidermal necrolysis with anti-TNF-alpha treatment. J Allergy Clin Immunol 2005;116:923–924.

72 Meiss F, Helmbold P, Meykadeh N, Gaber G, Marsch W, Fischer M: Overlap of acute generalized exanthematous pustulosis and toxic epidermal necrolysis: response to antitumour necrosis factor-alpha antibody infliximab: report of three cases. J Eur Acad Dermatol Venereol 2007;21:717–719.

73 Kamanabroo D, Schmitz-Landgraf W, Czarnetzki BM: Plasmapheresis in severe drug-induced toxic epidermal necrolysis. Arch Dermatol 1985;121: 1548–1549.

74 Lissia M, Figus A, Rubino C: Intravenous immunoglobulins and plasmapheresis combined treatment in patients with severe toxic epidermal necrolysis: preliminary report. Br J Plast Surg 2005;58:504–510.

75 Yamada H, Takamori K, Yaguchi H, Ogawa H: A study of the efficacy of plasmapheresis for the treatment of drug induced toxic epidermal necrolysis. Ther Apher 1998;2:153–156.

76 Furubacke A, Berlin G, Anderson C, Sjoberg F: Lack of significant treatment effect of plasma exchange in the treatment of drug-induced toxic epidermal necrolysis? Intensive Care Med 1999;25:1307–1310.

77 Frangogiannis NG, Boridy I, Mazhar M, Mathews R, Gangopadhyay S, Cate T: Cyclophosphamide in the treatment of toxic epidermal necrolysis. South Med J 1996;89:1001–1003.

78 Heng MC, Allen SG: Efficacy of cyclophosphamide in toxic epidermal necrolysis. Clinical and pathophysiologic aspects. J Am Acad Dermatol 1991;25:778–786.

79 Sheridan RL, Schulz JT, Ryan CM, Schnitzer JJ, Lawlor D, Driscoll DN, Donelan MB, Tompkins RG: Long-term consequences of toxic epidermal necrolysis in children. Pediatrics 2002;109:74–78.

80 Barrera JE, Meyers AD, Hartford EC: Hypopharyngeal stenosis and dysphagia complicating toxic epidermal necrolysis. Arch Otolaryngol Head Neck Surg 1998;124:1375–1376.

81 Herman TE, Kushner DC, Cleveland RH: Esophageal stricture secondary to drug-induced toxic epidermal necrolysis. Pediatr Radiol 1984;14: 439–440.

82 Romano A, Di Fonso M, Pocobelli D, Giannarini L, Venuti A, Garcovich A: Two cases of toxic epidermal necrolysis caused by delayed hypersensitivity to beta-lactam antibiotics. J Investig Allergol Clin Immunol 1993;3:53–55.

83 Tagami H, Tatsuta K, Iwatski K, Yamada M: Delayed hypersensitivity in ampicillin-induced toxic epidermal necrolysis. Arch Dermatol 1983;119:910–913.

84 Asensio-Sanchez VM: Toxic epidermal necrolysis following dorzolamide eyedrops (in Spanish). An Med Interna 2008;25:47–48.

85 Schmutz JL, Barbaud A, Trechot P: Polymorphous bullous erythema and trihexiphenidyl (or why police questioning is not always the most productive method) (in French). Ann Dermatol Venereol 2007;134:899.

86 Wolkenstein P, Chosidow O, Flechet ML, Robbiola O, Paul M, Dume L, Revuz J, Roujeau JC: Patch testing in severe cutaneous adverse drug reactions, including Stevens-Johnson syndrome and toxic epidermal necrolysis. Contact Dermatitis 1996;35: 234–236.

87 Pichler WJ, Tilch J: The lymphocyte transformation test in the diagnosis of drug hypersensitivity. Allergy 2004;59:809–820.

88 Kano Y, Hirahara K, Mitsuyama Y, Takahashi R, Shiohara T: Utility of the lymphocyte transformation test in the diagnosis of drug sensitivity: dependence on its timing and the type of drug eruption. Allergy 2007;62:1439–1444.

89 Beeler A, Zaccaria L, Kawabata T, Gerber BO, Pichler WJ: CD69 upregulation on T cells as an in vitro marker for delayed-type drug hypersensitivity. Allergy 2008;63:181–188.

90 Zawodniak A, Lochmatter P, Yerly D, Kawabata T, Lerch M, Yawalkar N, Pichler WJ: In vitro detection of cytotoxic T and NK cells in peripheral blood of patients with various drug-induced skin diseases. Allergy 2009;65:376–384.

91 Bastuji-Garin S, Fouchard N, Bertocchi M, Roujeau JC, Revuz J, Wolkenstein P: SCORTEN: a severity-of-illness score for toxic epidermal necrolysis. J Invest Dermatol 2000;115:149–153.

92 Yun SJ, Choi MS, Piao MS, Lee JB, Kim SJ, Won YH, Lee SC: Serum lactate dehydrogenase is a novel marker for the evaluation of disease severity in the early stage of toxic epidermal necrolysis. Dermatology 2008;217:254–259.
93 Yang Y, Xu J, Li F, Zhu X: Combination therapy of intravenous immunoglobulin and corticosteroid in the treatment of toxic epidermal necrolysis and Stevens-Johnson syndrome: a retrospective comparative study in China. Int J Dermatol 2009;48: 1122–1128.
94 Molgó M, Carreño N, Hoyos-Bachiloglu R, Andresen M, González S: Use of intravenous immunoglobulin for the treatment of toxic epidermal necrolysis and Stevens-Johnson/toxic epidermal necrolysis overlap syndrome. Review of 15 cases. Rev Med Chil 2009;137:383–389.
95 Chen J, Wang B, Zeng Y, Xu H: High-dose intravenous immunoglobulins in the treatment of Stevens-Johnson syndrome and toxic epidermal necrolysis in Chinese patients: a retrospective study of 82 cases. Eur J Dermatol 2010;20:743–747.

Prof. Lars E. French
Department of Dermatology, University Hospital Zurich
Gloriastrasse 31
CH–8091 Zurich (Switzerland)
Tel. +41 44 255 25 50, E-Mail lars.french@uzh.ch

French LE (ed): Adverse Cutaneous Drug Eruptions.
Chem Immunol Allergy. Basel, Karger, 2012, vol 97, pp 167–179

Phototoxic and Photoallergic Cutaneous Drug Reactions

Martin Glatz · Günther F.L. Hofbauer

Department of Dermatology, University Hospital Zurich, Zurich, Switzerland

Abstract

A variety of topical and systemic drugs can induce cutaneous photosensitive reactions. These drugs and their metabolites accumulate in the skin and increase photosensitivity of the skin typically in the UVA spectrum of light. Concerning the underlying biochemical mechanisms and the phenotype of reactions, photosensitivity can be divided into phototoxic and photoallergic reactions. In phototoxic reactions, often highly reactive oxygen molecules are formed that induce tissue damage. Skin changes resemble sunburn and develop within hours after incubation with the drug together with sunlight. In contrast, photoallergic reactions are type IV hypersensitivity reactions, and therefore resemble eczema. They usually develop within days and are less common than phototoxic reactions. Diagnosis is based on a synopsis of complete history, clinical examination, phototesting for minimal phototoxicity dose, patch testing including photopatch tests, and histopathology. Mainstays of treatment are the withdrawal of the culprit drug, and avoidance of sunlight by wearing protective clothing and broadband sunscreens with UVA filters.

Essentials in a Nutshell

- Phototoxic and photoallergic skin reactions can be triggered by a variety of topical and systemic medications, and are mainly due to UVA light
- Phototoxic reactions are frequent and resemble sunburn
- Photoallergic reactions are rare and resemble allergic contact eczema
- Avoidance of sunlight and withdrawal of the responsible drug are the mainstays of treatment

Introduction

Photosensitivity skin reactions can frequently be induced by systemically or topically administered drugs (photosensitizers). Drug classes with a high photosensitizing

Table 1. Topical medications causing phototoxicity and their action spectrum, selected

Drug class	Medication	Action spectrum
NSAIDs	ketoprofen	UVA
Antibiotics	erythromycin	unknown
Steroids	hydrocortisone	UVA
Dyes	eosin	unknown
	methylene blue	unknown
Others	coal tar	UVA
	psoralens	UVA
	tretinoin	UVA, UVB
	benzocaine	UVA
	benzoyl peroxide	UVB

From Stein and Scheinfeld [1] and Gould et al. [2], with modifications.

potential are for example antibiotics, diuretics and nonsteroidal anti-inflammatory drugs (NSAIDs; tables 1–4). Photosensitizers are chromophores that usually have a planar, tricyclic or polycyclic configuration with a low molecular mass of 200–500 Da [1]. Usually, they are excited by ultraviolet (UV) light or rarely visible light by absorbing radiant energy in form of photons [1, 2]. UVA light with a wavelength of 320–400 nm penetrates the skin deeply into the dermis and is the most common responsible wavelength in photosensitivity reactions of the skin. After absorbance of photons (excited stage), the photosensitizers undergo photochemical reactions with other molecules in the epidermal and/or dermal tissue. These reactions are the molecular substrate of photosensitivity reactions in the skin. Depending on the underlying pathophysiologic mechanism of this tissue reaction, photosensitivity drug reactions can be divided into phototoxic and photoallergic reactions. Phototoxic reactions are frequent, can occur in all individuals, and depend only on the dose of the photosensitizer and the exposure to activating wavelengths of light. Photoallergic reactions are type IV hypersensitivity reactions. They are seldom, require prior sensitization, and are independent of the dose of the photosensitizer (table 5) [1, 2].

Incidence of Drug-Induced Phototoxic and Photoallergic Reactions

Data on drug-induced photosensitivity are mostly collected by national reporting systems, for example the databases of the US Food and Drug Administration or of the Committee on Safety of Medicines in the UK, and only rarely by international

Table 2. Systemic medications causing phototoxicity and their action spectrum, selected

Drug class	Medication	Action spectrum
Antimicrobials	doxycycline	UVA
	minocycline	UVA
	ciprofloxacin	UVA
	levofloxacin	UVA
	voriconazole	unknown
Diuretics	furosemide	unknown
	hydrochlorothiazide	UVA
NSAIDs	ketoprofen	UVA
	naproxen	UVA
Antimalarials	chloroquine	unknown
	hydroxychloroquine	UVB
	quinidine	UVA
Others	psoralens	UVA
	retinoids	UVA, UVB
	calcium channel blockers	UVA
	chlorpromazine	UVA

From Stein and Scheinfeld [1] and Gould et al. [2], with modifications.

Table 3. Topical medications causing photoallergy and their action spectrum, selected

Drug class	Medication	Action spectrum
NSAIDs	ketoprofen	UVA
	benzophenone	UVA
	meloxicam	UVA
	piroxicam	UVA
Others	acyclovir	UVA
	hydrocortisone	UVA

From Stein and Scheinfeld [1] and Gould et al. [2], with modifications.

databases like the WHO Program for International Drug Monitoring. Moreover, reports are usually a voluntary process. Therefore data on drug-induced photosensitivity are often biased, inaccurate, and mostly concentrated on newly marketed drugs [3]. Apparently, drug-induced photosensitivity seems to be a frequent phenomenon, responsible for up to 8% of all adverse events during medication [1].

Table 4. Systemic medications causing photoallergy and their action spectrum, selected

Drug class	Medication	Action spectrum
NSAIDs	piroxicam	UVA
	celecoxib	UVA
Sulphur-containing drugs	hydrochlorothiazide	UVA
	sulfadiazine	UVB
	sulfonamides	UVB
	sulfonylureas	UVA
Antimalarials	chloroquine	unknown
	hydroxychloroquine	UVB
	quinidine	UVA
Antimicrobials	chloroamphenicol	unknown
	lomefloxacin	UVA, UVB
Phenotiazines	chlorpromazine	UVA
Others	dapsone	unknown
	amantadine	UVA
	ranitidine	UVA

From Stein and Scheinfeld [1] and Gould et al. [2], with modifications.

Table 5. Characteristics of drug-induced phototoxic and photoallergic reactions

	Phototoxicity	Photoallergy
Incidence	high	low
Dose dependent	yes	no
Prior exposure necessary	no	yes
Required amount of drug	high	low
Incubation period	minutes to hours	hours to days
Clinical appearance	sunburn	eczema
Hyperpigmentation	common	uncommon

From Stein and Scheinfeld [1], with modifications.

Around 10% of all patients receiving systemic drugs suffer from photosensitivity. From 260 to 400 different medications are reported to be potent photosensitizers, but only a small number of them are frequently found to be responsible, or have been well described [1].

Drug-Induced Phototoxic Cutaneous Reactions

Pathophysiology

Phototoxic reactions may develop in any person exposed to a photosensitizing medication in conjunction with sufficient levels of radiant energy. Phototoxicity of a given drug depends on environmental (e.g. wind, humidity, temperature) and host factors (e.g. gastrointestinal absorption and metabolism of the drug, skin tan, thickness of stratum corneum) [2]. To trigger phototoxicity, three conditions are required: (a) the photosensitizer must accumulate in skin cells, (b) light of the appropriate wave length must reach the skin, and (c) the photosensitizer must absorb the light energy [1]. Phototoxic tissue damage is caused by different mechanisms, each of which may occur alone or in combination. In general, these mechanisms depend on the presence (photodynamic mechanisms) or absence (non-photodynamic mechanisms) of oxygen. During photodynamic mechanisms, a photosensitizer is excited by radiation energy and usually forms a triplet state. This excited photosensitizer then reacts with oxygen and either forms free radicals (type I photodynamic reaction) or singlet oxygen (type II photodynamic reaction). These highly reactive oxygen molecules cause an oxidation of amino acids and unsaturated fatty acids, leading to tissue damage. Photodynamic phototoxicity is for example induced by chlorpromazine, quinolones, or NSAIDs [1]. In contrast to photodynamic reactions, non-photodynamic tissue damage occurs without the requirement of oxygen by at least three different pathways: (a) the excited photosensitizer binds covalently to tissue molecules, for example 8-methoxypsoralen binds to pyrimidine bases of DNA [4]; (b) the excited photosensitizer is a mediator for inflammation by induction of polymorphonuclear cells and/or prostaglandins which has been described for quinolones [5]; (c) the excited photosensitizer induces apoptosis of keratinocytes, a mechanism described for chlorpromazine [6].

The site of tissue damage by phototoxicity primarily depends on the biodistribution of the photosensitizer. Topically applied photosensitizers in creams or ointments accumulate preferentially in the upper layers of the epidermis and cause damage to keratinocytes. Orally or parenterally administered drugs reach the skin by the blood stream, and therefore accumulate in the vascular dermis. Hydrophilic molecules are arrested at the cell surface and preferably damage the cell membranes, whereas hydrophobic molecules often penetrate the cell membrane and damage cytoplasmatic and/or nuclear components [2].

Clinical Manifestations of Phototoxicity

Acute Phototoxicity

Acute phototoxic reactions usually begin within minutes to hours after sun exposure. An important exception is psoralen-induced phototoxicity which typically appears 24 h after light exposure with a peak reaction after 48–72 h. The symptoms of acute phototoxicity resemble exaggerated sunburn reactions. They comprise erythema and edema, in more severe cases accompanied by vesicles or bullae, followed by desquamation. Subjective complaints include burning and stinging sensations or pain. Skin lesions preferably develop on sun-exposed skin areas like the face, the V area of the chest, the nuchal region, and the dorsa of the hands. Typically, sun-protected skin areas like the submental area or areas covered by clothes are spared and usually present a sharp demarcation from affected areas [1, 2].

Chronic Phototoxicity

Chronic and repeated drug-induced phototoxic damage of the skin is probably best described in patients who received long-term UVA therapy together with psoralen (PUVA). Psoralen covalently binds to pyrimidine bases of the DNA. Over years, this leads to premature skin ageing with wrinkling, atrophy, hyper- and hypopigmentation. Other typical skin changes are PUVA lentigines that develop in 40–50% of patients as brown, unevenly pigmented lesions with irregular borders. Recently, a mutation in the BRAF pathway was identified in melanocytes of PUVA lentigines [7]. This may be responsible for the increased risk for the development of cutaneous melanoma in PUVA patients which has been reported at least in the US [8]. An increased risk for squamous cell carcinoma following PUVA is well confirmed [9]. Moreover, a variety of drugs has also been reported to be responsible for chronic phototoxicity during the last few years, for example diuretics, a frequently prescribed drug class. An increased risk for squamous cell carcinomas and even melanoma was found among patients receiving a therapy with amiloride/hydrochlorothiazide or indapamide [10]. Another example is voriconazole, a second-generation triazole antifungal. Apart from its well-known acute phototoxicity, accelerated photoageing and the development of multiple, extraordinary aggressive squamous cell carcinomas were observed even in very young patients as well as in immunocompromised patients after long-term voriconazole therapy [11]. Azathioprine, a frequently used immunosuppressant prodrug, is metabolized to 6-thioguanine. It is an UVA-sensitive chromophore that accumulates in human DNA and induces oxidative DNA damage. That may explain the high incidence of nonmelanoma skin cancer in patients treated with azathioprine [12].

Hyperpigmentation of Phototoxic Skin Reactions

Hyperpigmentation of affected skin areas is a common sequel of phototoxic reactions and may persist for several months. It is either a result of melanocytic proliferation and migration, which is the case in psoralen-induced phototoxicity [13]. Phototoxic hyperpigmentation may also be caused by deposition of the drug itself or its photoproducts in the skin. A well-known example is the lysosomal deposition of a phospholipid conjugate of amiodarone which causes a typical blue-brown to slate-grey skin color in up to 10% of patients [13].

Pseudoporphyria

Pseudoporphyria is a variant of drug-induced phototoxicity. It clinically and histologically resembles porphyria but is not associated with an abnormal heme biosynthetic pathway. It is most commonly caused by the NSAID naproxene but also by nalidixic acid, tetracyclines, pyridoxine, furosemide and voriconazole [1, 2, 14]. Cases of pseudoporphyria are also described after melanoma therapy using the tyrosine-kinase inhibitor imatinib [15]. Clinical symptoms comprise skin fragility, bullae, and easy bruising [1].

Photoonycholysis

This is another variant of phototoxicity, preferentially caused by tetracyclines, psoralens, quinolones, or several chemotherapies [1, 16, 17]. Explanations for this phototoxic nail affection are manifold. Perhaps the nail itself serves as a lens focusing UV light. Furthermore there are few melanocytes in the nail bed, and therefore it is not well protected against UV light [2]. Four clinical subtypes are proposed, characterized by a concave separation of several nails (type I), a circular notch at a single finger (type II), yellow staining of the nail bed (type III), and bullae under the nails (type IV) [18].

Lichenoid Phototoxic Reactions

The existence of this entity has been discussed controversially. It has for example been reported that thiazide diuretics, pyrazinamide, and quinine can cause lichenoid skin changes [1]. They are characterized by violaceous flat-topped papules distributed at sun-exposed areas. The oral mucosa is not involved. Skin lesions themselves are indistinguishable from lichen planus [1].

Telangiectatic Phototoxic Reactions

Telangiectasias are dilated dermal blood vessels. Some reports suggest that calcium channel blockers like nifedipine or amlodipine are predominantly responsible for phototoxic telangiectasias, but antibiotics like cefotaxime are also suspected. Although telangiectasias are quite common, they are apparent more frequently in sun-exposed areas, especially the face. Phototoxic telangiectasias may resolve after discontinuation of the responsible drug and may recur after resumption [1].

Histopathology of Phototoxic Skin Reactions

Acute phototoxic reactions cause apoptotic death of epidermal keratinocytes. Therefore, the characteristic histopathological features are individual necrotic keratinocytes (sunburn cells) or epidermal necrosis in severe reactions together with epidermal spongiosis. Within the first 24 h, epidermal eosinophilia can be noted. Epidermal changes are emphasized when the photosensitizer was administered topically. In the case of systemic application, the dermis may be the site of primary damage with dermal edema and an inflammatory infiltrate composed of neutrophils, lymphocytes, and macrophages [19].

Hyperpigmentation is histologically reflected by an increase in melanin and deposits of the drug or its metabolites in the dermis. Lichenoid reactions resemble the histopathologic characteristics of lichen planus. Pseudoporphyria is characterized by separation of epidermis and dermis in the lamina lucida and the deposition of immunoglobulins in the dermal-epidermal junction as well as in the wall of the surrounding blood vessels [13].

Drug-Induced Photoallergic Cutaneous Reactions

Pathophysiology

Fundamentally, photoallergy is a cell-mediated type IV hypersensitivity response. Like in phototoxic reactions, photoallergy requires both the photosensitizer and radiation of the eliciting wave length, mostly UVA. Nevertheless, photoallergic reactions show many differences compared to phototoxic reactions. Photoallergy is (a) less common, (b) it does not depend on the dose of either the photosensitizer or the radiation, (c) it usually develops more than 24 h after radiation, (d) it requires prior sensitization, and (e) it may be provoked by biochemically similar drugs in the sense of a cross-reaction [1]. The type IV hypersensitivity response is initiated by the formation of an antigen that is recognized by the host immune system. This antigen formation may be performed by two different mechanisms. (a) The drug is excited to a higher energy state by radiation. Thus, it can act as a hapten and conjugate with a carrier protein (e.g. albumin or γ-globulin) forming the antigen. This mechanism is hypothesized for chlorpromazine and sulfanilamide. (b) Alternatively, the drug is excited by radiation and by returning back to the resting state, the released energy promotes the conjugation with a protein resulting in an entirely new antigen. This is thought to be the mechanism in photoallergy to halogenated salicylanilides, para-aminobenzoic acid, and again chlorpromazine. Independently from the antigen-forming mechanism, the new antigen is processed by Langerhans cells and presented by the MHC II complex. Langerhans cells migrate to regional lymph nodes where they initiate the activation, differentiation and proliferation of nodal T lymphocytes. This step seems to be influenced by the MHC haplotype which may contribute to the different susceptibility of individuals to photoallergic reactions. The activated T lymphocytes then recirculate to the light-exposed skin, where they play a key role in the cell-mediated type IV hypersensitivity reaction [1, 2, 20]. Drugs that act as photoallergens are usually lipophilic molecules with a low molecular weight [2]. Today,

UV filters in sunscreens (especially benzophenone-3) and topically administered NSAIDs have been identified to be the most common causes of photoallergic drug reactions [1, 20].

Clinical Manifestations of Photoallergy

In sensitized patients, photoallergic drug reactions develop within 24 h after exposure to the photosensitizer and sunlight. Men seem to be affected more often than women. The reaction is pronounced at sun-exposed skin areas, but in severe cases or after repeated photoallergic events also sun-protected areas may be affected, albeit at a lower intensity. The clinical picture resembles eczematous dermatitis, initially with sharply demarcated erythema and rarely subsequent formation of vesicles or blisters and scaling. Patients complain of intense pruritus. After repeated or long-lasting photoallergic reactions, affected skin develops lichenification with reduced inflammation but pronounced scaling and thickening. Usually, photoallergy resolves after discontinuation of the responsible drug without postinflammatory hyperpigmentation [1, 2, 20].

Chronic Actinic Dermatitis

Occasionally, the photoallergic drug reaction persists months to years beyond the removal of the culprit drug. The persistence of a photoallergic reaction may evolve into chronic actinic dermatitis (CAD). Today, different entities previously described in the literature are summarized under the term CAD. A persistent photoallergic reaction was first described in 1962 in patients with ongoing usage of soaps containing halogenated salicylanilides [20]. The mechanism of the persistent photoallergic reaction is not completely understood, but some theories have been proposed. For example, small amounts of the photosensitizing drug may remain in the dermis [20]. Another explanation may be the modification of carrier proteins or other dermal components forming new and persistent immunogenic molecules. The responsible drugs have mostly been administered topically rather than systemically. Still today, major contributors seem to be halogenated salicylanilides and musk ambrette [2]. Interestingly, a change in eliciting wavelength of the radiation is observed during the course of CAD. Thus, UVB and visible light can cause skin eruptions in patients with CAD as well. CAD occurs most commonly in elderly men and is characterized by a spread of the eczematous skin lesions all over the sun-exposed areas. Also sun-protected skin areas can be affected during the course of the disease. Typically, affected skin shows pronounced lichenification. In more severe cases, skin edema or disfiguring nodules resembling cutaneous lymphomas may develop (facies leontina) [21]. A proposed subtype of CAD is the actinic reticuloid that is histologically characterized by atypical lymphocytes, which explains why actinic reticuloid used to be grouped with cutaneous lymphoma. The development of cutaneous lymphomas was described in some cases [22].

Lichen Planus-Like Photoallergic Skin Reactions

Some drug-induced photoallergic reactions are characterized by lichenoid eruptions rather than eczema. This clinical type is called lichen planus-like photoallergic reaction. It occurs more commonly in geographic regions with a high amount of sunlight. Most common responsible drugs are chloroquine and its derivates, quinine, quinidine, and thiazides. Characteristic skin lesions are lichenoid papules on violaceous erythematosus patches. They are restricted to sun-exposed areas of the skin, the oral mucosa is spared. Eruptions normally resolve after withdrawal of the responsible drug [2].

Histopathology of Photoallergic Skin Reactions

The histopathological changes in acute photoallergic skin reactions resemble allergic contact dermatitis with epidermal spongiosis and vesiculation. In the dermis, vascular dilatation and a perivascular infiltration of lymphohistiocytic cells with variable numbers of eosinophils is found. The papillary dermis often shows an edema. Histopathological changes in CAD are led by signs of lichenification with dermal thickening and hyperkeratosis. Lichen planus-like reactions resemble common lichenoid lesions on histopathology [19].

Evaluation of Patients with Phototoxicity and Photoallergy

A history of exposure is essential for the correct diagnosis of a photosensitive reaction. It has to include questioning regarding the possible exposure to various topical and systemic photosensitizers. It may be helpful to evaluate whether glass-filtered sunlight induced the skin changes, because window glass filters out UVB and a part of UVA in the UVA2 range [23]. In a next step, the inspection of the whole body is necessary. The distribution of skin eruptions may be a hint to the underlying trigger. The restriction of skin lesions to sun-exposed skin areas like the face, the neck or dorsa of hands raises suspicion for light-induced dermatoses. Widespread skin eruptions suggest the systemic application of a photosensitizer whereas skin lesions restricted to certain areas of the skin are typical with topically applied photosensitizers. The morphology of the individual lesion may suggest the pathophysiological mechanism. Vesicles and bullae together with burning sensations are commonly associated with phototoxicity, whereas eczema and pruritus suggest photoallergy [2, 23]. In a next step, a skin biopsy should be performed since phototoxicity and photoallergy can often be distinguished by their histopathologic features.

In case of suspected photosensitivity, phototesting should be performed [24]. In a first step, the susceptibility of the skin to UVA and UVB has to be determined by assessing the minimal erythema dose (MED) 24 h after irradiation. In the setting of drug-induced photosensitization, the minimal phototoxicity dose (MPD) at 72 h should be read as well with psoralens in PUVA treatment being a prime example for such MPD testing. For such phototesting, six small fields of the gluteal skin are irradiated with gradually increasing dosages of each UVA and UVB. The dosage of UV irradiation depends on the skin type. For UVA, dosages from 0.5 to 5 J/cm^2 for skin types I and II and 10–45 J/cm^2 for skin types III–VI may be applied. For UVB, the dosage is lower and may range from 0.01 to 0.09 J/cm^2. Evaluation is performed immediately after irradiation and during the following 4 days. Although the interpretation of the MED and MPD are more straightforward in phototoxicity, a decreased MED and MPD may be found in photoallergy as well [2, 13]. In a second step, a photopatch test may be performed, which is especially useful to assess photoallergy [2]. Here, a set of potential photosensitizers in non-irritant dose and formulation is patched in duplicate on the dorsum of the patient. The applied photosensitizers consist of a standardized set amended by substances that may be relevant for the particular patient (e.g. cosmetics, sunscreens) chosen based on a careful evaluation of his/her history. One of the two sets of test samples is covered to protect it completely from light, whereas the other set is irradiated with UVA the following day. The dosage of UVA irradiation is between 5 and 10 J/cm^2, and needs adjusting in case of a decreased MED. The non-irradiated patches are removed 48 h after application, and both sites are evaluated over the next 4 days. Several scenarios are possible (table 6) [24]. Sometimes it is helpful to seek histopathologic confirmation by biopsy of fresh lesions from a reactive phototest site. Laboratory tests should be routinely performed, including full blood count (eosinophilia), liver function tests and auto-antibody screening (ANA, dsDNA, SSA, SSB) [23].

Differential Diagnoses of Phototoxicity and Photoallergy

Allergic contact dermatitis is the most important differential diagnosis in the case of suspected photosensitivity and can be differentiated by localization of skin lesions. It affects both sun-exposed and sun-protected areas of the skin. Even airborne allergic contact dermatitis involves areas of the skin protected by skinfolds like the retroauricular or submental region. Other important differential diagnoses are polymorphous light eruption and solar urticaria. Polymorphous light eruption appears within a few hours or days after excess light exposure on intermittently exposed areas of the skin such as décolleté and upper arms, and resolves after a few days. Symptoms typically decrease over the course of the summer with increasing habituation of the skin to

Table 6. Interpretation of photopatch test results

		Non-irradiated side	
		Reaction	No reaction
Irradiated side	Reaction	– irritation – allergic contact dermatitis (with photoaggravation)	– phototoxic: decrescendo pattern – photoallergic: crescendo pattern – false positive result
	No reaction	– no interpretation	– no photosensitivity – photosensitizer was not tested – photosensitizer did not penetrate the epidermis – tested substance was not converted to photosensitizing metabolite

From Neumann et al. [24], with modifications.

solar radiation. Solar urticaria appears within minutes after light exposure with typical itching hives and resolves within hours.

Management of Patients with Phototoxicity and Photoallergy

The mainstays of treatment in case of phototoxicity and photoallergy are the avoidance of sun light and of the offending drug after its identification [2]. This includes protective clothing and daily application of sunscreen. As UVA is the responsible light quality in most cases, patients should be instructed to apply sunscreens with high UVA filters, also indoors behind window glass. In patients recurrently suffering from photosensitivity, a change in lifestyle, recreational activities and even occupation may need to be considered [23]. After removal of drugs, remnants or metabolites may persist in the skin for days or weeks, maintaining skin reactions. In those cases, a medical intervention is often necessary. Topical steroids together with soothing and cooling lotions are appropriate to decrease local inflammatory response and itching or burning sensations. Sometimes systemic antihistamines provide added relief. Systemic application of steroids in a dosage of 1 mg per kilogram body weight daily during one week should be restricted to severe cases [2, 23]. Occasionally, artificial hardening using low doses of narrow-band UVB (311 nm) or PUVA can be performed [25].

The use of antioxidants is discussed controversially. Some authors state that the application of flavonoids or the vitamins A, C, and E may positively interfere with the pathogenetic mechanisms of photosensitive reactions [3]. In case of hyperpigmentation after phototoxic events or lichenoid eruptions, patients should be informed that it can take several months after discontinuation of the responsible drug for the skin changes to resolve [2].

References

1 Stein KR, Scheinfeld NS: Drug-induced photoallergic and phototoxic reactions. Expert Opin Drug Saf 2007;6:431–443.

2 Gould JW, Mercurio MG, Elmets CA: Cutaneous photosensitivity diseases induced by exogenous agents. J Am Acad Dermatol 1995;33:551–573.

3 Moore DE: Drug-induced cutaneous photosensitivity: incidence, mechanism, prevention and management. Drug Saf 2002;25:345–372.

4 Song PS, Tapley KJ Jr: Photochemistry and photobiology of psoralens. Photochem Photobiol 1979;29: 1177–1197.

5 Shimoda K: Mechanisms of quinolone phototoxicity. Toxicol Lett 1998;102–103:369–373.

6 Kurita M, Shimauchi T, Kobayashi M, Atarashi K, Mori K, Tokura Y: Induction of keratinocyte apoptosis by photosensitizing chemicals plus UVA. J Dermatol Sci 2007;45:105.

7 Lassacher A, Worda M, Kaddu S, Heitzer E, Legat F, Massone C, Cerroni L, Kerl H, Ananthaswamy HN, Wolf P: T1799A BRAF mutation is common in PUVA lentigines. J Invest Dermatol 2006;126: 1915–1917.

8 Stern RS, Nichols KT, Väkevä LH, for the PUVA Follow-up Study: Malignant melanoma in patients treated for psoriasis with methoxsalen (psoralen) and ultraviolet A radiation (PUVA). N Engl J Med 1997;336:1041–1045.

9 Chuang TY, Heinrich LA, Schultz MD, Reizner GT, Kumm RC, Cripps DJ: PUVA and skin cancer. A historical cohort study on 492 patients. J Am Acad Dermatol 1992;26:173–177.

10 Jensen AØ, Thomsen HF, Engebjerg MC, Olesen AB, Sørensen HT, Karagas MR: Use of photosensitising diuretics and risk of skin cancer: a population-based case-control study. Br J Cancer 2008;99: 1522–1528.

11 Cowen EW, Nguyen JC, Miller DD, McShane D, Arron ST, Prose NS, Turner ML, Fox LP: Chronic phototoxicity and aggressive squamous cell carcinoma of the skin in children and adults during treatment with voriconazole. J Am Acad Dermatol 2010;62:31–37.

12 O'Donovan P, Perrett CM, Zhang X, Montaner B, Xu YZ, Harwood CA, McGregor JM, Walker SL, Hanaoka F, Karran P: Azathioprine and UVA light generate mutagenic oxidative DNA damage. Science 2005;309:1871–1874.

13 Epstein JH: Phototoxicity and photoallergy. Semin Cutan Med Surg 1999;18:274–284.

14 Miller DD, Cowen EW, Nguyen JC, McCalmont TH, Fox LP: Melanoma associated with long-term voriconazole therapy: a new manifestation of chronic photosensitivity. Arch Dermatol 2010;146:300–304.

15 Timmer-de Mik L, Kardaun SH, Kramer MH, Hayes DP, Bousema MT: Imatinib-induced pseudoporphyria. Clin Exp Dermatol 2009;34:705–707.

16 Gilbar P, Hain A, Peereboom VM: Nail toxicity induced by cancer chemotherapy. J Oncol Pharm Pract 2009;15:143–155.

17 Piraccini BM, Iorizzo M, Starace M, Tosti A: Drug-induced nail diseases. Dermatol Clin 2006;24:387–391.

18 Baran R, Juhlin L: Photoonycholysis. Photodermatol Photoimmunol Photomed 2002;18:202–207.

19 Crowson AN, Magro CM: Recent advances in the pathology of cutaneous drug eruptions. Dermatol Clin 1999;17:537–560.

20 Kerr A, Ferguson J: Photoallergic contact dermatitis. Photodermatol Photoimmunol Photomed 2010; 26:56–65.

21 Dawe RS: Chronic actinic dermatitis in the elderly: recognition and treatment. Drugs Aging 2005;22: 201–207.

22 Zak-Prelich M, Schwartz RA: Actinic reticuloid. Int J Dermatol 1999;38:335.

23 Bylaite M, Grigaitiene J, Lapinskaite GS: Photodermatoses: classification, evaluation and management. Br J Dermatol 2009;161(suppl 3):61–68.

24 Neumann NJ, Fritsch C, Lehmann P: Photodiagnostic test methods. 1. Stepwise light exposure and the photopatch test. Hautarzt 2000;51:113.

25 Man I, Dawe RS, Ferguson J: Artificial hardening for polymorphic light eruption: practical points from ten years' experience. Photodermatol Photoimmunol Photomed 1999;15:96–99.

Dr. Günther F.L. Hofbauer
Department of Dermatology, University Hospital Zurich
Gloriastrasse 31
CH–8091 Zurich (Switzerland)
Tel. +41 44 255 1111, E-Mail hofbauer@usz.ch

French LE (ed): Adverse Cutaneous Drug Eruptions.
Chem Immunol Allergy. Basel, Karger, 2012, vol 97, pp 180–190

Immediate and Delayed Cutaneous Reactions to Radiocontrast Media

Knut Brockow

Department of Dermatology and Allergy Biederstein, Technische Universität München, Munich, Germany

Abstract

Hypersensitivity reactions to contrast media (CM) are frequent causes of anaphylaxis and drug exanthemas. Adverse events after CM exposure are classified into immediate (≤1 h) and non-immediate reactions (>1 h), with differing mechanisms. In the majority of patients with immediate reactions, IgE-mediated allergy cannot be demonstrated, and the underlying mechanism remains unknown. However, recent data have provided evidence for skin test positivity and/or specific IgE in some patients. T cell-mediated hypersensitivity is the responsible mechanism for the majority of non-immediate skin eruptions. These insights have consequences for diagnosis and prevention. Skin testing evolves to be a useful tool for diagnosis of CM allergy. Skin tests have been employed to confirm this hypersensitivity. Previous reactors have an increased risk to develop new reactions upon repeated exposure; however, other risk factors are poorly defined. The use of skin tests for the selection of a 'safe' CM is under investigation with promising results. In vitro tests to search for CM-specific cell activation include flow cytometric approaches, lymphocyte cultures and construction of cell lines and hybridomas. Premedication of previous reactors is common practice among radiologists; however, breakthrough reactions are a concern, and physicians should not rely on the efficacy of pharmacological premedication.

Essentials in a Nutshell

- Modern radiocontrast media (RCM) lead to hypersensitivity reactions in 1–3% of applications
- Adverse reactions to RCM may be classified into toxic, unrelated/unspecific and immediate or non-immediate hypersensitivity reactions
- The manifestation of immediate hypersensitivity reactions is anaphylaxis
- Exanthemas are the predominant clinical picture of non-immediate RCM hypersensitivity and resemble those to other drugs
- There is growing evidence that the mechanism of immediate hypersensitivity to RCM may be IgE mediated, and that of non-immediate skin eruptions is T cell mediated. Allergy to iodine does not play a major role

- Skin tests are of value as a screening test for allergy to RCM hypersensitivity, and may be used to select a radiographic contrast medium (CM) for future use
- Provocation tests are recommended to validate skin tests in non-immediate exanthemas
- As prevention, a different skin test-negative RCM should be chosen for future examinations. Doctors should not rely on the efficacy of premedication

Epidemiology of Hypersensitivity Reactions to Radiocontrast Media

RCM are concentrated solutions of tri-iodinated benzene derivatives. Non-ionic monomers are most commonly used, whereas the older ionic monomers are not available any more in many countries, and only one non-ionic dimeric preparation is available for intravenous use. RCM are used for the diagnosis and treatment of vascular disease and enhancement of radiographic contrast [1]. Adverse reactions after application of RCM are common [2]. The frequency hypersensitivity reactions differs between different types of RCM. Mild immediate reactions, such as urticaria and pruritus have been reported to occur in up to 12.7% of patients receiving the older ionic monomeric RCM, but only in 0.7–3.1% of patients receiving the modern non-ionic RCM [3]. Severe immediate adverse reactions to ionic RCM have been reported in 0.1–0.4% of procedures, but only in 0.02–0.04% of applications of nowadays non-ionic RCM [reviewed in 4]. Fatal hypersensitivity reactions still occur in 1–3 per 100,000 CM administrations to both ionic and non-ionic preparations. The frequency of reported non-immediate reactions varies greatly between publications. Skin exanthemas (skin rash, skin eruptions) account for the majority of the RCM-induced non-immediate hypersensitivity reactions, and can be estimated to affect 1–3% of RCM-exposed patients [5]. There appears to be a higher incidence of exanthemas associated with dimeric non-ionic RCM. The only well-established risk factor for immediate as well as non-immediate hypersensitivity reactions are a previous hypersensitivity reaction [5, 6]. It is of interest that immediate reactions are not risk factors for developing a non-immediate reaction and vice versa.

Classification of Radiographic Contrast Media Hypersensitivity Reactions

Not all symptoms after RCM exposure resemble real hypersensitivity reactions (fig. 1). Toxic reactions to RCM are well known, e.g. nephrotoxicity or neurotoxicity. The unspecific feeling of warmth should also not be confused with a real hypersensitivity reaction. Unspecific reactions of unknown origin and or unrelated diseases may also occur after application of RCM, such as unrelated chronic idiopathic

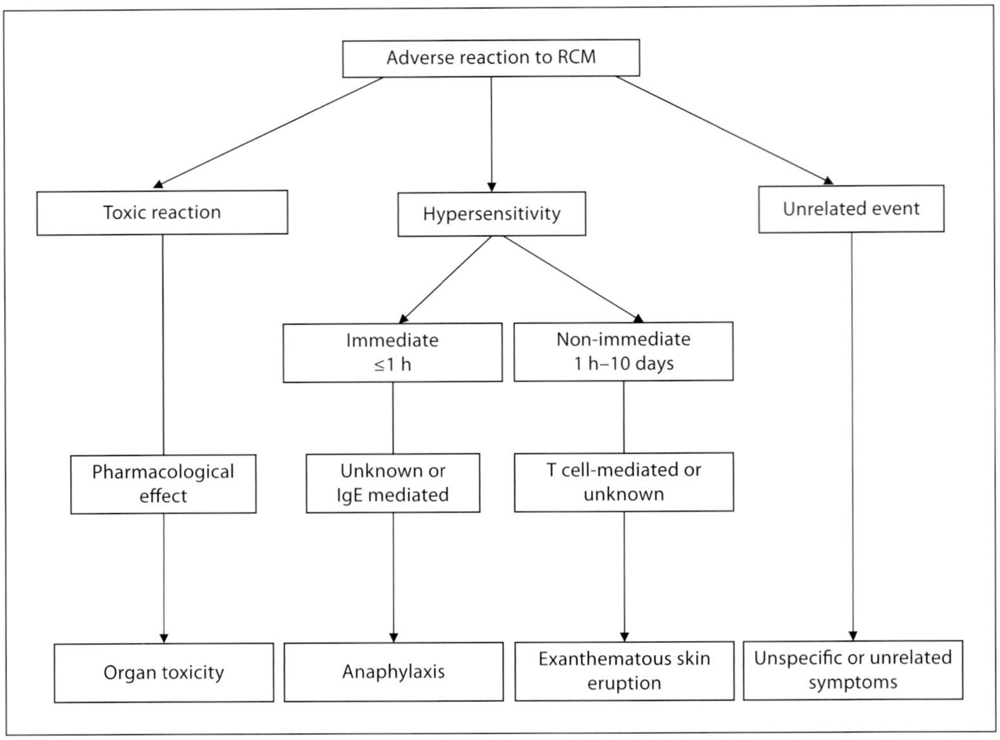

Fig. 1. Classification of adverse reactions to RCM. Adapted from Brockow et al. [2].

urticaria [2]. In a recent study on 539 patients receiving either computed tomography unenhanced or enhanced with iohexol, also 2.5% of 281 with no CM application reported reactions [7]. Typical hypersensitivity reactions to RCM may either present under the clinical picture of anaphylaxis, or as delayed occurring exanthema. In an attempt for classification, they have been differentiated with regard to the time interval between administration and the first appearance of symptoms as immediate, when they occur within 1 h after RCM administration, or non-immediate, when they occur 1 h up to 10 days after RCM application [2]. The present review will give an update on our present understanding of immediate and non-immediate hypersensitivity reactions to RCM.

Clinical Presentations of Immediate and Non-Immediate Hypersensitivity

Immediate RCM hypersensitivity reactions manifest as anaphylaxis (table 1). The majority of patients with immediate reaction present with pruritus and urticaria; sometimes angioedema occurs [4]. For several other frequent reactions, such as nausea, and vomiting, however, it remains unclear, if these reactions represent hypersensitivity or rather toxic reactions. Gastrointestinal symptoms such as

Table 1. Clinical pictures of typical immediate and non-immediate hypersensitivity reactions to RCM

Anaphylactic immediate reactions	Exanthematic non-immediate reactions
Urticaria	Exanthema (mostly maculopapular drug eruptions)
Angioedema/facial edema	Urticaria, angioedema (facial edema)
Abdominal pain, nausea, or diarrhea	DRESS
Rhinitis (sneezing, rhinorrhea)	SDRIFE
Hoarseness, cough	Erythema multiforme minor
Dyspnea (bronchospasm, laryngeal edema)	Fixed drug eruption
Respiratory arrest	Stevens-Johnson syndrome
Hypotension, cardiovascular shock	Toxic epidermal necrolysis
Cardiac arrest	Graft-versus-host reaction
	Vasculitis

abdominal pain and diarrhea may occur. More severe reactions involve the respiratory and cardiovascular systems and present with dyspnea, bronchospasm, and/or a sudden drop in blood pressure. Hypotension is mostly combined with reflex tachycardia and can be associated with a loss of consciousness (anaphylactic shock) [2]. About 70% of those reactions occur within 5 min after injection [8], and 96% of severe or fatal reactions manifest within 20 min [4]. The grading system published by Ring and Messmer is helpful for scoring the severity of anaphylaxis regardless of the mechanism [9].

Most patients with a non-immediate RCM reaction present with a macular or maculopapular exanthema (fig. 2a). It may occur only some hours, but also several days after the RCM administration (table 1) [5, 8]. More specific exanthemas after RCM exposure include symmetrical drug-related intertriginous and flexural exanthema (SDRIFE; fig. 2b), or drug-related eosinophilia with systemic symptoms (DRESS). Other skin reactions have been described, such as fixed drug eruption, erythema exsudativum multiforme, scaling skin eruption, graft-versus-host reaction, pruritus and pompholyx [1, 4]. Most non-immediate RCM hypersensitivity reactions are mild to moderate in severity and are self-limited [8]. Some rare cases of severe reactions have also been reported, presenting with cutaneous vasculitis, DRESS syndrome, Stevens-Johnson syndrome, toxic epidermal necrolysis and papulopustular eruptions [2]. Sometimes mild non-immediate anaphylactoid symptoms are reported, such as erythema, urticaria, or angioedema occurring hours after RCM application. Most of these may be regarded as exanthemas, such as the facial angioedema typical for DRESS syndrome. Systemic symptoms with delayed more anaphylactoid manifestations such as hypotension, fever, abdominal pain, dyspnea after several hours and biphasic reactions had been reported when dimeric non-ionic RCM had been introduced. However, even in dimeric non-ionic RCM they do appear to be very uncommon [2].

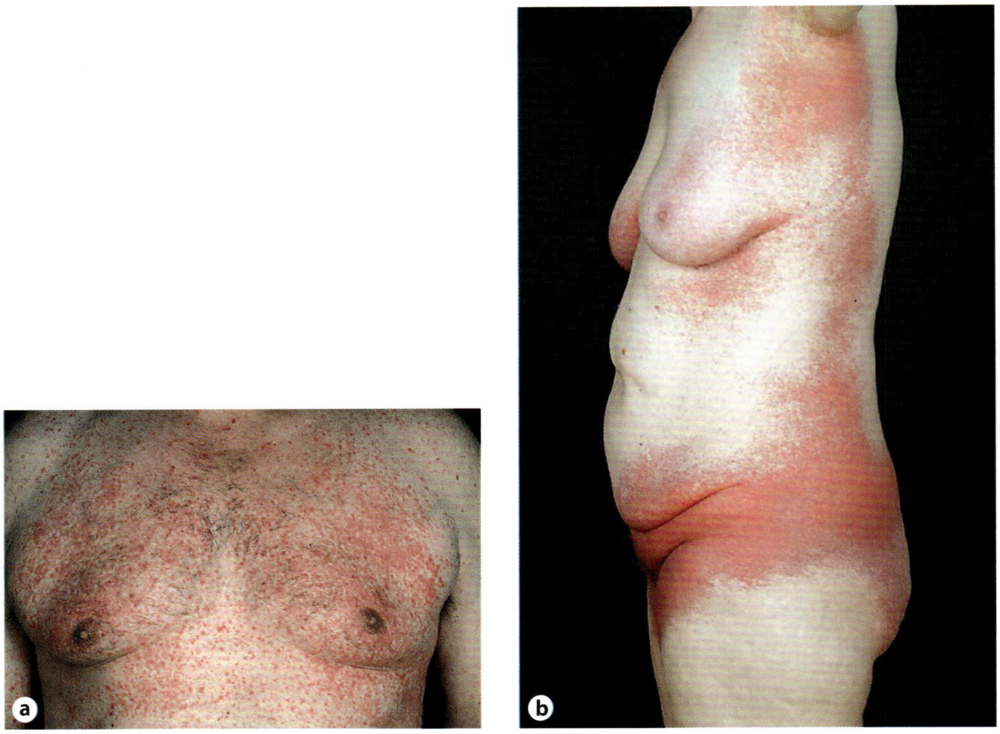

Fig. 2. Clinical pictures of cutaneous non-immediate RCM reactions showing a typical maculopapular exanthema developing 7 days after application of iomeprol (**a**) and a SDRIFE 2 days after application of iomeprol (**b**).

Pathophysiology

Immediate Radiocontrast Media Hypersensitivity

The mechanisms of the allergy-like reactions to RCM are still under investigation [4]. Anaphylaxis to RCM has been discussed to be due either to a direct membrane effect related to the osmolality of the CM or the chemical structure of the CM molecule (pseudoallergy), complement activation, bradykinin formation, or an IgE-mediated mechanism [4].

There is some indirect evidence that immediate hypersensitivity reactions may be caused by an IgE-mediated allergic mechanism. First, immediate hypersensitivity reactions to CM are associated with histamine release from basophils and mast cells, and extensive mast cell activation in vivo associated with clinical symptoms has been demonstrated by Laroche et al. [10]. Patients with hypersensitivity reactions after CM exposure had increased plasma levels of both histamine and tryptase, and levels correlated with severity [10, 11].

Second, several groups have reported positive skin test results for patients with severe immediate reactions to either ionic or non-ionic RCM [8]. Some of these patients were shown to react not only to the skin test of the culprit CM but also to other CM [8]. The frequency of positive skin tests has been investigated in a European multicenter study in patients with RCM hypersensitivity and in 82 controls [8]. The intradermal test (IDT) showed specificity in 96.3% of controls, but was positive in only 26% of patients. Another recent French prospective clinical study on 38 patients with immediate hypersensitivity reactions to RCM as determined by a reaction at the Radiology Department examined clinical data, serum and plasma analysis of tryptase and histamine as well as skin test reactivity to RCM [12]. In this study employing higher (undiluted) RCM concentrations, positive skin test reactions were even found in 73% of patients. Patients with more severe reactions had more positive skin test reactions and higher plasma histamine and tryptase levels after the reaction. Cross-reactivity between different RCM was rare, supporting the non-irritative character of the skin tests; however, control patients as a proof of specificity of the reactions were missing.

In vitro, positive basophil activation tests were reported in patients with immediate RCM hypersensitivity reactions, which may be regarded as another indirect indication for an IgE-mediated allergy [13]. Older studies also demonstrated CM-specific IgE by immunoassays [reviewed in 4]. Unfortunately, these results have not been confirmed by newer studies and/or for the modern non-ionic RCM, as it is difficult to bind non-ionic RCM to a solid phase, limiting research in this field.

Pathophysiology of Non-Immediate Reactions

The majority of these reactions appear to be T cell-mediated reactions. First, the most common clinical picture of non-immediate RCM reactions is a maculopapular exanthema, which resembles other drug-induced allergic T cell-mediated hypersensitivity reactions. The reported onset of skin eruptions 2–10 days after the first exposure to an RCM and 1–2 days after reexposure to the same substance is compatible with an allergic drug reaction and with a sensitization phase. Previous reactors are at risk for a new reaction compatible with a sensitization. In many cases, readministration of the culprit CM to patients with a previous non-immediate exanthema resulted in a repeat reaction [1].

Second, the histopathology of those exanthemas and of positive skin test sites provides evidence for an involvement of T cells [14, 15]. The perivascular infiltrate of positive skin test site biopsies consist mainly of CD4+ and CD8+ (CD45RO+) T cells accompanied by eosinophils [14, 15]. Also skin biopsies obtained from the site of positive skin tests to the culprit RCM showed similar results, with high expression of CD69 in lymphocytes [15–17].

Positive delayed skin tests in patients with CM-induced non-immediate skin reactions have been frequently reported [summarized in 1]. In a European multicenter study with 220 patients, 37% of patients with non-immediate reactions were positive in delayed IDTs and/or patch tests [8]. The majority of the patients reacted to the culprit CM and also to other CM indicating cross-reactivity.

The presence of RCM-specific T cells in patients with non-immediate exanthematous skin eruptions has been demonstrated in vitro in the lymphocyte transformation test [14], and by increased T lymphocyte activation markers (CD69, CD25 and HLA-D) by flow cytometric analysis, as well as by skin homing receptors (CLA) in CD4-positive lymphocytes. Perforin expression was increased in the CD8-positive cytotoxic lymphocytes [15]. When RCM-specific T cell clones were generated from human blood of three RCM-allergic patients and a specific T cell receptor was transfected into a mouse T cell hybridoma, RCM were stimulatory for T cells either by direct bridging of the major histocompatibility complex T cell receptor structure or by binding after uptake and processing by antigen-presenting cells [18]. This hapten-independent model would also better explain the cross-reactivity observed between different compounds, and challenges the assumed inert nature of RCM.

Role of Iodine in Contrast Media Hypersensitivity

In 19 patients with immediate or non-immediate RCM hypersensitivity reactions to RCM, skin tests with several RCM and iodine were done and oral provocation with Lugol's solution was performed [19]. Out of 9 patients with immediate hypersensitivity, skin tests to RCM were positive in 3 (33%). Skin tests to iodine preparations remained negative, but one skin test-negative patient reacted twice to oral iodine with urticaria. All 10 patients (100%) with non-immediate reactions showed positive skin tests to RCM. Even though in 7/10 (70%) additional positive skin tests to the iodine formulations were found, only 2 patients (20%) with extensive cross-reactivity between RCM developed a mild exanthema after oral provocation with Lugol's solution. This study confirmed that iodine is rarely the eliciting agent in RCM hypersensitivity.

Diagnosis

Immediately after the reaction, an RCM-induced anaphylaxis may be confirmed by blood samples for histamine analysis drawn as soon as possible after the reaction and/or by tryptase analysis of a sample drawn 1–2 h after onset of symptoms [10]. Tryptase values have to be compared to baseline levels and significant increases indicate anaphylaxis. In non-immediate reactions, hematology and clinical chemistry should be considered in more severe exanthema to exclude systemic involvement [1]. A skin biopsy may sometimes help in the differential diagnosis.

The further allergologic workup is recommended to be performed between 2 and 6 months after the reaction, as this is associated with a much higher frequency of positive skin test reactions as compared with longer time intervals (table 2) [8].

Table 2. Currently recommended skin test concentrations

Test	Concentration[a]	Readings	
		immediate reaction	non-immediate reaction
Skin prick test	Undiluted	20 min	20 min, 48 h, 72 h[b]
Intradermal test	1/10 diluted[c]	20 min	20 min, 48 h, 72 h[b]
Patch test	Undiluted		20 min, 48 h, 72 h[b]

[a] Undiluted RCM with an iodine concentration of 300–320 mg/ml.
[b] The reading times are tentative: if the patient notices a positive reaction (pruritus, erythema) at the skin test site at other time points, additional readings may be performed (e.g. after 24 or 96 h).
[c] For non-severe non-immediate reactions, also undiluted RCM may be used.

Skin Tests

A skin prick test (SPT) should be performed with undiluted RCM. As skin test reactions resemble the original reaction, for immediate reactions readings after 20 min are indicated, whereas for non-immediate reactions additional readings after 48 and 72 h have to be done. A positive reaction in the SPT is rare, but it is a good screening test for a strong sensitivity. Systemic reactions to IDT have been described. Afterwards, IDTs with RCM (300–320 mgI/ml) diluted 10-fold in sterile saline and reading after 20 min have been recommended [8]. IDTs with undiluted RCM had been reported in non-severe reactions to increase sensitivity; however, at the cost of an undetermined specificity [12]. As cross-reactivity is frequent, a panel of several different RCM should be tested in an attempt to find a skin test-negative product, which might be tolerated in future RCM examinations. Both delayed IDTs and patch tests are frequently positive, when read after 48 and 72 h, but the best time points for readings have not been compared, and in the case of local pruritus or erythematous plaques additional readings at other time points are advisable, e.g. 24, 96 h. Patch tests should be conducted with undiluted CM. Since rare patients tested positive with either IDT or patch test only, it is recommended to use both tests in parallel (table 2). In summary, skin tests are best screening tests to demonstrate an immunological mechanism in patients with RCM hypersensitivity. When used with the concentrations recommended, they have a high specificity and only a moderate sensitivity.

Laboratory Tests

In immediate RCM hypersensitivity, there is no assay for routine measurement of serum levels of RCM-specific IgE antibodies available. The reliability of other in vitro tests, such as the basophil activation test has not yet been established. Highly increased CD63 expressions in patients with immediate hypersensitivity reactions in vitro indicate that the basophil activation test may be helpful in individual patients [13]. RCM-related T cell activity in non-immediate hypersensitivity may be assessed in vitro by lymphocyte transformation test [14, 15]. This, however, appears to have a lower sensitivity as compared to skin tests [own unpubl. obs.]. In addition, CD69 upregulation (lymphocyte activation test) was observed in patients with positive lymphocyte transformation tests [15]. These tests appear to be a promising tool to identify drug-reactive T cells in the peripheral blood of patients with RCM-induced drug hypersensitivity reactions. Further research on the specificity and sensitivity is indicated.

Provocation Tests

Whereas in immediate hypersensitivity provocation is not generally recommended, as intravenous applications of as low as 0.5–1 ml RCM have led to severe anaphylaxis, in non-severe non-immediate hypersensitivity, provocation tests can validate skin test results and are recommended. Until further results are available, a positive skin test to a given RCM dictates that this RCM should not be chosen for a future exposure as alone the epicutaneous or intradermal application was able to lead to a local reaction, but a negative test does not necessarily guarantee tolerance. Here, provocation tests are helpful, depending on the time course of the primary reaction: e.g. 1/10 of the full dose on day 1, 1/2 of this volume on day 2 and the full dose on day 3 at the Radiology Department [20]. Provocation tests should be performed only in centers with experience to perform monitoring and emergency treatment. Noteworthy, a previous non-immediate exanthematous reaction does not pose a higher risk for a subsequent immediate anaphylactic reaction. In one study, safe readministration of a skin test-negative CM has been published in a series of 15 patients with non-immediate skin eruptions [20]. In this study, however, non-serious skin symptoms after exposure to the dimeric agents iodixanol (n = 4) or ioxaglate (n = 1) were described despite negative skin tests for these agents. In contrast, in a more recent study, a negative predictive value of 96.6% was calculated, when skin tests had been negative [21]. Out of 159 patients who had been skin tested and advised to use a skin test-negative RCM for further procedures, 29 patients were identified who had been reexposed to RCM after they had experienced an immediate (n = 24) or non-immediate (n = 4) hypersensitivity reaction. Of those patients, only 2 reported mild reactions to the subsequent examination. Thus, skin tests are probably helpful in the selection of a tolerable RCM in a patient with previous hypersensitivity reaction, but preliminary results should be further validated in a European multicenter follow-up study by provocation tests and reexposure data.

Prevention

In patients with a previous immediate hypersensitivity reaction to an RCM, the culprit preparation should be avoided in a new contrasted examination because of growing evidence that the hypersensitivity reaction may be structure dependent. Skin tests (SPT and IDT) with RCM are recommended [1]. RCM with positive skin tests should be avoided because of cross-reactivity among RCM [8]. In those patients who develop no positive skin test reaction to the culprit or other RCM, a negative skin test does not guarantee tolerance. However, the overall risk of a repeat reaction was very low according to a recent study, indicating a high negative predictive value. The use of premedication in patients at high risk for immediate RCM reactions has recently been challenged [22]. Corticosteroids and H1 and H2 antihistamines are the most frequently used agents with different protocols and administration routes. However, severe reactions still may develop in patients who receive corticosteroid premedication and the recurrence rate of RCM reaction after corticosteroid administration has been estimated to be almost 10% in one study [23]. In a recent study in 30 patients who had been pretreated with corticosteroid and H_1 antihistamines and/or H_2 blockers, immediate hypersensitivity reactions were not prevented in 5 of 30 patients (17%) with prior RCM reactions with similar severity and clinical manifestations [24]. In unselected patients, the usefulness of premedication is doubtful [22]. Sufficient data supporting the use of premedication in patients with a history of allergic reactions only are lacking. In summary, physicians dealing with these patients should not rely on the efficacy of premedication [22].

Similarly, patients with previous non-immediate skin exanthemas to RCM are at risk for developing new eruptions upon reexposure to the RCM [1], and another RCM should be chosen if reexposure is required. Due to frequent cross-reactivity between different RCM, an unselected change of product is no guarantee against a repeat reaction. PT and delayed IDT are recommended [8]. In case of positive skin tests, the substances that are able to elicit test reactions should be avoided. At present, the administration of skin test-negative CM in previous reactors does not guarantee tolerability, but appears to be associated with high negative predictive value even without pretreatment. In non-severe hypersensitivity (e.g. not in blistering reactions, systemic symptoms), a fractionated provocation test is indicated. In current practice, steroid prophylaxis is given in patients with previous serious non-immediate adverse reactions with partial success. However, repeated non-immediate reactions, including a case of toxic epidermal necrolysis, have been reported despite corticosteroid premedication [25]. A more intensive immunosuppressant protocol used intramuscular 6-methyl-prednisolone (40 mg daily) and oral cyclosporine (100 mg twice daily) in a patient with two previous episodes of maculopapular reactions after RCM administration, the last despite steroid premedication [25]. No studies have been performed to establish the optimum pretreatment regimen.

References

1 Brockow K: Contrast media hypersensitivity-scope of the problem. Toxicology 2005;209:189–192.

2 Brockow K, Christiansen C, Kanny G, et al: Management of hypersensivity reactions to iodinated contrast media. Allergy 2005;60:150–158.

3 Katayama H, Yamaguchi K, Kozuka T, et al: Adverse reactions to ionic and nonionic contrast media. A report from the Japanese Committee on the Safety of Contrast Media. Radiology 1990;175:621–628.

4 Brockow K, Ring J: Classification and pathophysiology of radiocontrast media hypersensitivity. Chem Immunol Allergy 2010;95:157–169.

5 Hosoya T, Yamaguchi K, Akutsu T, et al: Delayed adverse reactions to iodinated contrast media and their risk factors. Radiat Med 2000;18:39–45.

6 Katayama H, Yamaguchi K, Kozuka T, et al: Full-scale investigation into adverse reaction in Japan. Risk factor analysis. The Japanese Committee on the Safety of Contrast Media. Invest Radiol 1991; 26(suppl 1):S33–S36.

7 Loh S, Bagheri S, Katzberg RW, et al: Delayed adverse reaction to contrast-enhanced CT: a prospective single-center study comparison to control group without enhancement. Radiology 2010;255: 764–771.

8 Brockow K, Romano A, Aberer W, et al: Skin testing in patients with hypersensitivity reactions to iodinated contrast media – a European multicenter study. Allergy 2009;64:234–241.

9 Ring J, Messmer K: Incidence and severity of anaphylactoid reactions to colloid volume substitutes. Lancet 1977;1:466–469.

10 Laroche D, Aimone-Gastin I, Dubois F, et al: Mechanisms of severe, immediate reactions to iodinated contrast material. Radiology 1998;209: 183–190.

11 Brockow K, Vieluf D, Puschel K, et al: Increased postmortem serum mast cell tryptase in a fatal anaphylactoid reaction to nonionic radiocontrast medium. J Allergy Clin Immunol 1999;104:237–238.

12 Dewachter P, Laroche D, Mouton-Faivre C, et al: Immediate reactions following iodinated contrast media injection: a study of 38 cases. Eur J Radiol 2011;77:495–501.

13 Trcka J, Schmidt C, Seitz CS, et al: Anaphylaxis to iodinated contrast material: nonallergic hypersensitivity or IgE-mediated allergy? AJR Am J Roentgenol 2008;190:666–670.

14 Kanny G, Pichler W, Morisset M, et al: T cell-mediated reactions to iodinated contrast media: evaluation by skin and lymphocyte activation tests. J Allergy Clin Immunol 2005;115:179–185.

15 Torres MJ, Mayorga C, Cornejo-Garcia JA, et al: Monitoring non-immediate allergic reactions to iodine contrast media. Clin Exp Immunol 2008;152: 233–238.

16 Brockow K, Becker EW, Worret WI, Ring J: Late skin test reactions to radiocontrast medium. J Allergy Clin Immunol 1999;104:1107–1108.

17 Kanny G, Marie B, Hoen B, et al: Delayed adverse reaction to sodium ioxaglic acid-meglumine. Eur J Dermatol 2001;11:134–137.

18 Keller M, Lerch M, Britschgi M, et al: Processing-dependent and -independent pathways for recognition of iodinated contrast media by specific human T cells. Clin Exp Allergy 2010;40:257–268.

19 Scherer K, Harr T, Bach S, Bircher AJ: The role of iodine in hypersensitivity reactions to radio contrast media. Clin Exp Allergy 2010;40:468–475.

20 Vernassiere C, Trechot P, Commun N, et al: Low negative predictive value of skin tests in investigating delayed reactions to radio-contrast media. Contact Dermatitis 2004;50:359–366.

21 Caimmi S, Benyahia B, Suau D, et al: Clinical value of negative skin tests to iodinated contrast media. Clin Exp Allergy 2010;40:805–810.

22 Tramer MR, von Elm E, Loubeyre P, Hauser C: Pharmacological prevention of serious anaphylactic reactions due to iodinated contrast media: systematic review. BMJ 2006;333:675.

23 Freed KS, Leder RA, Alexander C, et al: Breakthrough adverse reactions to low-osmolar contrast media after steroid premedication. AJR Am J Roentgenol 2001;176:1389–1392.

24 Kim SH, Lee SH, Lee SM, et al: Outcomes of premedication for non-ionic radio-contrast media hypersensitivity reactions in Korea. Eur J Radiol 2011;80:363–367.

25 Romano A, Artesani M, Andriolo M, et al: Effective prophylactic protocol in delayed hypersensitivity to contrast media: report of a case involving lymphocyte transformation studies with different compounds. Radiology 2002;225:466–470.

Dr. Knut Brockow
Department of Dermatology and Allergy Biederstein, Technische Universität München
Biedersteiner Strasse 29
DE–80802 Munich (Germany)
Tel. +49 89 4140 3182, E-Mail knut.brockow@lrz.tum.de

French LE (ed): Adverse Cutaneous Drug Eruptions.
Chem Immunol Allergy. Basel, Karger, 2012, vol 97, pp 191–202

Cutaneous Drug Eruptions Associated with the Use of New Oncological Drugs

Benedetta Belloni · Nicola Schönewolf · Sima Rozati · Simone M. Goldinger · Reinhard Dummer

Department of Dermatology, University Hospital Zurich, Zurich, Switzerland

Abstract

There is a variety of adverse effects and toxicities of newer and older chemotherapeutic agents which emerge in the skin, mucosa and adnexa. Common skin reactions while undergoing chemotherapy include alopecia, changes in skin pigmentation, palmoplantar erythrodysesthesia, nail dystrophies and stomatitis. Extravasation injuries or hypersensitivity reactions may be severe. New oncologic agents have led to the development of different, class-specific cutaneous side effects. Epidermal growth factor receptor (EGFR) inhibitors induce papulopustular rashes in a high percentage of patients as well as, to a smaller degree, xerosis cutis, hair and nail changes, hyperpigmentation and enhancement of radiation dermatitis. Multikinase inhibitors will often cause hand-foot syndrome, but may also induce facial erythema, subungual splinter hemorrhages and other less frequent skin changes. BRAF inhibitors can lead to rash and development of cutaneous keratinocytic neoplasias for which patients should be closely monitored. Finally, MEK/ERK inhibitors induce similar skin toxicities to EGFR inhibitors such as papulopustular rashes, xerosis cutis and paronychia. Our chapter will focus on the clinical picture, histopathology and treatment options of these new class-specific cutaneous side effects.

Essentials in a Nutshell

- Chemotherapeutic agents generally target rapidly dividing cells and thus may often affect skin and mucosal tissue, as well as adnexal structures such as hair and nails
- New oncologic agents have led to the development of class-specific cutaneous side effects, such as papulopustular rashes under epidermal growth factor receptor (EGFR) inhibitor therapy, hand-foot syndrome (HFS) under multikinase inhibition, and development of keratinocytic neoplasias under BRAF inhibitor therapy
- Knowledge of these cutaneous side effects and their management can improve the patient's quality of life and prevent unnecessary treatment interruptions

Introduction

There are a variety of adverse effects and toxicities of newer and older chemotherapeutic agents which emerge in the skin, mucosa and adnexa. These reactions are more often toxic in nature than allergic.

Regarding older chemotherapeutic agents, one can distinguish a series of common skin reactions which can be either dose dependent or occur sporadically.

Alopecia is one of the most common manifestations, and occurs in numerous agents targeting rapidly dividing cells such as those found in the hair follicle. Chemotherapy-induced alopecia is reversible, but hair may subsequently regrow with a change in color or texture.

Changes in skin pigmentation such as hyperpigmentation are often noticed especially in patients undergoing treatment with busulfan.

The HFS, also known as palmoplantar erythrodysesthesia, was originally described in patients receiving cytarabine therapy, but is also a common side effect of liposome-encapsulated doxorubicin or 5-fluorouracil as well as newer agents such as kinase inhibitors.

Nail dystrophies include ridging and separation of the nail from the nail bed and are especially common in patients receiving docetaxel.

Chemotherapy often affects mucous membranes especially in patients undergoing treatment with doxorubicin and can result in very painful stomatitis.

Extravasation injuries caused by leakage of intravenously administered chemotherapeutics can range from erythema to severe necrosis depending on the agent and amount. The most toxic drugs are anthracyclines, vinca alkaloids, paclitaxel and cisplatin.

Chemotherapeutic agents such as doxorubicin can not only enhance radiation sensitivity, but in some cases may also induce a recall phenomenon of radiation dermatitis weeks to years after radiation took place. Newer agents such as EGFR inhibitors are also suggested to enhance the severity of radiation dermatitis.

Finally, hypersensitivity reactions can be caused by any medication including chemotherapy. Especially before administration of L-asparaginase, paclitaxel, and docetaxel, prophylactic use of corticosteroids as well as H1 and H2 blockers is recommended [1, 2].

In the following chapter, class-specific cutaneous toxicities of new oncologic agents will be discussed.

Epidermal Growth Factor Receptor Inhibitors

The EGFR is a member of the human EGFR family, and is expressed in a large number of human tissues. It belongs to a family of receptor tyrosine kinases which can subsequently activate multiple signal transduction pathways, including the mitogen-

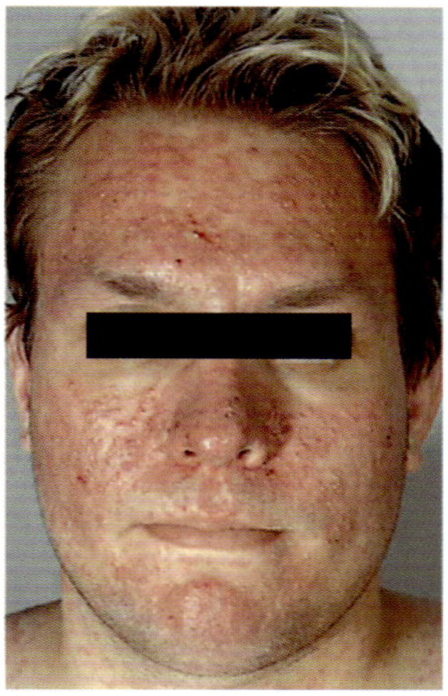

Fig. 1. Papulopustular rash unter anti-EGFR treatment in a colon cancer patient.

activated protein kinase (MAPK) pathway and the phosphatidylinositol 3-kinase/AKT pathway.

Overexpression of EGFR, resulting from gene amplification or activating mutations, is a common feature in a variety of solid tumors such as colon carcinoma, and plays an important role in tumor cell proliferation, angiogenesis and metastasis [3].

Therefore, inhibition of EGFR is an effective treatment approach to these tumors, and has led to the development of several agents. Currently, either monoclonal antibodies (cetuximab, panitumumab) that target the extracellular ligand-binding domain of the EGFR, or small molecule tyrosine kinase inhibitors (gefitinib, erlotinib) that target the EGFR intracellularly are used in the treatment of various types of cancer [4, 5].

As the EGFR is widely expressed in the epidermis, class-specific toxicities of these agents include above all cutaneous eruptions which can cause great discomfort and severely reduce the patient's quality of life. The incidence of skin toxicities under treatment with EGFR inhibitors ranges from 50 to 90% in reported clinical trials. Other toxicities include hypomagnesemia, diarrhea, infusion reactions and ocular symptoms with varying incidence rates [6].

Papulopustular rashes are the most common and earliest cutaneous side effects of EGFR inhibitors. They usually develop during the first weeks of treatment beginning in the seborrheic areas of the head and trunk, and gradually spreading over the integument, sparing however the palms and soles and the periorbital region. Monoclonal antibodies seem to induce more severe reactions as compared to small molecule tyrosine kinase inhibitors, but independently of the agent used, skin reactions will clear completely within weeks of stopping the treatment. The skin eruptions are comprised of follicular erythematous pustules and papules that resemble certain clinical aspects of acne or rosacea, and are therefore often referred to as acneiform rash, even though comedones do not occur (fig. 1). Histologically, a superficial folliculitis and perifolliculitis with hyperkeratotic and ectatic infundibula can be detected [7]. Treatment consists of topical application of emollients containing 1–2% erythromycin, and in severe cases the oral administration of tetracyclines or retinoids [4].

Xerosis cutis or excessive dryness of the skin is the second most common cutaneous side effect associated with scaling, atrophic and vulnerable skin as well as pulpitis sicca and painful fissures on palms and soles. Patients under treatment with EGFR inhibitors should generally be advised to avoid mechanical trauma, as well as excessive exposure to water and soap, even before symptoms occur. Treatment of xerosis and eczema should include emollients and topical steroids [6].

Paronychia and nail changes are described in 10–20% of patients and usually arise later during therapy. They can be characterized by slower nail growth, changes to the nail structure, painful, erythematous swelling of the nail folds, pyogenic granuloma-like inflammation and ingrown nails. In spite of prophylactic care with emollients, such as petroleum jelly, local disinfectants or antibiotics may have to be administered, as well as surgical debridement in severe cases [8].

Hair changes include trichomegaly, curling and trichorrhexis of eyelashes and eyebrows, as well as alopecia and inflammation of the scalp. There exists no adequate therapy, except for careful trimming of the eyelashes [4, 9].

Teleangiectasias and hyperpigmentation may appear in a small number of patients undergoing anti-EGFR treatment, usually as a result of photosensitivity, which is why these patients should generally be counseled to practice sun protection [6].

Furthermore, combining anti-EGFR therapy with radiation therapy has been suggested to enhance the severity of radiation dermatitis in several studies, and may also lead to discontinuation of treatment [10].

Multikinase Inhibitors

Adverse cutaneous drug eruptions have been noted to have a high incidence under multikinase treatment. In the following, we will explain relevant side effects of sorafenib (Nexavar, BAY 43-9006, Bayer, Leverkusen, Germany) and sunitinib (SU011248; Sutent, Pfizer, New York, N.Y., USA).

Sorafenib is a multikinase inhibitor approved by the Food and Drug Administration for the treatment of renal cell and hepatocellular carcinoma. The mode of action involves inhibition of RAF serine/threonine kinases (Raf-1, wild-type and V600E-mutated BRAF). RAF is located in the MAPK pathway. Deregulations in this pathway lead to tumorigenesis. Additional targets are the vascular endothelial growth factors (VEGFR-2 and -3), platelet-derived growth factor-β, FMS-like tyrosine kinase 3 (FLT-3), c-KIT and RET receptor tyrosine kinases. Inhibition of the latter results in reduced tumor angiogenesis and proliferation [11].

Sunitinib is approved as multikinase inhibitor for the treatment of gastrointestinal stromal tumors and advanced renal cell carcinoma, and also shows efficacy in colon

Table 1. NCI-CTCAE version 3.0 grading of HFS adjusted according to National Cancer Institute, 2008

Grade	Description
I	Minimal skin changes/dermatitis, no pain
II	Skin changes (e.g. blisters, peeling, bleeding, edema) or pain; no impairment on patient's daily activities
III	Ulcerative dermatitis or skin changes with pain; patient's daily activities impaired

and breast cancers. The main targets of sunitinib are angiogenic receptor tyrosine kinases such as VEGFR and PDGFR [12]. As for sorafenib, cKIT, RET and FLT-3 can also be targeted by sunitinib. The colony-stimulating factor 1 is an additional target [13].

Both drugs are small molecule tyrosine kinase inhibitors, interfering with specific molecular targets. Thus, they induce less severe side effects known from regular chemotherapeutics. However, adverse skin reactions are found for both drugs.

In several preclinical and clinical trials, the incidence of sorafenib- and sunitinib-induced adverse skin effects was investigated, and ranges between 74 and 91%. The HFS occurred with the highest frequency (20–78%) [14–19].

The HFS usually affects the palms and soles symmetrically. In some cases, the lateral sides of fingers or periungual zones are also affected. Furthermore, edematous lesions, desquamation and fissures have been observed in some patients [14]. Intolerance of contact to (hot) objects is often an additional manifestation. Burning and painful sensations are described by patients, mostly preceding the clinical signs. Furthermore, walking and holding things can be restricted [14, 15]. Large painful and tense blisters may develop [17].

The pathophysiological mechanisms are not yet well understood. However, the preference of small vessel traumatization in areas with pressure (nails, sole or palm contact areas) hints to a correlation of direct VEGFR or PDGFR inhibition [14]. Depending on the grading (I–III), symptoms are more or less severe (table 1).

Histologically, the epidermis is thickened and shows hyperkeratosis. Nonspecific dermal cell infiltrates and dilated vessels can be detected [14, 17]. In a number of cases, characteristic vacuolar degeneration of keratinocytes is found. The keratinocytic damage is presented by intracytoplasmic eosinophilic bodies, vacuolar degeneration and necrosis, and can lead to intraepidermal cleavage. Intracytoplasmic eosinophilic bodies have not been described before and are thus specific for sorafenib-induced HFS. An acceleration of epidermal cell replication is observed in active HFS lesions. This is represented by papillomatosis and acanthosis [17].

In contrast to the classical HFS (acral erythema or palmoplantar dysesthesia) induced by older cytostatic drugs, sorafenib-induced HFS is less severe. HFS is accompanied more often by hyperkeratosis, localized to pressure areas, whereas the

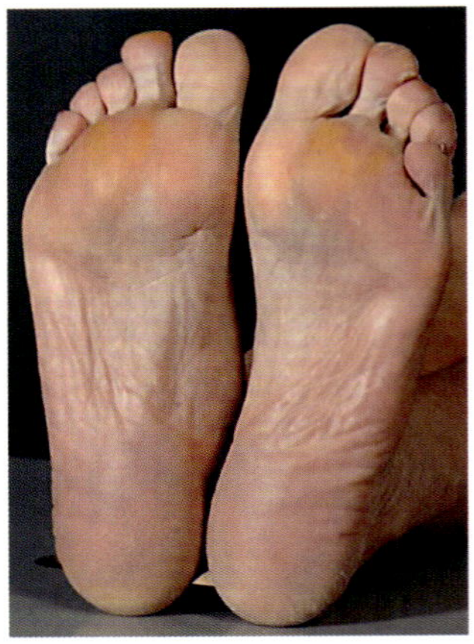

Fig. 2. Hyperkeratotic yellowish plaques on the foot soles after 1 cycle of sorafenib treatment in a melanoma patient.

Table 2. Patient-led practical prevention and management of HFS (adjusted to Robert et al. [15])

Treatment type	Apply/Dos	Don'ts
Patient-led practical prevention	alcohol-free moisturizer (cream) after bathing, moisturizer under cotton gloves/socks overnight, wear open shoes with padded soles during treatment, pedicure treatment of hyperkeratosis	exposure to hot water
Patient-led practical management	soak hands in cool water, dry well, petroleum jelly when skin still moist, foot bath and pumice stone to exfoliate feet, immediately apply moisturizer, use shock-absorbing soles to relieve painful pressure	
Chemical	urea or salicylic acid-containing treatments for skin exfoliation, topical steroids 2×/day – under medical supervision	
Other	analgesics if pain too strong	

distribution is more diffuse in classic HFS. However, sorafenib-induced HFS can also affect non-pressure areas (toes, finger webs, lateral sides of the soles and even perianal skin). Hyperkeratotic plaques are yellowish and painful, and can present as the only sign of HFS (fig. 2) [14, 17].

Topical treatment is appropriate for grade I severity. Table 2 offers recommendations for the patient-led prevention and management. Since sorafenib-induced HFS seems to be dose dependent, a reduction in the dose is recommended in higher grade severities. Oftentimes, reinitiation of the treatment with the same dose after temporary discontinuation is possible [14]. A broad literature search by Anderson et al. [18] revealed the reasonable need of prophylactic removal of hyperkeratosis prior to treatment. By doing so, unwanted side effects can be significantly reduced.

Facial erythema presents usually 1–2 weeks after treatment in up to 63% of patients treated with sorafenib. Preceding symptoms can present as scalp dysesthesia. Sometimes, superficial desquamation is associated similar to classical seborrheic dermatitis. Exacerbation is observed under hot temperatures [14, 15].

Histopathological investigation of a few patient lesions shows compact hyperkeratosis. The typical basket-weave configuration of the eosinophilic stratum corneum is lost. Usually, facial erythema does not require specific treatment. However, symptomatic therapy can include topical emollients, imidazole derivatives or steroids [15]. Spontaneous disappearance is observed within 8 weeks after treatment in most of the patients [14].

Between 60 and 70% of patients experience painless subungual splinter hemorrhages occurring during the first 1–2 weeks of treatment. Usually, the lesions are distally located and grow with the nail. They present as painless straight black or red lines under the fingernails. Interestingly, toe nails are only rarely affected [14]. These side effects hint to the antiangiogenic effects by sunitinib and sorafenib.

Thrombotic, embolic or simple traumatic events can present identically. However, they might rather affect only one digit in contrast to splinter hemorrhages that occur on several fingers [15]. No treatment is required, since these lesions are asymptomatic and disappear spontaneously.

Alopecia or hair loss can occur in up to 44% of the patients between 3 and 15 weeks of sorafenib treatment. Characteristically, the hair is thinned and grows patchy. A slowdown of beard growth in men is observed. Typically, this side effect does not occur under imatinib or sunitinib treatment [20]. For most patients, the symptoms resolve after cessation of the treatment or already during the treatment. In some cases, an increase in pigmentation is observed by the patients after cessation of the treatment [15].

In particular, sunitinib leads to pigmentation changes of the skin. These changes can vary between skin darkening and yellowish coloration. Strangely, local or diffuse hypopigmentation can be observed as well [16]. Transient yellow skin coloration can be observed after 3–4 weeks of 50 mg treatment per day.

Furthermore, hair depigmentation occurs in 60–64%, approximately 5–6 weeks after treatment. However, the hair shaft is not affected. Unchanged melanocytes imply that migration and survival of the melanocytes are not affected. Resolution is correlated to cessation of the treatment and appears 2–3 weeks afterwards [5]. Upon treatment cessation, hair is darker pigmented in some cases. No particular management is necessary.

Less frequent cutaneous events include xerosis cutis, which is mainly located on the inferior limbs and occurs in 10–20% of patients. A disseminated exanthematous rash is observed in several cases (fig. 3). It occurs within a few days after initial treatment. Independent of sun exposure or other treatments, eruptive benign naevi can be experienced. Furthermore, in an unknown frequency papular, pustular, cystic and keratotic lesions appear, mainly located in the face. Cases with keratoacanthoma or inflammation of actinic keratoses and squamous cell carcinoma have been reported.

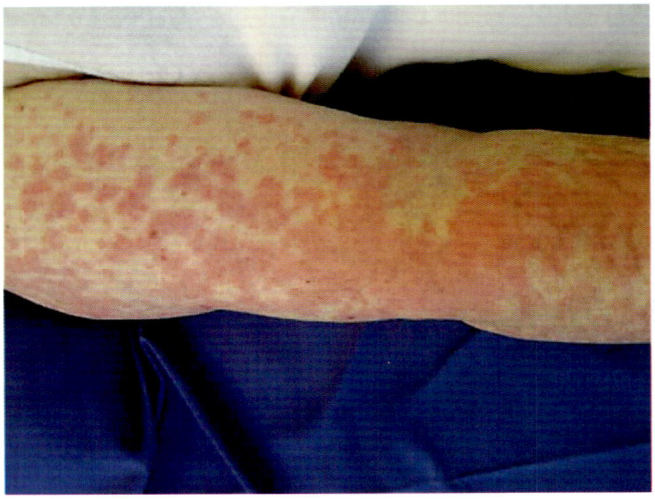

Fig. 3. Maculopapular exanthema after 14 days of treatment with the multikinase inhibitor sorafenib + DTIC in a melanoma patient.

Stomatitis, cheilitis and painful hyperkeratosis of the nipples, or facial lesions presenting as different kinds of cysts are experienced in a few patients [14, 16]. Interestingly, in a study by Lee et al. [16], stomatitis was the main adverse cutaneous event in combination with HFS under sunitinib treatment.

Even though adverse skin reactions occur with a remarkable frequency under both sorafenib and sunitinib treatment, they are usually well manageable.

Whether sorafenib induced adverse skin reactions correlate with treatment outcome still remains unclear [14, 21]. To date, clear guidelines presenting optimal prevention and management tips for cutaneous side effects are missing. It is important to establish general guidelines in order to maintain the patient's quality of life and prevent unnecessary treatment interruptions due to side effects.

BRAF Inhibitors

Significant scientific advances in the development of BRAF inhibitors were made after the identification of mutations in the gene encoding the BRAF serine-threonine kinase, which is part of the MAPK pathway. BRAF is found to be the most frequent oncogenic protein kinase mutation found in human cancer cells. The presence of a BRAF mutation in 40–70% of melanomas, and the dependence of these tumors on this pathway has led to clinical trials administrating BRAF inhibitors such as Vemurafenib (PLX 4032) that target mutated BRAF in advanced stages of melanoma with significant success [22].

However, dose-limiting side effects are observed in clinical trials, and include arthralgia, rash, nausea, photosensitivity, fatigue, pruritus and palmoplantar dysesthesia. Furthermore, keratinocytic proliferations are observed, including mostly

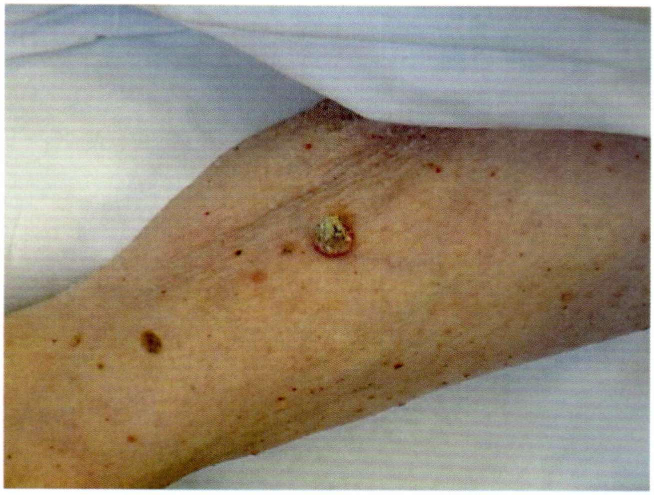

Fig. 4. Keratoacanthoma under treatment with the BRAF inhibitor Vemurafenib (PLX4032).

keratoacanthomas and rarely invasive squamous cell carcinomas. In recent studies, 89% of all side effects were grade 1 or 2, and only 5% of patients reported drug-related adverse events of grade 3 or higher. The grading was performed according to the Common Terminology Criteria for Adverse Events (version 3.0).

The skin eruption is usually evenly distributed on the face or neck, trunk and extremities. Unfortunately, as of now there is no detailed pathohistological description of the rash seen with the treatment of selective BRAF inhibitors [23].

The occurrence of keratoacanthomas which was noticed in 20–30% of patients in clinical trials has also been seen in other BRAF inhibitor studies [23–24] (fig. 4). This has prompted investigations to elucidate the development of these tumors during/after therapy. Although the detailed mechanisms are beyond the scope of this chapter, recently it has been shown that BRAF inhibitors can actually activate the RAS-RAF-MEK-ERK pathway in cancers that have the RAS mutant together with wild-type BRAF, as is seen in 20% of squamous cell carcinomas (SCC) and also in actinic keratosis (precursor of keratoacanthoma and SCC). This might be partly responsible for the growth of such tumors in patients exposed to BRAF inhibitors, and underscores the importance of further investigation and better patient population selection [25].

MEK Inhibitors

The kinases involved in the RAS-RAF mitogen-activated protein/extracellular signal-regulated kinase (MEK/ERK) signaling pathway are activated in most human cancer cells, including most melanomas. This pathway mediates proliferation and tumor growth. AZD6244 is a MEK inhibitor that inhibits phosphorylation of ERK 1/2, which is a critical step in the pathway downstream of EGFR [26].

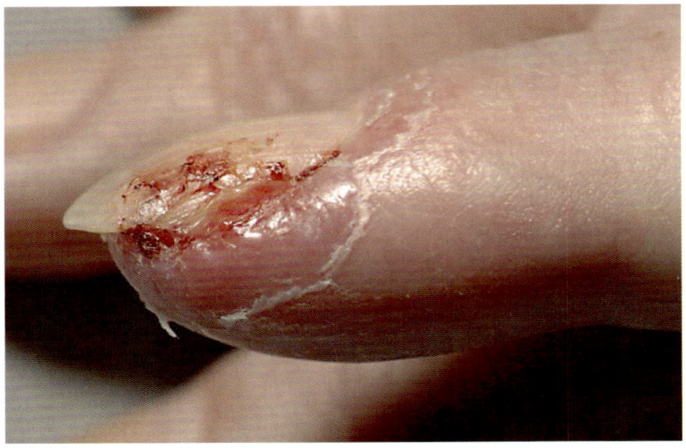

Fig. 5. Paronychia under treatment with the MEK/ERK inhibitor AZD6244.

The most common dose-limiting toxicities seen with AZD6244 administration are rash, diarrhea, nausea, vomiting, fatigue, blurred vision and other less frequent toxicities [27]. In one recently conducted clinical trial, up to 86% of patients undergoing this treatment presented with at least one cutaneous symptom [26].

The clinical manifestations can be classified according to the treatment duration into acute changes (<6 weeks of treatment) including a papulopustular rash, and chronic changes (>6 weeks of treatment) including xerosis cutis, paronychia, fissured finger tips, reduced pigmentation and hair abnormalities similar to the symptoms observed upon EGFR inhibition.

Acute Changes

Over 75% of patients develop a papulopustular rash within the first 6 weeks of therapy, which is described as papulopustules without comedones. The rash is distributed predominantly on the face, upper chest and back. The palms, soles and mucosa are usually spared. The rash peaks during the second and third week of treatment and diminishes over the following 6 weeks.

Chronic Changes

Patients may also experience xerosis cutis (erythematous skin with fine scaling and papules associated with itching) mainly on the extremities and trunk, often associated with fissured finger tips.

Paronychia is described in some patients as periungual inflammation with redness, swelling, and exudative granulation tissue (fig. 5).

In addition, reduced hair pigmentation can be observed in a few patients during the AZD6244 treatment period.

Histologically, apoptotic keratinocytes with sunburn cell morphology and focal infiltrates of neutrophils and lymphocytes with destruction of adnexal structures can be seen in acute lesions. The number of melanocytes is not reduced in acute or chronic skin lesions.

Cutaneous toxicity may be interpreted as a stress response that affects epidermal homeostasis. Also an inflammatory response is induced by the transmission of stress signals to the effectors in the cell. It seems that acute skin damage is mainly caused by neutrophils, suggesting the importance of an anti-inflammatory approach such as topical steroids. As UV may mediate additional stress signals to keratinocytes, use of UV protection is recommended. Considering the explanation above, this rash is not acneiform, and therefore the usual acne treatment can worsen it [26].

References

1 Alley E, Green R, Schuchter L: Cutaneous toxicities of cancer therapy. Curr Opin Oncol 2002;14:212–216.

2 Remlinger KA: Cutaneous reactions to chemotherapy drugs: the art of consultation. Arch Dermatol 2003;139:77–81.

3 Sun QM, Miao ZH, Lin LP, Gui M, Zhu CH, Xie H, Duan WH, Ding J: BB, a new EGFR inhibitor, exhibits prominent anti-angiogenesis and antitumor activities. Cancer Biol Ther 2009;8:1640–1647.

4 Reck M, Gutzmer R: Management of the cutaneous side effects of therapeutic epidermal growth factor receptor inhibition. Onkologie 2010;33:470–479.

5 Hammond-Thelin LA: Cutaneous reactions related to systemic immunomodulators and targeted therapeutics. Dermatol Clin 2008;26:121–159, ix.

6 Fakih M, Vincent M: Adverse events associated with anti-EGFR therapies for the treatment of metastatic colorectal cancer. Curr Oncol 2010;17(suppl 1): S18–S30.

7 Gerber PA, Buhren BA, Kurle S, Homey B: Therapy with epidermal growth factor receptor inhibitors. Clinical spectrum of cutaneous adverse effects (in German). Hautarzt 2010;61:654–661.

8 Fox LP: Nail toxicity associated with epidermal growth factor receptor inhibitor therapy. J Am Acad Dermatol 2007;56:460–465.

9 Gerber PA, Homey B: Images in clinical medicine. Erlotinib-induced hair alterations. N Engl J Med 2008;358:1175.

10 Giro C, Berger B, Bolke E, Ciernik IF, Duprez F, Locati L, Maillard S, Ozsahin M, Pfeffer R, Robertson AG, Langendijk JA, Budach W: High rate of severe radiation dermatitis during radiation therapy with concurrent cetuximab in head and neck cancer: results of a survey in EORTC institutes. Radiother Oncol 2009;90:166–171.

11 Wilhelm SM, Carter C, Tang L, Wilkie D, et al: BAY 43-9006 exhibits broad spectrum oral antitumor activity and targets the RAF/MEK/ERK pathway and receptor tyrosine kinases involved in tumor progression and angiogenesis. Cancer Res 2004;64: 7099–7109.

12 Laird AD, Christensen JG, Li G, Carver J, Smith K, Xin X, Moss KG, Louie SG, Mendel DB, Cherrington JM: SU6668 inhibits Flk-1/KDR and PDGFRbeta in vivo, resulting in rapid apoptosis of tumor vasculature and tumor regression in mice. FASEB J 2002;16: 681–690.

13 Arora A, Scholar EM: Role of tyrosine kinase inhibitors in cancer therapy. J Pharmacol Exp Ther 2005; 315:971–979.

14 Autier J, Escudier B, Wechsler J, Spatz A, Robert C: Prospective study of the cutaneous adverse effects of sorafenib, a novel multikinase inhibitor. Arch Dermatol 2008;144:886–892.

15 Robert C, Mateus C, Spatz A, Wechsler J, Escudier B: Dermatologic symptoms associated with the multikinase inhibitor sorafenib. J Am Acad Dermatol 2009;60:299–305.

16 Lee WJ, Lee JL, Chang SE, Lee MW, Kang YK, Choi JH, Moon KC, Koh JK: Cutaneous adverse effects in patients treated with the multitargeted kinase inhibitors sorafenib and sunitinib. Br J Dermatol 2009; 161:1045–1051.

17 Yang CH, Lin WC, Chuang CK, Chang YC, Pang ST, Lin YC, Kuo TT, Hsieh JJ, Chang JW: Hand-foot skin reaction in patients treated with sorafenib: a clinicopathological study of cutaneous manifestations due to multitargeted kinase inhibitor therapy. Br J Dermatol 2008;158:592–596.

18 Anderson R, Jatoi A, Robert C, Wood LS, Keating KN, Lacouture ME: Search for evidence-based approaches for the prevention and palliation of hand-foot skin reaction (HFSR) caused by the multikinase inhibitors (MKIs). Oncologist 2009;14:291–302.

19 Lacouture ME, Wu S, Robert C, Atkins MB, Kong HH, Guitart J, Garbe C, Hauschild A, Puzanov I, Alexandrescu DT, Anderson RT, Wood L, Dutcher JP: Evolving strategies for the management of hand-foot skin reaction associated with the multitargeted kinase inhibitors sorafenib and sunitinib. Oncologist 2008;13:1001–1011.

20 Robert C, Soria JC, Spatz A, Le Cesne A, Malka D, Pautier P, Wechsler J, Lhomme C, Escudier B, Boige V, Armand JP, Le Chevalier T: Cutaneous side-effects of kinase inhibitors and blocking antibodies. Lancet Oncol 2005;6:491–500.

21 Strumberg D, Awada A, Hirte H, Clark JW, Seeber S, Piccart P, Hofstra E, Voliotis D, Christensen O, Brueckner A, Schwartz B: Pooled safety analysis of BAY 43-9006 (sorafenib) monotherapy in patients with advanced solid tumours: is rash associated with treatment outcome? Eur J Cancer 2006;42:548–556.

22 Bollag G, Hirth P, Tsai J, Zhang J, et al: Clinical efficacy of a RAF inhibitor needs broad target blockade in BRAF-mutant melanoma. Nature 2010;467:596–599.

23 Flaherty K, Puzanov I, Kim K, Ribas A, McArthur G, Sosman J, O'Dwyer P, Lee R, Grippo J, Nolop K, Chapman P: Inhibition of mutated, activated BRAF in metastatic melanoma. N Engl J Med 2010;363:809–819.

24 Sosman J, Kim K, Schuchter L, Gonzalez R, Pavlick A, Weber J, McArthur G, Hutson T, Lawrence D, Moschos S, Flaherty K, Hersey P, Kefford R, Chmielowski B, Amaravadi R, Puzanov I, Li J, Bhattacharya S, Nolop K, Lee R, Joe A, Ribas A: An open-label, multicenter Phase II study of continuous oral dosing of RG7204 (PLX4032) in previously treated patients with BRAF V600E mutation-positive metastatic melanoma. Oral abstract, Society for Melanoma Research meeting 2010. Pigment Cell Melanoma Res 2010;23:912.

25 Cichowski K, Jänne P: Drug discovery: inhibitors that activate. Nature 2010;464:358–359.

26 Schad K, Baumann Conzett K, Zipser M, Enderlin V, Kamarashev J, French L, Dummer R: Mitogen-activated protein/extracellular signal-regulated kinase kinase inhibition results in biphasic alteration of epidermal homeostasis with keratinocytic apoptosis and pigmentation disorders. Clin Cancer Res 2010;16:1058–1064.

27 Adjei A, Cohen R, Franklin W, Morris C, Wilson D, Molina J, Hanson L, Gore L, Chow L, Leong S, Maloney L, Gordon G, Simmons H, Marlow A, Litwiler K, Brown S, Poch G, Kane K, Haney J, Eckhardt S: Phase I pharmacokinetic and pharmacodynamic study of the oral, small-molecule mitogen-activated protein kinase kinase 1/2 inhibitor AZD6244 (ARRY-142886) in patients with advanced cancers. J Clin Oncol 2008;26:2139–2146.

Prof. Reinhard Dummer
Department of Dermatology, University Hospital Zurich
Gloriastrasse 31
CH–8091 Zurich (Switzerland)
Tel. +41 44 255 25 07, E-Mail Reinhard.Dummer@usz.ch

French LE (ed): Adverse Cutaneous Drug Eruptions.
Chem Immunol Allergy. Basel, Karger, 2012, vol 97, pp 203–216

Cutaneous Drug Eruptions Associated with the Use of Biologics and Cutaneous Drug Eruptions Mimicking Specific Skin Diseases

Julien Seneschal · Brigitte Milpied · Alain Taieb

Department of Dermatology, Saint-André Hospital, Bordeaux University, Bordeaux, France

Abstract

Drug eruptions are common adverse events affecting approximately 3% of hospitalized patients, and can be seen with the use of almost any medication. Making a diagnosis could be challenging because no pattern is specific for a particular drug. A study of clinical aspects, histopathology and history of drug intake is usually necessary to establish the diagnosis, and discontinue the offending agent when feasible. The pathomechanisms of drug-related skin reactions remain unclear. However, the induction of drug reactions by a new class of biologics which block a specific target should help to better understand the pathogenesis of these eruptions.

Essentials in a Nutshell

- Drug eruptions mimicking specific skin diseases are common
- Because of the absence of specific patterns, a clinicopathologic confrontation is always necessary for a definitive diagnosis
- The emergence of skin eruptions mimicking specific inflammatory skin diseases with the use of biologics which target specific proteins or pathways will help to better understand the pathomechanisms of these eruptions

Introduction

Cutaneous drug eruptions are common side effects of drug therapy. They can reproduce a variety of inflammatory skin diseases and may thus be difficult to distinguish from these. While the exact mechanism of cutaneous adverse reactions to drugs remains unclear, a deregulation of the immune/inflammatory system as a consequence of the culprit drug seems to be a common denominator. The emergence of adverse skin reactions associated with the use of modern therapies called biologics which target a specific protein should help us to better understand in the future the mechanism of these skin reactions. In this chapter, we will review the clinical and pathological features of inflammatory skin conditions induced by drugs and discuss the therapies implicated including biologics.

Psoriasiform Eruptions

Drug-induced psoriasiform eruptions appear morphologically similar to idiopathic psoriasis. They usually present with erythematous plaques with thick, large, dry silvery scales. However, drug-associated psoriasiform reactions can also present as other psoriatic variants, such as limited plaque, generalized plaque with palmoplantar pustular lesions, erythroderma, nail or scalp involvement. The period between initiation of treatment and onset of the eruption varies among drugs from less than 1 month up to more than 3 months. Histologically, psoriasis exacerbated by drugs is similar to idiopathic psoriasis. In contrast, drug-induced psoriasiform eruptions associated with drugs show certain pathological features of psoriasis such as psoriasiform hyperplasia, decreased granular cell layer and neutrophils within parakeratosis, but can also be associated with inflammatory infiltrates of lymphocytes with lichenoid/spongiotic pattern, apoptotic keratinocytes, and rare eosinophils [1, 2].

Medications can either induce lesions de novo or exacerbate preexisting disease in patients with psoriasis. The most common drugs are listed in table 1. Recently, biologics such as anti-TNF-α agents and anti-CD11a have been reported to induce psoriasiform eruptions.

TNF-α blocker therapies are indicated for the treatment of arthritis, inflammatory bowel diseases and psoriasis. These treatments have been associated with the development of paradoxical psoriasiform eruptions (fig. 1). All TNF-α inhibitors currently available have been implicated in the induction of these eruptions. Most patients have no personal or family history of psoriasis. No predilection for age or sex could be statistically proven. The time to induction of cutaneous adverse effects varies considerably between patients (from the first injection to several months). Eruptions are treated in most patients by local treatments including topical steroids, vitamin D analogues or keratolytics and/or systemic antipsoriatic therapy like UV irradiation, methotrexate or occasional use of cyclosporine [3]. The pathogenesis remains elusive but a local production of type I interferons such as IFN-α, induced by the blocking of the TNF-α seems to play a role in the emergence of the eruptions. IFN-α is known to induce expression of the chemokine receptor CXCR3 on T cells, inducing T cell migration to the skin [4, 5]. Increased IFN-α expression does not fully explain the development of psoriasiform eruptions under anti-TNF-α treatment, and the role of others cytokines such as IL-17 and IL-22 needs to be defined [6].

Table 1. Drug eruptions mimicking skin disorders

Clinical presentation	Pattern and distribution of skin lesions	Mucous membrane involvement	Implicated drugs
Psoriasiform	Erythematous plaques with sick, large, dry silvery scale, pustular, erythrodermic, palmoplantar, nail or scalp involvement	Absent	IFN-α, anti-TNF-α, anti-CD11a (efalizumab), lithium, beta-blocker, anticonvulsant drugs, metformin, terbinafine, rGM-CSF, captopril, digoxin
Lichenoid	Violaceous flat-topped polygonal papules, trunk and extremities involvement	Present	Beta-blocker, thiazides, captopril, methyl-dopa, oral hypoglycemics, NSAIDs, quinidine, gold, anti-TNF-α, imatinib
Vasculitis	Purpuric papules, urticaria, hemorrhagic bullae, ulcers, nodules, Raynaud's syndrome, digital necrosis	Absent	All pharmacology class ANCA positive: propylthiouracil, hydralazine, allopurinol, minocycline, penicillamine, and phenytoin ANCA negative: rGM-CSF, isotretinoin, methotrexate, biologics as anti-TNF-α
Lupus-like eruptions	SLE symptoms, vasculitis, purpuric lesions, Raynaud's syndrome SCLE Chronic cutaneous lupus: discoid lupus	Present	SLE: hydralazine, procainamine, isoniazid, methyldopa, chlorpromazine, quinidine and minocycline SCLE: antihypertensive treatment: calcium channel blockers, angiotensin-converting enzyme inhibitors and thiazide diuretics; more recently, terbinafine, bupropion, acebutolol, proton pump inhibitors such as lansoprazole and pantoprazole, leflunomide and biologics (anti-TNF-α) Chronic cutaneous lupus: fluorouracil and anti-TNF-α
Bullous disorders			
Pemphigus	Flaccid bullae, chest	Present/absent	Thiol drugs: penicillamine, captopril and enalapril Non-thiol drugs: piroxicam, penicillin, rifampicin, propranolol, imiquimod
Bullous pemphigoid	Tense bullae, widespread	Present/absent	Furosemide, amoxicillin, ampicillin, penicillamine, cephalexin, phenacetin, penicillamine, psoralen-UVA light, beta-blockers, captopril

Table 1. Continued

Clinical presentation	Pattern and distribution of skin lesions	Mucous membrane involvement	Implicated drugs
Pseudo-porphyria	Skin fragility, blister formation in photodistribution	Absent	NSAIDs such as propionic acid derivatives (naproxen, diflunisal, ketopren, nabumetone, oxaprozin, mefenamic acid, rofecoxib), antibiotics (tetracycline, ampicillin, sulbactam and cefepime), voriconazole, diuretics (furosemide, chlorthalidone, butamide, hydrochlorothiazide) amiodarone, 5-fluorouracil, cyclosporine, vitamin A derivatives, flutamide, oral contraceptive pills (levonorgestrel and ethinyl estradiol)
Linear IgA eruptions	Varied bullous dermatosis	Present/absent	Vancomycin, lithium, antibiotics (ampicillin, cephalosporins, metronidazole and rifampicin), diclofenac, piroxicam, amiodarone, captopril, phenytoin, furosemide, ACE inhibitors, GM-CSF
Acneiform	Monomorphic follicular eruption on face and trunk	Absent	Corticosteroids, androgens, oral contraceptives, lithium, haloperidol, isoniazid, phenytoin, tetracyclines, vitamins B_1, B_6, B_{12}, quinidine, azathioprine, cyclosporine, sirolimus, iodides, bromides, EGFR inhibitors
Interstitial granulomatous dermatitis	Erythematous erythematoviolaceous papules or plaques/ annular lesions	Absent	Calcium channel blockers, ACE inhibitors, lipid-lowering agents, beta-blockers, antihistamines, anticonvulsants, antidepressants, anti-TNF-α, methotrexate
Pseudolymphoma	Erythematous or erythematoviolaceous papules or nodules/ mycosis fungoides-like eruptions	Absent	Anticonvulsants, antipsychotics, or ACE inhibitors Calcium channel blockers, antihistamines and antidepressants and imatinib
Pigmentation disorders			
Hyper pigmentation	Acquired and progressive Affect sun exposed areas	Present/absent	Minocycline, antimalarials, amiodarone, oral contraceptives, imipramine, chemotherapeutic agents such as cytostatic dugs, and clofazimine, tacrolimus
Hypo pigmentation	Acquired, area where treatment was applied	Absent	Topical agents: retinoic acid, corticosteroids, monobenzyl ether of hydroquinone
Hair disorders			
Hair loss	Anagen or telogen effluvium: non-scarring alopecia	Absent	Antineoplastic drugs, antiepileptic drugs, beta-blockers, antidepressants, antithyroid drugs, IFN agents, oral contraceptives and lipid-modifying agents

Table 1. Continued

Clinical presentation	Pattern and distribution of skin lesions	Mucous membrane involvement	Implicated drugs
Hair growth	Hirsutism/ hypertrichosis	Absent	Hirsutism: anabolic steroids, oral contraceptives of the nonsteroid progesterone group, testosterone, and corticotropin Hypertrichosis: streptomycin, steroids, vasodilator, diuretics, phenytoin) immunosuppressive agents, psoralens and zidovudine
Hair structure	Brittle, fine, curly hair	Absent	EGFR inhibitors

Flares of psoriasis can also occur during anti-CD11a treatment (efalizumab). Efalizumab was initially approved for the treatment of psoriasis before being suspended in the US and the European market because of safety concerns [7]. Moreover, there have been reports of patients whose psoriasis seemingly changed in character during therapy. Some cases of inverse psoriasis and some cases of pustular psoriasis have been reported. Some patients would develop an erythematous papular eruption during the course of the treatment. These lesions were called Papp's papules by a number of dermatologists, and may represent a drug-induced eruption or a disease modification. These lesions resolved without additional treatment or after application of topical corticosteroids [8].

Lichenoid Eruptions

Lichenoid drug eruptions appear very similar to idiopathic lichen planus with violaceous flat-topped polyglonal papules with or without oral involvement. However, drug-induced eruption generally has a more extensive symmetrical involvement of the trunk and extremities when compared with lichen planus, which classically involves flexural areas. The eruptions generally develop insidiously weeks to months after the beginning of the treatment. Histologically, lichenoid drug eruptions are very similar to pathological features of lichenoid dermatitis with epidermal hyperplasia, hyperkeratosis, hypergranulosis, basilar vacuolar change, scattered necrotic keratinocytes, and a dermal lichenoid mononuclear cell infiltrate with melanophages. However, a drug-induced lichenoid eruption can be associated with more necrotic keratinocytes and eosinophils in the infiltrate [1]. Drugs implicated in lichenoid drug eruptions are listed in table 1.

Anti-TNF-α agents can also be associated with the induction of lichenoid eruptions. According to recent data, no predilection for age and sex has been found. Clinical features similar to idiopathic lichen planus have been described. Other skin

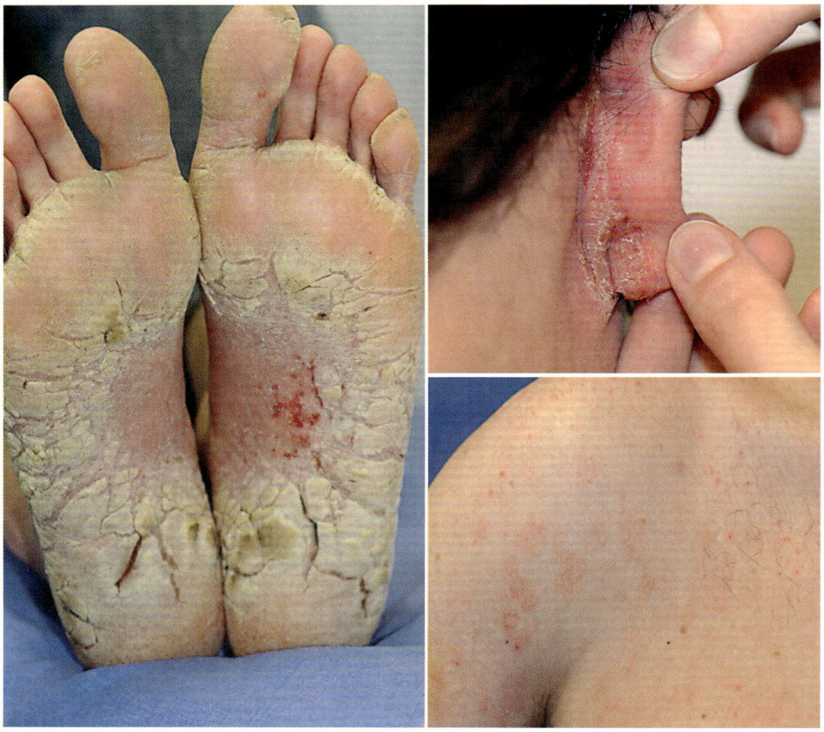

Fig. 1. Psoriasiform eruptions under anti-TNF-α treatment.

lesions might be less specific, described as erythematous papular rashes, macular exanthema, erythematosquamous exanthema or white oral plaques, but all biopsy specimens show a lichenoid interface dermatitis. In most cases, anti TNF-α treatment has been stopped with complete recovery. Some patients may experience a complete recovery despite the continuation of the treatment. Topical corticosteroids can be used with partial improvement [9].

Vasculitis

The term vasculitis refers to inflammation targeted to the blood vessels resulting in vessel wall damage. It is estimated that about 20–30% of all cases of vasculitis can be attributed to the ingestion/administration of drugs. Clinically, drug-associated vasculitis is localized to the skin. Symptoms include palpable purpuric papules, sometimes pruritic and usually confined to the lower extremities. Urticaria can be a manifestation of small vessel vasculitis. Other clinical features include hemorrhagic bullae, ulcers, nodules, Raynaud's syndrome, and digital necrosis. Systemic vasculitis with serious complications may also occur but remains a rare event.

Although drug-related vasculitis has been reported to occur within hours to a year after culprit drug intake, it usually occurs 7–10 days after administration of the offending treatment. Identifying the offending drug is the most important aspect of treatment as its discontinuation is followed by a rapid improvement of the vasculitis in most cases. Histopathologic findings of drug-induced vasculitis are similar to those of leukocytoclastic vaculitis, namely, an inflammatory infiltrate rich in neutrophils targeting the post-capillary venules resulting in damage of the vessel wall. According to certain studies, the presence of eosinophils in the sample could help to distinguish drug-induced vasculitis from other causes [10].

The list of medications reported to induce vasculitic reactions is large, including almost every pharmacological class, and biologics such as anti-TNF-α as well. The offending drugs are listed in table 1.

Lupus Erythematous-Like Eruptions

As for psoriasiform eruptions, drugs may either cause an exacerbation of preexisting lupus, or provoke drug-induced lupus.

Clinically, in a similar manner to for idiopathic lupus, drug-induced lupus can be divided into systemic (SLE), subacute cutaneous (SCLE) and chronic cutaneous lupus. The time to development of clinical disease after initiation of the drug ranges from 1 month to almost 8–10 months. SCLE represents the most common presentation of drug-induced cutaneous lupus. Drug-induced SCLE is similar to idiopathic SCLE in terms of both clinical and serologic characteristics. Characteristic skin symptoms include erythematous papules or plaques covered with fine scale on sun-exposed areas. However, a frequent involvement of the lower legs and a bullous presentation are more frequently seen in drug induced SCLE than in the idiopathic form. Vasculitic skin lesions can also develop in drug-induced SCLE, usually on the lower leg. Systemic symptoms are usually absent. Blood analysis frequently reveals the presence of anti-Ro/SSA antibodies, together with antinuclear antibodies (ANA) and sometimes with anti-La/SSB antibodies. Skin biopsy will show vacuolar alteration of the epidermis, associated with a thickened basement membrane.

Drug-induced SLE has been shown to resemble a milder version of idiopathic SLE. However, no sex predilection is found. Skin involvement is considered to be less frequent in drug-induced SLE compared with idiopathic SLE: the classic cutaneous manifestations including malar rash, mucosal ulcers, scalp involvement and Raynaud's symptoms are absent. Purpuric lesions, erythema nodosum, and photosensitivity are more frequent. Vasculitis can also be found. Systemic symptoms are frequent including fever, arthralgia and myalgia. The typical laboratory profile of drug-induced SLE consists of positive ANA and antihistone antibodies (+ve in 95% of patients). Histological findings show vacuolar alterations along the dermoepidermal junction, necrotic keratinocytes with a lymphocytic infiltrate. Papillary dermis can be subjected to edema with dilated blood vessels and scattered melanophages [11].

Drugs implicated in the induction of lupus erythematous-like eruptions are listed in table 1. Moreover biologics such as TNF-α antagonists have been described as offending drugs. Symptoms of the lupus-like syndrome associated with TNF-α blockers include fever, malaise, and asthenia. Cutaneous signs include malar rash, photosensitivity, and/or discoid lupus, oral ulcers. ANA are found in 95% of the patients. Cytopenia, antiphospholipid, anti-Sm, anti SSA/SSB and anti-RNP antibodies can be found in 10–20% of patients. The treatment of the lupus-related syndrome requires anti-TNF therapy to be stopped in the majority of cases. Corticosteroids and immunosuppressive agents can also be used if needed [12].

Vesiculobullous Drug Eruptions

This category of vesiculobullous reactions includes drug-induced pemphigus, bullous pemphigoid, pseudoporphyria cutanea tarda, and drug-induced linear IgA eruptions.

Drug-Induced Pemphigus

Drug-induced pemphigus usually presents with scaling and crusting as in pemphigus foliaceus. Moreover, drug-induced pemphigus frequently presents with a prodromal morbilliform or urticarial eruption as seen in other drug eruptions. Lesions of drug-related pemphigus usually develop within several weeks or months after beginning of the offending treatment. Histological findings in drug-related pemphigus are very similar to idiopathic pemphigus with acantholytic cells in a blister in the upper part of the spinous zone, in the granular zone, or in both. These pathological features can vary according to the time at which the skin sample is taken. Immunofluorescence of perilesional epidermis shows intercellular IgG. Blood analysis reveals circulating antibodies in 70% of the patients. These antibodies can be directed against desmoglein 1 or 3 or both. The offending drugs are listed in table 1.

Drug-Induced Bullous Pemphigoid

Drug-induced bullous pemphigoid can encompass a wide variety range of presentations, from the classical features of bullous pemphigoid, erythema multiforme lesions, pemphigus-like lesions or scarring plaques as seen in cicatricial pemphigoid. However, in contrast with patients affected by the idiopathic form, patients with drug-induced bullous pemphigoid are generally younger and symptoms generally resolve after discontinuation of the drug.

Bullous pemphigoid-like lesions can occur weeks or several months after the beginning of the culprit agent. Like in idiopathic bullous pemphigoid, skin biopsy analysis reveals subepidermal bullae with an abundant number of eosinophils and preserved dermal papillae. Dermal edema and a lymphocytic infiltrate are also present. Direct immunofluorescence shows linear IgG and C3 in the basement membrane zone of the dermoepidermal junction. But a possible lack of tissue-bound and circulating antibasal membrane zone IgG is also possible [13, 14].

A variety of medications have been reported to induce bullous pemphigoid including sulphur-containing drugs such as furosemide. Other agents known to cause drug-induced pemphigoid are listed in table 1.

Drug-Induced Pseudoporphyrias

Pseudoporphyria is a cutaneous phototoxic disorder that can resemble either porphyria cutanea tarda in adults or erythropoietic protoporphyria in children. However, porphyrin profiles are normal. Moreover, pseudoporphyria is rarely associated with other clinical features observed in porphyria cutanea tarda in adults such as hypertrichosis, hyperpigmentation, and sclerodermoid changes. Pseudoporphyria of the porphyria cutanea tarda variety is characterized by skin fragility, blister formation and scarring in photodistributed zones. The other clinical pattern mimics erythropoietic protoporphyria and manifests as cutaneous burning, erythema, and vesiculation. The eruption may begin within 1 day of initiation of therapy or may be delayed for as long as 1 year. Just like porphyria cutanea tarda, a supepidermal blister beneath which the dermal papillae are usually preserved characterizes pseudoporphyria histopathologically. There is an accumulation of PAS-positive eosinophilic hyalinized material around the venules and capillaries of the upper dermis. A mild lymphocytic infiltrate is generally observed. Solar elastosis generally associated with porphyria cutanea tarda is usually absent in pseudoporphyria [15]. The most common medications implicated in drug-induced pseudoporphyria are listed in table 1.

Drug-Induced Linear IgA Bullous Eruption

The clinical, histological and immunofluorescence features of drug-induced linear IgA disease are impossible to differentiate from the idiopathic form. Both have varied clinical presentations as erythema multiforme-like lesions, bullous pemphigoid-like lesions, or dermatitis herpetiformis-like lesions. Drug-induced like lesions are usually transient and disappear within weeks after discontinuation of the offending agent [16].

The eruption typically appears 1–15 days (average 8 days) after the beginning of intake of the culprit agent. Pathology shows in early lesions a predominantly neutrophilic interface dermatitis with a mixed infiltrate containing eosinophils around the vessels of the superficial vascular plexus. Direct immunofluorescence, as in its idiopathic counterpart, shows a linear band of IgA along the dermoepidermal junction. The most common medication reported to induce drug induced linear IgA bullous reaction is intravenous vancomycin. Other medications are listed in table 1.

Acneiform Eruptions

The term acneiform eruption applies to any eruption resembling acne vulgaris. Clinically, the follicular eruption starts with an inflammatory papule or pustule. In contrast to acne vulgaris, acneiform eruptions due to drugs tend to be monomorphic and comedones are generally absent. The face and trunk are generally involved. These reactions generally appear after 7–14 days of treatment. Histopathologic features show a keratin-filled follicular plug within a widened infundibulum. Infundibular spongiosis, perifollicular edema with mild perivascular and peri-infundibular infiltrates of neutrophils and lymphocytes can also be associated [17].

The most common drugs implicated in the emergence of acneiform eruptions are listed in table 1. More recently, new agents targeting epidermal growth receptors have been identified as frequent inducers of papulopustular eruptions or acneiform eruptions. Members of the human epidermal receptor (HER/ErbB) family, in particular epidermal growth factor receptor (EGFR or HER1/ErbB1) and HER2/neu/ErbB2, are receptor tyrosine kinases that play a key role in the pathogenesis of many cancers. Drugs designed to target EGFR and/or HER2 receptors include small molecule tyrosine kinase inhibitors and anti-EGFR monoclonal antibodies (cetuximab, panitumumab, matuzumab, zalutumumab, nimotuzumab). EGFR inhibitors are approved to treat non-small cell lung cancer, pancreatic cancer, colorectal cancer and head and neck cancer. The papulopustular eruption is the most common adverse cutaneous reaction associated with EGFR inhibitors (fig. 2). It affects the sebaceous areas in the scalp, face, and upper trunk, and can extend to other parts of the body in severe cases. The eruption starts as skin redness and swelling, and then progresses to papulopustular eruptions that affect primarily the sebaceous areas. In general, patients treated with monoclonal antibodies have more frequent and severe skin rash than those treated with small molecules. No predilection for sex has been reported. Skin biopsy specimens show a superficial dermal infiltrate dominated by neutrophils surrounding hyperkeratotic and ectatic follicular infundibula, and a suppurative superficial folliculitis. Culture of pustules for bacteria and fungi is negative [18]. The pathogenesis of these eruptions remains unclear: inhibition of EGFR-mediated signaling pathways affects keratinocytes by inducing growth arrest and apoptosis, decreasing cell migration, increasing cell attachment and differentiation, and stimulating inflammation. It was recently shown that blocking EGFR signaling results in the overexpression of inflammatory chemokines in keratinocytes

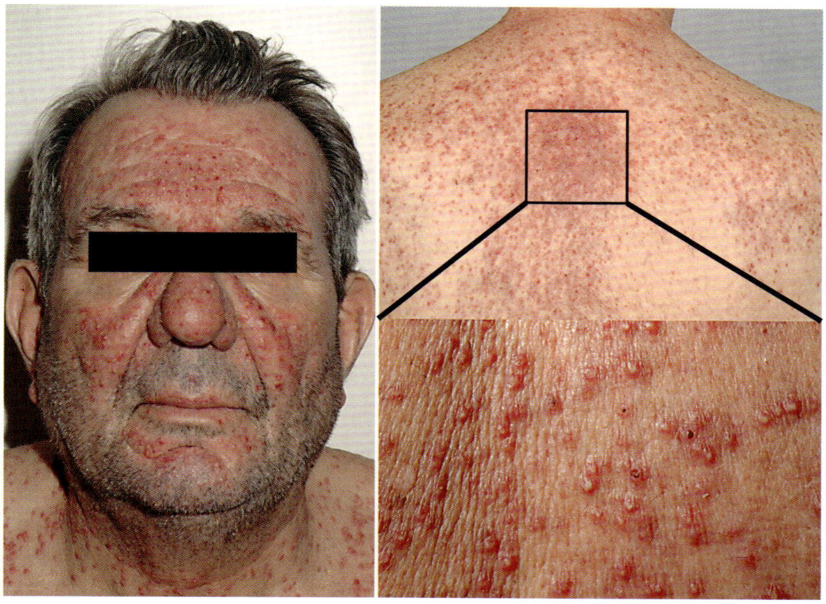

Fig. 2. Acneiform eruptions under EGFR inhibitors.

such as TNF-α-driven CCL2, CCL5, and CXCL10 [19–21]. Unfortunately, there is currently no evidence-based treatment guideline to prevent or treat the EGFR inhibitor-associated skin rash. All skin rashes usually resolve within one month after discontinuation of EGFR inhibitors.

Drug-Induced Interstitial Granulomatous Dermatitis

The interstitial granulomatous drug eruption was first described in 1998 in a study of 20 patients [22]. Clinically, patients presented erythematous or erythematoviolaceous papules or plaques in annular array over the skin folds. The major differential diagnosis is granuloma annulare or interstitial granulomatous dermatitis with arthritis. Histopathological features show interstitial lymphocytes and histiocytes with elastic and collagen fiber fragmentation and vacuolar interface dermatitis. Sometimes, atypical lymphocytes may be observed. The most common implicated treatments are listed in table 1.

Lymphomatoid Drug Eruptions

Lymphomatoid drug eruptions define eruptions clinically and histopathologically resembling lymphoma. Clinically, these eruptions are characterized by the emergence of localized erythematous or erythematoviolaceous papules or nodules. Other symptoms observed are patch and plaque-like mycosis fungoides or erythroderma. The eruption can appear from weeks to months or years after starting the culprit agent. Histopathological features generally include a lymphocytic infiltrate involving the papillary and reticular dermis [23]. The infiltrating lymphocytes may have atypical nuclei. Plasma cells and eosinophils can be encountered. Mucinous degeneration of follicles can also be observed. The most common drugs associated with the development of lymphomatoid drug eruptions are listed in table 1.

Skin Pigmentation Disorders

Clinical features of drug-induced hyperpigmentation are not specific. However, in drug-associated hyperpigmentation, generally, the pigmentation disorder is by definition acquired and progressive. It affects generally the sun-exposed areas and may also involve the mucous membranes. Finally the pigmentation usually fades slowly and incompletely when the offending drug is stopped. The pigmentation disorder usually occurs 4–6 months after starting the culprit drug. Histopathological features are not specific, but pattern of accumulation of melanin can distinguish specific offending drugs. Accumulation of melanin can be associated with inflammatory lesions [24]. Presence or accumulation of an unusual pigment be it free or included in dermal macrophages can also be observed with drugs such as silver or gold salts. The most common drugs implicated in drug-induced hyperpigmentation are listed in table 1.

Drug-Induced Hypopigmentation

Hypopigmentation can occur with the long-term use of several topical medications including retinoic acid, corticosteroids, and monobenzyl ether of hydroquinone [24].

Hair Disorders

Drug-Induced Hair Loss

Drug-induced hair loss can be categorized into two different modalities: (1) anagen effluvium: hair loss occurs within days to weeks of drug administration, and (2) telogen effluvium: hair loss starts 2–4 months after administration of the offending drug. Clinically, the hair loss is characterized by diffuse non-scarring alopecia. The differential diagnosis with other causes of hair loss is generally difficult, and the improvement of the hair disorder after withdrawal of the culprit treatment can be an argument for the diagnosis of drug-induced hair loss. Normalization of hair loss may require 2–3 months after drug discontinuation. Many agents listed in table 1 can induce hair loss [25].

Drug-Induced Hirsutism or Hypertrichosis

Hirsutism is an excessive growth of coarse hair with masculine characteristics observed in females. Hair growth is the result of an androgenic stimulation of hormone-sensitive hair follicles. Anabolic steroids, oral contraceptives of the non-steroid progesterone group, testosterone, and corticotropin can induce hirsutism.

Drug-induced hypertrichosis is mainly localized on the forehead and temporal areas of the face. The main drugs responsible for hypertrichosis are listed in table 1 [25].

Drug-Induced Changes in Hair Structure

Changes in hair structure were recently reported with new agents such as EGFR inhibitors: scalp hair can become more brittle, fine and curly, and this generally occurs 2–3 months after treatment administration.

Conclusion

Drugs can induce or reproduce various types of inflammatory skin disorders. Clinical and histological similarities with the idiopathic conditions can make the diagnosis difficult to establish. However, it is commonly assumed that the diagnosis of drug-induced skin diseases should be made in patients where the skin reaction occurs after administration of the treatment and disappears after discontinuation of the drug. Consideration of clinical and pathological features can also be helpful in the diagnosis. For example, the presence of eosinophils in the inflammatory infiltrate on skin sections can be an argument for a drug-related event.

In conclusion, because of their frequency, physicians should be aware of drug reactions mimicking skin inflammatory disorders in which besides the usual drugs, biologics have become more and more implicated. Because of the more selective effect of biologics, new pathomechanisms are emerging, which may pertain to other drug reactions and common inflammatory skin disorders.

References

1 Justiniano H, Berlingeri-Ramos AC, Sanchez JL: Pattern analysis of drug-induced skin diseases. Am J Dermatopathol 2008;30:352–369.

2 Sehgal VN, Dogra S, Srivastava G, Aggarwal AK: Psoriasiform dermatoses. Ind J Dermatol Venereol Leprol 2008;74:94–99.

3 Wollina U, Hansel G, Koch A, Schonlebe J, Kostler E, Haroske G: Tumor necrosis factor-alpha inhibitor-induced psoriasis or psoriasiform exanthemata: first 120 cases from the literature including a series of six new patients. Am J Clin Dermatol 2008;9:1–14.

4 Seneschal J, Lepreux S, Milpied B, Schaeverbeke T, Taieb A: Psoriasiform eruptions during anti TNF-alpha treatment: psoriasis or not? Arch Dermatol 2007;143:1593–1595, author reply 5.

5 Seneschal J, Milpied B, Vergier B, Lepreux S, Schaeverbeke T, Taieb A: Cytokine imbalance with increased production of interferon-alpha in psoriasiform eruptions associated with antitumour necrosis factor-alpha treatments. Br J Dermatol 2009;161:1081–1088.

6 Ma HL, Napierata L, Stedman N, et al: Tumor necrosis factor alpha blockade exacerbates murine psoriasis-like disease by enhancing Th17 function and decreasing expansion of Treg cells. Arthritis Rheum 2010;62:430–440.

7 Carson KR, Focosi D, Major EO, et al: Monoclonal antibody-associated progressive multifocal leucoencephalopathy in patients treated with rituximab, natalizumab, and efalizumab: a review from the Research on Adverse Drug Events and Reports (RADAR) Project. Lancet Oncol 2009;10:816–824.

8 Thielen AM, Kuenzli S, Saurat JH: Cutaneous adverse events of biological therapy for psoriasis: review of the literature. Dermatology 2005;211:209–217.

9 Asarch A, Gottlieb AB, Lee J, et al: Lichen planus-like eruptions: an emerging side effect of tumor necrosis factor-alpha antagonists. J Am Acad Dermatol 2009;61:104–111.

10 Wiik A: Drug-induced vasculitis. Curr Opin Rheumatol 2008;20:35–39.

11 Marzano AV, Vezzoli P, Crosti C: Drug-induced lupus: an update on its dermatologic aspects. Lupus 2009;18:935–940.

12 Callen JP: Complications and adverse reactions in the use of newer biologic agents. Semin Cutan Med Surg 2007;26:6–14.

13 Brenner S, Wolf R, Ruocco V: Drug-induced pemphigus. I. A survey. Clin Dermatol 1993;11:501–505.

14 Ruocco V, De Angelis E, Lombardi ML: Drug-induced pemphigus. II. Pathomechanisms and experimental investigations. Clin Dermatol 1993;11:507–513.

15 Schanbacher CF, Vanness ER, Daoud MS, Tefferi A, Su WP: Pseudoporphyria: a clinical and biochemical study of 20 patients. Mayo Clin Proc 2001;76:488–492.

16 Kuechle MK, Stegemeir E, Maynard B, Gibson LE, Leiferman KM, Peters MS: Drug-induced linear IgA bullous dermatosis: report of six cases and review of the literature. J Am Acad Dermatol 1994;30:187–192.

17 Momin SB, Peterson A, Del Rosso JQ: A status report on drug-associated acne and acneiform eruptions. J Drugs Dermatol 2010;9:627–636.

18 Li T, Perez-Soler R: Skin toxicities associated with epidermal growth factor receptor inhibitors. Target Oncol 2009;4:107–119.

19 Mascia F, Cataisson C, Lee TC, et al: EGFR regulates the expression of keratinocyte-derived granulocyte/macrophage colony-stimulating factor in vitro and in vivo. J Invest Dermatol 2010;130:682–693.

20 Pastore S, Mascia F, Mariani V, Girolomoni G: The epidermal growth factor receptor system in skin repair and inflammation. J Invest Dermatol 2008;128:1365–1374.

21 Pastore S, Mascia F, Mariotti F, Dattilo C, Mariani V, Girolomoni G: ERK1/2 regulates epidermal chemokine expression and skin inflammation. J Immunol 2005;174:5047–5056.

22 Magro CM, Crowson AN, Schapiro BL: The interstitial granulomatous drug reaction: a distinctive clinical and pathological entity. J Cutan Pathol 1998;25:72–78.

23 Albrecht J, Fine LA, Piette W: Drug-associated lymphoma and pseudolymphoma: recognition and management. Dermatol Clin 2007;25:233–244, vii.

24 Dereure O: Drug-induced skin pigmentation. Epidemiology, diagnosis and treatment. Am J Clin Dermatol 2001;2:253–262.

25 Valeyrie-Allanore L, Sassolas B, Roujeau JC: Drug-induced skin, nail and hair disorders. Drug Saf 2007;30:1011–1030.

Dr. Julien Seneschal
Department of Dermatology, Saint-André Hospital, Bordeaux University
1 rue Jean Burguet
FR–33075 Bordeaux (France)
Tel. +33 5 56 79 47 05, E-Mail julien.seneschal@chu-bordeaux.fr

French LE (ed): Adverse Cutaneous Drug Eruptions.
Chem Immunol Allergy. Basel, Karger, 2012, vol 97, pp 217–233

Desensitization for Hypersensitivity Reactions to Medications

Maria del Carmen Sancho · Rebecca Breslow · David Sloane · Mariana Castells

Harvard Medical School, Division of Rheumatology, Allergy and Immunology, Department of Medicine, Brigham and Women's Hospital, Boston, Mass., USA

Abstract

Rapid drug desensitization (RDD) is a technique that induces temporary tolerance to a drug, allowing a medication-allergic patient to receive the optimal agent for his or her disease. Through RDD, patients with IgE and non-IgE hypersensitivity reactions (HSRs) including anaphylaxis can safely be administered important medications while minimizing or completely inhibiting adverse reactions. Adverse reactions to drugs are increasingly recognized as important contributors to disease as well as impediments to the best treatment of dermatological, infectious, autoimmune, and neoplastic disorders. With the development of novel pharmacologic agents and the evolution of personalized treatments based on pharmacogenetic profiling, clinicians must decide which agent is the best for a particular patient with a given disease. Biological agents have greatly improved the treatment of chronic inflammatory diseases and malignancies while limiting some medication-associated toxicities. Because of better outcomes, longer patient survival, and extended treatment courses, patients are exposed to drugs more frequently and for longer time periods, increasing the risk of sensitization and the potential for HSRs. The frequency of adverse drug reactions has therefore increased in the last 10 years. Because of the severity of some reactions and the fear of inducing a potentially lethal reaction in highly sensitized patients, first-line treatments are sometimes abandoned, relegating hypersensitive patients to secondary, less effective, therapy. Some of these reactions are mast cell-mediated HSRs, a subset of which occur through an IgE-dependent mechanism, and are thus true allergies. Others involve mast cells, but an IgE mechanism cannot be demonstrated. Both types of reactions are amenable to RDD, and our group has successfully performed several hundred desensitizations to chemotherapy, antibiotics and biological agents including monoclonal antibodies with a standardized 12-step protocol that can be universally applied to all desensitizations. The molecular basis of RDD has now been studied, and an in vitro mouse mast cell model has shown that RDD is an antigen-specific process that does not induce subclinical mast cell mediator release, and that blocks the release of acute and late mast cell mediators by preventing calcium influx and antigen/IgE/and IgE receptor internalization.

Essentials in a Nutshell

- Rapid desensitizations are safe and effective for the treatment of type I IgE-dependent and IgE-independent hypersensitivity reactions (HSRs), including anaphylaxis
- In vitro rapid drug desensitization (RDD) is an antigen-specific process that does not induce subclinical mast cell mediator release and prevents antigen/IgE/IgE receptor internalization
- Antibiotic desensitizations can be safely performed in cystic fibrosis patients with very low pulmonary function before or after lung transplant
- A 12-step RDD protocol developed at BWH is the safest and most effective universal protocol that can be used for antibiotics, chemotherapy and biological agent desensitizations based on several hundred cases

Introduction

Adverse reactions to drugs are increasingly recognized as important contributors to disease as well as impediments to the best treatment of various maladies, including dermatological, infectious, autoimmune, and neoplastic disorders. With the development of novel pharmacologic agents and the evolution of personalized treatments based on pharmacogenetic profiling, clinicians must decide which agent is the best for a particular patient with a given disease. Biological agents have greatly improved the treatment of chronic inflammatory diseases and malignancies while limiting some medication-associated toxicities. Because of better outcomes, longer patient survival, and extended treatment courses, patients are exposed to drugs more frequently and for longer time periods, increasing the risk of sensitization to medications. The frequency of adverse drug reactions has increased in the last 10 years. Because of the severity of some reactions and the fear of inducing a potentially lethal reaction in highly sensitized patients, first line treatments are sometimes abandoned, relegating hypersensitive patients to secondary, less effective, therapy. Some of these reactions are mast cell-mediated HSRs, a subset of which occur through an IgE-dependent mechanism, and are thus true allergies. Others involve mast cells, but an IgE mechanism cannot be demonstrated. RDD is a technique that induces temporary tolerance to a drug, allowing a medication-allergic patient to receive the optimal agent for his or her disease. Through RDD, patients with IgE and non-IgE HSRs can safely be administered important medications while minimizing or completely inhibiting adverse reactions.

General Principles and Proposed Mechanisms of Rapid Drug Desensitization

Exposure of IgE-sensitized patients to medication can cause the sudden systemic release of inflammatory mediators from activated mast cells, leading to anaphylaxis

[1, 2], and medication avoidance, while effective for circumventing an HSR, may lead to significant morbidity and mortality due to suboptimal treatment of disease. RDD is a process by which mast cells are rendered hyporesponsive to an agent that, when administered in typical fashion, induces mast cell activation and degranulation. RDD provides temporary tolerization for drug-hypersensitive patients, protecting them from anaphylaxis. Desensitization protocols have been developed to help deliver full therapeutic doses of drug allergens, in an incremental, stepwise fashion without eliciting life-threatening symptoms [3–5]. Most IgE-sensitized patients present with a positive skin test to the medication, indicating that mast cells (likely through drug-specific IgE) are the main cells responsible for these reactions. After rapid desensitization, specific skin test reactivity is abolished, implying a complete inhibition of the mechanisms that induced mast cell activation [6].

Mast cells activated by antigen crosslinking of IgE-bound FcεRI receptors display aggregation of these receptors, recruitment and activation of target molecules, calcium mobilization, degranulation, arachidonic acid metabolism, and cytokine and chemokine gene transcription [7, 8]. RDD then induces mast cell tolerization to antigen via Internalization of FcεRI. This may occur through progressive crosslinking at low antigen concentration, sub-threshold depletion of mediators, and depletion of activating signal transduction components such as Syk kinase, all of which have been postulated as mechanisms for cellular unresponsiveness to specific activating doses of allergen [9, 10].

To test these hypotheses, we and others developed a reproducible in vitro model of antigen specific, rapid mast cell/IgE desensitization in the presence of physiologic levels of calcium (fig. 1). Increasing doses of antigen delivered at fixed time intervals induced a highly specific and prolonged hyporesponsiveness to triggering doses of the desensitizing antigen. Mast cells desensitized to DNP or OVA antigens demonstrated almost complete inhibition of β-hexosaminidase and preformed TNF-α release, calcium flux, and arachidonic acid metabolism, suggesting a complete abolition of the acute phase of mast cell activation and demonstrating that the subclinical release of mediators was unlikely during human desensitizations. Desensitized mast cells did not release significant amounts of newly generated IL-6 or TNF-α, confirming that during rapid desensitization, patients were not at risk for a delayed reaction due to the lack of late-phase mediator generation.

When mast cells were sensitized to both DNP and OVA antigens, DNP-desensitized cells responded fully to OVA and vice versa, proving antigen specificity and providing evidence that the activating signal transduction pathways are intact for a second allergen. Therefore, the hypothesis that activating signaling molecules are exhausted during rapid desensitization is not supported.

Importantly, antigen-specific IgE bound to the α-chain of FcεRI remained at the membrane level after rapid desensitization, indicating that the lack of reactivity during desensitization was not due to the disappearance of surface IgE and FcεRI when bound to small doses of antigen (fig. 2). Thus, the biochemical mechanism(s) by

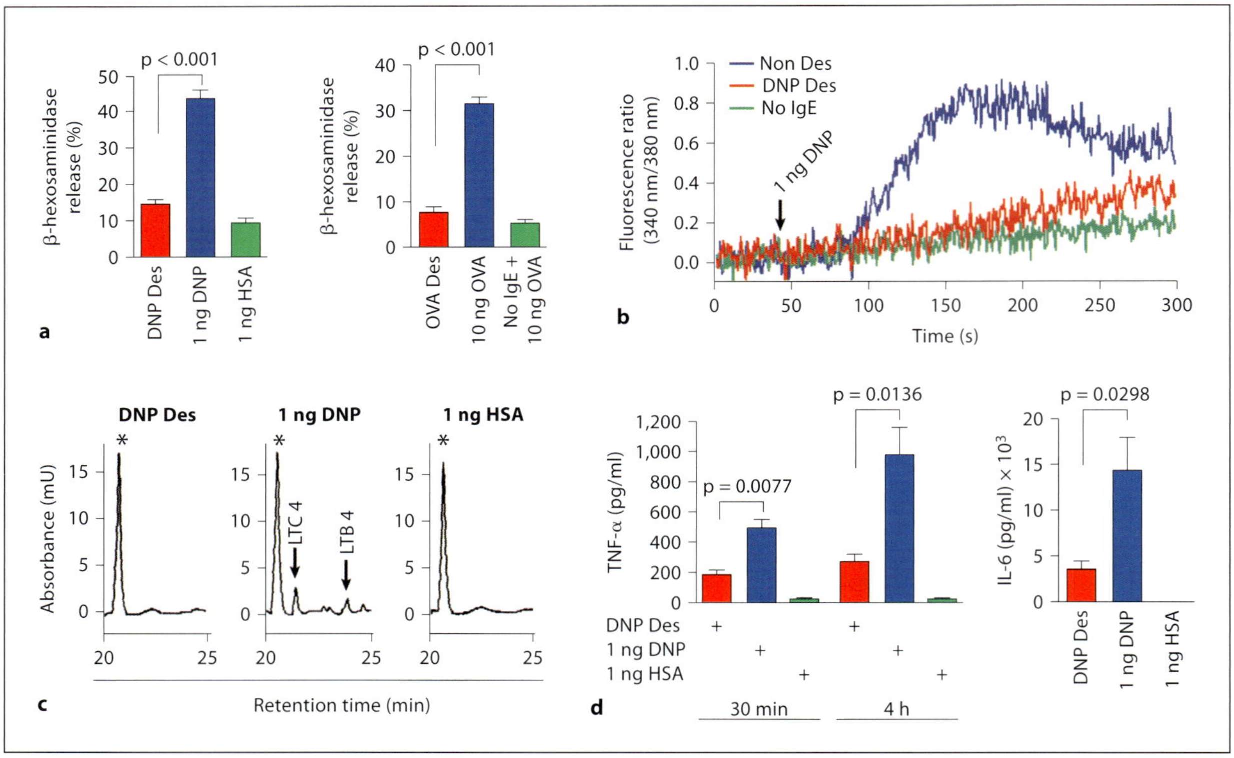

Fig. 1. Rapid desensitization impairs early- and late-phase mast cell activation responses. **a** Percent β-hexosaminidase release after desensitization (DNP Des or OVA Des) or DNP-HSA or OVA challenge (1 ng DNP or 10 ng OVA) and negative control HSA. **b** Calcium flux when 1 ng DNP-HSA is added to cells treated as indicated. **c** RP-HPLC analysis of arachidonic acid products (LTC4 and LTB4) in supernatants of cells treated as indicated. Asterisk signifies internal standard. **d** TNF-α and IL-6 secretion from mast cells during the early (30 min) and late (4 h) phases of antigen activation and during rapid desensitization. Adapted from Sancho-Serra et al. [62].

which RDD induces mast cell tolerance are still unclear. However, this in vitro model provided an optimal dose-time relationship, leading to almost complete abrogation of early- and late-phase activation events, providing a basis for a modified human rapid desensitization protocol that has been used successfully in hundreds of desensitizations, illustrating the profound inhibition of acute and delayed mast cell responses and the protection against anaphylactic reactions [4, 5].

Clinical Rapid Desensitization: Protocols and Agents

The BWH Desensitization Program devised a 12- to 20-step standard protocol based on the above in vitro mouse mast cell model, in which unresponsiveness to a triggering antigen dose was achieved by delivering doubling doses of antigen at fixed time

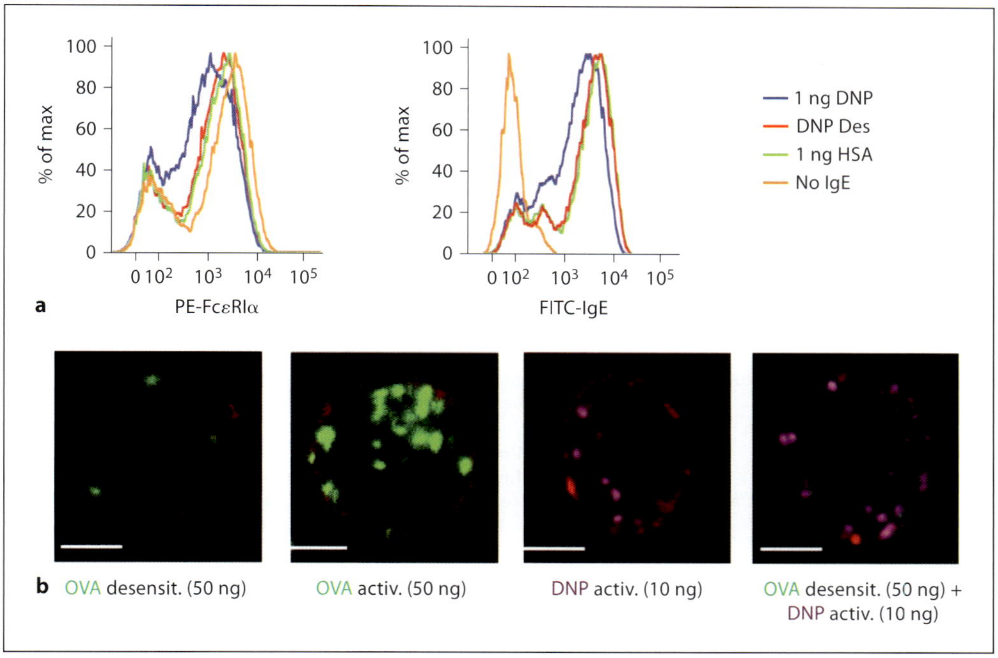

Fig. 2. Mast cell antigen/IgE/FcεRI complex internalization is inhibited during rapid desensitization but does not impair specific activation. **a** Cells were treated as indicated and the FcεRIα and IgE surface expression were analyzed by flow cytometry. The blue line shows the internalization of the antigen/IgE/FcεRI during activation as opposed to the red line in which no internalization occurs during desensitizations. **b** Confocal microscopy of cells treated as indicated. Cells activated with OVA (second panel) presented intracellular green fluorescence indicative of antigen internalization while desensitized cells (first panel) presented little internalization. Cells desensitized to OVA responded to DNP (fourth panel), indicating that the desensitization process is highly specific. Adapted from Sancho-Serra et al. [62].

intervals starting at 1/1,000 dilution of the final dose [11]. The most commonly used protocol has 12 steps, using three ten-fold diluted solutions at escalating rates (fig. 3). Patients who have had severe anaphylactic reactions to the given agent, or who have reacted early in the standard 12-step desensitization may experience fewer symptoms if desensitized using a 16-step protocol, which adds another bag containing a 1/10,000 dilution of the full dose. The use of a 16-step (4 bags) or 20-step (5 bags) protocol is reserved for high-risk patients (see below). Drug desensitization is more than a protocol; it is an approach to specialized patient care. It thus starts with an allergy evaluation of the patient, including an in-depth historical analysis of the patient's HSR, skin testing when available, design and testing of an initial desensitization protocol, and adjustment of this protocol in an iterative fashion based on the patient's response.

Below, we summarize our experience with rapid desensitization to four different classes of drugs: antibiotics, taxane chemotherapy agents, platinum-based chemotherapeutic agents, and monoclonal antibodies and other miscellaneous medications.

Name of medication:		**Infliximab**	
Target dose (mg)			800.0
Standard volume per bag (ml)			250
Final rate of infusion (ml/h)			80
Calculated final concentration (mg/ml)			3.2
Standard time of infusion (min)			187.5

					Total mg per bag
Solution 1	250	ml of	0.032	mg/ml	8.000
Solution 2	250	ml of	0.320	mg/ml	80.000
Solution 3	250	ml of	3.175	mg/ml	793.704

*** PLEASE NOTE *** The total volume and dose dispensed are more than the final dose given to patient because many of the solutions are *not completely infused*

Step	Solution	Rate (ml/h)	Time (min)	Volume infused per step (ml)	Dose administered with this step (mg)	Cumulative dose (mg)
1	1	2.0	15	0.50	0.0160	0.0160
2	1	5.0	15	1.25	0.0400	0.0560
3	1	10.0	15	2.50	0.0800	0.1360
4	1	20.0	15	5.00	0.1600	0.2960
5	2	5.0	15	1.25	0.4000	0.6960
6	2	10.0	15	2.50	0.8000	1.4960
7	2	20.0	15	5.00	1.6000	3.0960
8	2	40.0	15	10.00	3.2000	6.2960
9	3	10.0	15	2.50	7.9370	14.2330
10	3	20.0	15	5.00	15.8741	30.1071
11	3	40.0	15	10.00	31.7482	61.8553
12	3	80.0	174.375	232.50	738.1447	800.0000
		Total time (min) =	339.375	= 5.66 h		

Fig. 3. The standard 12-step, 3-bag desensitization protocol from the Brigham and Women's Hospital Rapid Drug Desensitization Program. Adapted from Castells et al. [5].

Rapid Drug Desensitization to Antibiotics

Despite a wide selection of antibiotics available for treatment of inpatient and outpatient infections, a single antibiotic often emerges as the preferred choice in a given situation. If the chosen antibiotic is one to which the patient has a history of HSR, but drug resistance, prohibitive intolerances, limited bactericidal or bacteriostatic activity, and poor bioavailability of alternatives pose a risk of uncontrolled infection, desensitization is the best course. Unlike chemotherapy and monoclonal antibodies, antibiotics are usually administered in doses scheduled 6–24 h apart for several days to weeks. This discussion focuses on intravenous rapid desensitization to antibiotics for immediate-type HSRs, and does not include slow oral desensitization regimens that have been described for delayed-type hypersensitivities to multiple antimicrobials, including trimethoprim/sulfamethoxazole, metronidazole, isoniazid, and antiretrovirals.

Experience with antibiotic desensitization, primarily with penicillins and cephalosporins, has accumulated over several decades following a case series describing penicillin desensitization in penicillin-sensitive pregnant women with syphilis [12]. Only immediate-type HSRs consistent with an IgE- and/or mast cell-mediated mechanism are considered amenable to desensitization. Such reactions include dermatologic (flushing, pruritus, urticaria, angioedema), upper and lower respiratory tract (sneezing, sinus and nasal congestion, cough, dyspnea, wheezing), gastrointestinal (abdominal pain, nausea, vomiting, diarrhea), and cardiovascular manifestations (hypotension) during anaphylaxis. Patients with other reactions, including maculopapular rashes, fixed drug eruptions, Stevens-Johnson syndrome, toxic epidermal necrolysis, bullous erythema, drug reaction with eosinophilia and systemic symptoms, transaminitis, acute interstitial nephritis, serum sickness, hemolytic anemia, thrombocytopenia, or neutropenia, are not candidates for rapid intravenous desensitization.

Once an evaluation of the patient determines that the initial reaction is consistent with a mast cell-/IgE-mediated HSR, determining the severity of and the time since the initial reaction makes an assessment of the patient's risk. Penicillin skin testing [reviewed in 13–17] helps in risk-stratifying patients with a history of reaction to penicillin. Such testing has high sensitivity and specificity in estimating the likelihood of reacting to penicillin derivatives and moderate utility in assessing the risk for reacting to cephalosporins, especially first-generation cephalosporins [18, 19]. Following earlier data suggesting high rates of cross-sensitization to carbapenems in penicillin skin test positive patients as measured by imipenem skin testing without challenge [20], systematic imipenem challenge in penicillin skin test positive patients has demonstrated very low true cross-reactivity between these classes [21]. While other studies have described the use of skin testing with non-penicillin antibiotics with increasing data for nonirritating concentrations, none of these testing protocols has been standardized or validated.

The literature on rapid desensitization to antibiotics largely consists of case reports, but several case series in the last decade in cystic fibrosis patients [22–24], a population disproportionately affected by recurrent infections (particularly by *Pseudomonas aeruginosa*), antibiotic allergies, resistant organisms, and therefore in need of antibiotic desensitization, have established the safety and efficacy of desensitization to various antibiotics. Three studies, including one at our institution, were retrospective chart reviews of patients who underwent desensitization. Success rates ranged from 58 to 100%. Mild to moderate reactions during desensitization did not preclude completion of desensitizations, and could be followed by full scheduled doses. Most patients required multiple desensitizations over time. In our case series, 15 patients completed 100% of 52 desensitizations, 45 without any reaction. Six patients experienced limited symptoms consistent with immediate type HSRs. One patient had acute respiratory failure requiring intubation following ceftazidime desensitization, which was attributed to preexisting infection-related declining respiratory status, and later had uneventful desensitizations to ceftazidime. In another group of patients, nafcillin, penicillin, cefazolin, and ceftriaxone were among the antibiotics to which patients were successfully desensitized using our protocol [3].

Current recommendations for patients with a history of penicillin reactions who may require penicillin or cephalosporin suggest penicillin skin testing with major and minor determinants when available [25]. Patients with negative skin testing should not require desensitization, and those with positive skin tests are recommended to avoid penicillins and cephalosporins, particularly first-generation agents. If these medications are deemed necessary, desensitization to penicillins and cephalosporins is useful.

Vancomycin is often used in infections with β-lactam resistant Gram-positive organisms or in β-lactam allergic patients. Its use continues to rise with the spread of community and hospital-acquired methicillin-resistant *Staphylococcus aureus* as well as in persistent and moderate-to-severe cases of *Clostridium difficile* colitis. Much more common than type I HSRs to vancomycin is red man syndrome (RMS), characterized by flushing, warmth, pruritus, and hypotension. RMS results from direct mast cell and basophil histamine release, can occur without prior exposure, and is not accompanied by an increase in tryptase [26]. While slowing the infusion rate usually ameliorates RMS, true hypersensitivity does not respond to this measure and may require desensitization. Multiple series have been published on successful vancomycin desensitization regimens, both rapid (over hours) and slow (over days) [27–31].

A few reports of ciprofloxacin desensitization exist in the literature [32]. Of the cystic fibrosis patient series described above, our series and that from The Children's Hospital in Boston each include a successful ciprofloxacin desensitization [23, 24]. The Prince Charles Hospital series includes a ciprofloxacin desensitization that was aborted because of an urticarial rash [22].

Hypersensitivity to trimethoprim/sulfamethoxazole most commonly presents as a delayed type cutaneous eruption, and it is a frequent culprit in Stevens-Johnson syndrome. These toxicities are thought to be mediated by reactive metabolites that cannot be fully metabolized by glutathione stores [33]. Slow outpatient oral desensitizations are well-described in patients with HIV/AIDS, who have a disproportionately high prevalence of hypersensitivity to this drug. We have limited experience with patients with the rarer immediate-type HSR, and have successfully performed rapid intravenous desensitizations in such patients [23].

Immediate HSRs to aminoglycosides are also relatively rare. We have described successful intravenous desensitization to tobramycin in a cystic fibrosis patient [23], and the Children's Hospital of Boston series includes a single case of failed gentamicin desensitization [24]. Tobramycin desensitizations via the intravenous and inhaled route have been described previously [34, 35].

Following desensitization, each scheduled full dose of the antibiotic must be administered in a timely fashion in order to prevent loss of the temporary desensitized state.

Rapid Drug Desensitization to Chemotherapeutic Agents: Taxanes

Paclitaxel and docetaxel are widely used in the treatment of ovarian, breast, non-small cell lung, and other solid tumors. HSRs to these taxanes are common: in early trials of paclitaxel, up to 30% of patients developed acute infusion reactions. Premedication with antihistamines and glucocorticoids as well as slower infusion rates have reduced the rate of severe HSRs to less than 10% [36–39]. Similarly, approximately 30% of patients receiving docetaxel without premedication developed acute HSRs, and premedication reduces this rate to less than 10% [40].

Acute HSRs to taxanes are characterized by dyspnea, urticaria, flushing, back or chest severe pain, gastrointestinal symptoms, hypo- or hypertension, and erythematous rashes. Symptoms typically develop within the first few minutes of the infusion, and most often occur on the first or second exposure to the drug [38, 41]. The mechanisms of taxane infusion reactions are not completely understood and may be multifactorial. Proposed mechanisms include complement activation, direct mast cell and/or basophil activation, and IgE-mediated anaphylaxis [42]. Taxane reactions are unlikely to be due solely to an IgE response, because a majority of reactions (56% in one study) occur with the first exposure to paclitaxel, without the prior sensitization necessary for an IgE-mediated reaction [41]. There is evidence that both the taxane moiety itself and the vehicles in which these agents are solubilized can contribute to infusion reactions. Specifically, paclitaxel is stabilized with Cremophor, which is derived from castor oil and is also used as the vehicle for other drugs, such as cyclosporine and vitamin K, which have been associated with similar adverse reactions [41, 43–46]. An albumin-based formulation of paclitaxel, devoid of Cremophor, has also been implicated in HSRs, providing further evidence for taxane moiety-based HSRs.

Desensitization to taxanes is generally well tolerated. In a series of 17 patients who underwent a total of 77 desensitizations to paclitaxel or docetaxel, 72 desensitizations occurred without reactions. Four patients had a total of 5 reactions during desensitization, all of which were much less severe than their original reactions. On the other hand, 5 patients who underwent rechallenge (i.e. readministration of the culprit taxane by regular infusion) prior to desensitization experienced recurrent reactions, despite additional premedication and a reduced infusion rate [47]. In our series of 98 patients undergoing a total of 413 desensitizations to various chemotherapeutic agents, the majority of desensitizations had mild or no reactions, and most reactions occurred during the final, most concentrated solution, and specifically during the last step of the protocol [5].

Rapid Drug Desensitization to Chemotherapeutic Agents: Platins

The platinum-containing compounds are extensively employed in the treatment of ovarian cancer and other malignancies. Cisplatin was the first to be used, but it was the relatively low toxicity profile of the second-generation carboplatin that was largely responsible for its increased popularity in the past decade [48]. The third-generation platinum derivative oxaliplatin is widely administered for the treatment of metastatic colorectal cancer. As the use of platinum-containing compounds has increased, so has the incidence of HSRs: cisplatin hypersensitivity varies from 5 to 20%, carboplatin from 9 to 27%, and oxaliplatin from 10 to 19% [49–51]. Unlike the situation with taxanes, repeated exposures are typically required prior to the onset of hypersensitivity to platins. In one study, 50% of the initial HSRs to a platin occurred during the eighth course [52]. Likewise, we found that 40 out of 55 patients with carboplatin HSRs reacted between the 7th and 10th exposure [5]. Cisplatin and oxaliplatin have similar characteristics in that reactions mostly occur between the 4th and 8th course or after the 6th exposure, respectively [51].

The characteristics of HSRs to platinum agents vary widely. In the case of carboplatin, most patients develop cutaneous symptoms, notably palmar or facial flushing. However, half of patients may progress to moderate to severe reactions, and cardiac arrests and deaths have been reported [5]. In our report of 413 desensitizations, of the 60 patients who had carboplatin HSR, 100% had cutaneous symptoms, 57% had cardiovascular symptoms, 40% had respiratory symptoms, and 42% had gastrointestinal manifestations [5].

Oxaliplatin HSRs are often similar to those seen in response to carboplatin and cisplatin, but there have been fewer reports of severe anaphylaxis. However, in contrast to carboplatin, respiratory symptoms are common, and other reactions such as Gell and Coombs type II-mediated thrombocytopenia and Gell and Coombs type III immune-complex-mediated symptoms of chronic urticaria, joint pain, and proteinuria associated, have been reported in response to oxaliplatin. Idiosyncratic reactions to oxaliplatin, including cytokine release syndrome and pulmonary fibrosis, make adverse responses to oxaliplatin heterogeneous and unpredictable [51, 53, 54].

There is a well-recognized association between the interval of carboplatin-free period and the risk of HSR, especially a severe reaction. Schwartz et al. [55] in a study looking at 126 patients with HSR to carboplatin noted that the risk of severe reactions was 47% if the platinum free interval was >24 months, versus only 6.5% if it was <12 months. All 8 patients receiving their third carboplatin regimen had severe reactions.

Skin testing has been used to predict platinum hypersensitivity, but methods vary widely from institution to institution. Our group skin tested 60 patients referred for previous HSRs to carboplatin. Of these, 53 were skin test positive. Of the 7 patients with negative skin tests, 2 converted to positive skin tests after several infusions, one skin test was considered delayed positive, and 4 patients experienced HSRs during infusion [5]. Hesterberg's group recently published a report of 38 women with carboplatin HSR who were skin tested and desensitized. Thirteen patients were skin test negative to carboplatin, and 7 of those patients had reactions during a rapid desensitization protocol. Interestingly, they found that when dividing the negative skin test group using the time from the HSR to skin testing, those with recent history of HSR

(<3 months) and negative skin tests did not react, whereas all 7 of the reactors had remote history of HSR (>9 months). Of note, this group uses a maximum carboplatin skin test dose of 3 mg/ml, while our group uses 10 mg/ml.

Patients hypersensitive to a platinum-containing compound or with a positive skin test may be treated by an attempt to readminister the same agent, or the decision may be to change to a different platinum drug, or to be desensitized. The first two choices have produced mixed results, and deaths have been reported. Polyzos et al. [56] reported a series of 32 patients rechallenged with carboplatin after HSRs. Four of the 20 patients with mild reactions again had erythema but were able to finish the medication infusions. However, 12 patients with initial severe reactions including hyper- or hypotension were unable to complete subsequent carboplatin infusions despite prophylaxis. Interestingly in this report, 4 of the 12 were switched to cisplatin and tolerated infusions, but the true incidence of cross-reactivity among platinum-based chemotherapeutic agents is not known. Attempts to circumvent a reaction by switching to another platinum-based chemotherapeutic can be dangerous [56], as exemplified by Dizon et al. [57] who reported the death of one patient due to anaphylaxis in a series of 7 patients switched from carboplatin to cisplatin.

Desensitization has proven to be a safe and effective way to allow a patient to continue carboplatin chemotherapy (see below). Variability in the success rates of desensitization is believed to be due to heterogeneity of methods and protocols.

Rapid Drug Desensitization to Monoclonal Antibodies

Monoclonal antibodies are generally well tolerated treatments for a broad array of diseases, including malignancies and chronic inflammatory conditions. However, a subset of patients experience HSRs following administration of these drugs [58]. Symptoms of such HSRs range from mild (fever, rash, pruritus) to severe, including severe life-threatening anaphylaxis [58].

The rates of HSRs clinically consistent with immediate hypersensitivity to specific monoclonal antibodies have been reported to be 5–10% for rituximab, 2–3% for infliximab, and 0.6–5% for trastuzumab [59]. Immediate HSRs have also been reported for omalizumab, natalizumab, basiliximab, abciximab, and cetuximab. Almost 70% of initial HSRs to monoclonal antibodies include a cutaneous component, the most frequently observed type of reaction overall, followed by cardiovascular, respiratory, and throat tightness [58]. The intensity of reactions to monoclonal antibody infusions is variable. Recent studies have reported that 26% of initial reactions are mild, 48% are moderate, and 26% are severe [59].

Patients with a history suggestive of a mast cell, possibly IgE-mediated HSR should be skin tested with the offending agent as previously described by Lee et al. [6]. HSRs are then classified as mild, moderate, or severe according to the classification system proposed by Brown [60]. Signs and symptoms of HSRs are classified as cutaneous

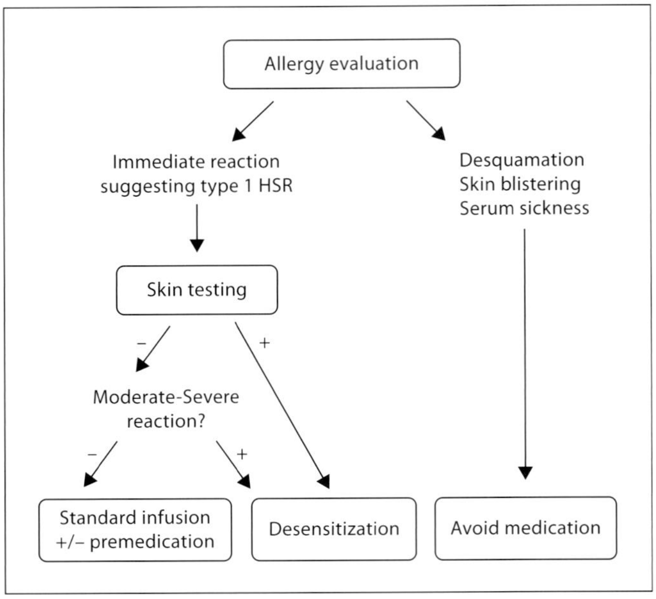

Fig. 4. Algorithm for assessment and treatment of patients with HSRs to medications. Adapted from Brennan et al. [59].

(flushing, pruritus, urticaria, angioedema), cardiovascular (chest pain, tachycardia, sense of impending doom, presyncope, syncope, and hypotension), respiratory (dyspnea, wheezing, and oxygen desaturation), throat tightness, gastrointestinal (nausea, vomiting, diarrhea, and abdominal pain), neurological/muscular (vision disturbances, back and neck pain, and numbness/weakness), and fever/chills [60].

Protocols for most monoclonal antibodies are generated using the same principles as previously discussed above. Despite its general success, some patients experience HSRs during RDD. In general, these reactions are less intense than the patient's original reaction. Treatment of such HSRs is aimed at blocking mast cell mediators including histamine, prostaglandins, and leukotrienes [59]. In the event of a reaction during RDD, the infusion is promptly held and the reaction treated. Once the reaction resolves, the protocol can almost always be resumed and completed. The algorithm in figure 4 describes the current approach to monoclonal antibodies hypersensitivity reactions since skin testing positive and negative predictive values are not available for all antibodies. Severe reactions will require desensitization despite negative skin testing.

Overall Safety and Efficacy

In 2008, our group reported the largest case series of rapid desensitizations, in which 98 patients with HSRs to chemotherapy underwent 413 desensitizations [5]. In this series, 67% of desensitizations proceeded without HSR, and 27% had only mild reactions (classified as absence of chest pain, changes in blood pressure, dyspnea, oxygen desaturation or throat tightness), even though 77% of patients had experienced a severe initial HSR. The remaining 6% of desensitizations were characterized by severe HSRs; however, epinephrine was only administered during one desensitization, and there were no transfers to a more acute-care setting, intubations, or deaths. All patients in the case series were able to receive their full target dose.

We subsequently published a case series of 105 desensitizations to monoclonal antibodies in 23 patients [59]. Seventy-four percent of the initial HSRs were moderate to severe. During desensitization, reactions were observed in 29% of desensitizations and 90% of these were mild. Antibiotic desensitization using our protocol is also exceedingly safe [23]: in our case series of 52 antibiotic desensitizations in 15 patients with cystic fibrosis (and a mean FEV1 of 44.1% of predicted), 96.2% of desensitizations were completed without severe adverse events. One patient developed severe acute respiratory failure requiring intubation; however, this was felt to be secondary to worsening pulmonary infection and not a manifestation of a severe HSR during his desensitizations. All desensitizations in this series were completed, suggesting that even markedly impaired baseline lung function is not a contraindication to rapid desensitization.

Treatment of Reactions during Desensitization

In our experience, reactions during desensitization manifest as a wide range of symptoms characteristic of HSRs [59]. Cutaneous reactions may include flushing, pruritus, urticaria and angioedema. More severe reactions may encompass cardiovascular manifestations, such as chest pain, tachycardia, a sense of impending doom, presyncope, syncope and hypotension, as well as respiratory symptoms, including sneezing, nasal congestion, dyspnea, coughing, wheezing, and oxygen desaturation. Severe reactions may also be characterized by throat tightness or gastrointestinal complaints, including nausea, vomiting, diarrhea and abdominal pain. Less common signs and symptoms may include neuromuscular symptoms, such as visual changes, back and neck pain, and numbness/weakness, or, in some cases, fever and chills.

In our 2008 case series of 413 desensitizations in 98 patients, there were a total of 180 reactions, all of which subsided when the infusion was paused and treated appropriately [5]. The majority of reactions (75%) occurred during infusion of solution 3, and 51% of reactions occurred during step 12 of the desensitization protocol. In our monoclonal antibody case series, in which a similar rate of reactions was reported (29%), cutaneous reactions were the most common and, again, the majority of reactions (70%) occurred during step 12. Our approach to treating reactions during desensitization is aimed at blocking local and systemic effects of mast cell mediators, including histamine, prostaglandins, and leukotrienes [59].

At our institution, all reactions during desensitization are treated by pausing the infusion and administering either diphenhydramine or hydroxyzine (25–50 mg administered intravenously) and/or ranitidine (50 mg intravenously). For severe reactions, we most commonly use methylprednisolone sodium succinate (0.5 mg/kg administered intravenously). We keep epinephrine, 0.3 ml (1 mg/ml) at the bedside. On resolution of the reaction, we restart the protocol from the step at which it had been paused. Patients who experience reactions are then presented and discussed at a weekly meeting of the physicians in our department who perform rapid desensitizations.

We have adopted a two-pronged approach to protocol modification for subsequent desensitizations for patients who react during a prior desensitization [59]. The first component includes administration of additional premedications prior to the start of the protocol or between specific steps during desensitization. Most commonly, these are H1 and sometimes H2 blockers and/or methylprednisolone. These are generally added at least one full step before the point at which the reaction occurred. The second component of our protocol modification involves adding or lengthening steps before the step at which a reaction occurred. This second component is used only when a patient reacts despite additional premedications. By using this approach, we have been able to markedly reduce the rate of reactions over multiple successive desensitizations [5, 59].

Unfortunately, there remains a subset of patients who continue to react during desensitization despite protocol modification and addition of high-dose histamine receptor blockade and corticosteroids. In another case series, we prophylactically treated these patients with oral acetylsalicylic acid (ASA), 325 mg and oral montelukast 10 mg, and were able to successfully treat those patients with refractory mast cell mediator-related symptoms during rapid desensitization [61]. In this study, 78 desensitizations were performed in 14 patients with HSR to platinum chemotherapy that had cutaneous symptoms, many also with associated systemic reactions, during rapid desensitization. Pretreatment with ASA and montelukast 2 days before and on the day of RDD allowed 86% of the patients to tolerate subsequent desensitizations with a less severe or no HSR (fig. 5). Interestingly, only 62% of patients in a control group that received adjunctive methylprednisolone premedication were able to tolerate further desensitizations with a less severe or with no reaction. The greatest benefit of ASA/montelukast pretreatment was seen in patients with skin and respiratory symptoms, suggesting a dominant role for prostaglandins and leukotrienes in these manifestations of HSR to platinum chemotherapies. We have subsequently also treated patients with only one dose of ASA/montelukast 60 min prior to RDD, and have expanded this treatment for use during monoclonal antibody and antibiotic desensitization, and have successfully blocked refractory skin and systemic reactions using this regimen [23, 59].

Conclusions

At our institution, we have had success using an intravenous RDD protocol to treat HSRs to a wide range of medications, including chemotherapeutics, monoclonal antibodies, and antibiotics. Over the past 10 years, more than 99.9% of nearly 800 patients have received the full dose of their first-line medication in thousands of

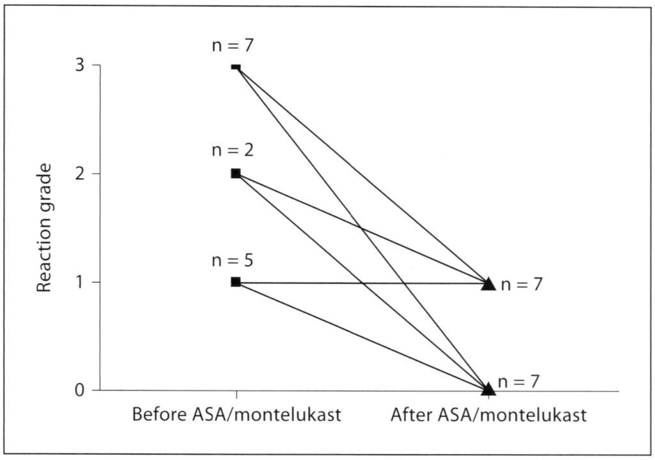

Fig. 5. Evolution of severity of reactions during desensitization before and after ASA/montelukast pretreatment. Under the ASA and montelukast protocol, 86% of patients were able to tolerate further desensitizations, with a less severe HSR or no reaction (grade 2.14 vs. grade 0.5, $p < 0.001$). Adapted from Breslow et al. [61].

desensitizations to a wide variety of agents in each of these three classes, and there have been no deaths. Although the molecular basis of RDD remains incompletely understood, an in vitro mast cell model has provided evidence of profound inhibitory mechanisms of mast cell activation during desensitization, which correlates with the remarkable success of the desensitization protocols when used by trained allergists. These safety and efficacy outcomes provide grounds for the continued and expanded use of this RDD approach for all patients for whom a drug hypersensitivity would prevent the administration of first-line pharmacologic therapy.

References

1 Schwartz LB, Metcalfe DD, Miller JS, et al: Tryptase levels as an indicator of mast-cell activation in systemic anaphylaxis and mastocytosis. N Engl J Med 1987;316:1622–1626.

2 Vadas P, Gold M, Perelman B, et al: Platelet-activating factor, PAF acetylhydrolase, and severe anaphylaxis. N Engl J Med 2008;358:28–35.

3 Castells M: Desensitization for drug allergy. Curr Opin Allergy Clin Immunol 2006;6:476–481.

4 Lee CW, Matulonis UA, Castells MC: Rapid inpatient/outpatient desensitization for chemotherapy hypersensitivity: standard protocol effective in 57 patients for 255 courses. Gynecol Oncol 2005;99: 393–399.

5 Castells MC, Tennant NM, Sloane DE, et al: Hypersensitivity reactions to chemotherapy: outcomes and safety of rapid desensitization in 413 cases. J Allergy Clin Immunol 2008;122:574–580.

6 Lee CW, Matulonis UA, Castells MC: Carboplatin hypersensitivity: a 6-h 12-step protocol effective in 35 desensitizations in patients with gynecological malignancies and mast cell/IgE-mediated reactions. Gynecol Oncol 2004;95:370–376.

7 Kraft S, Kinet JP: New developments in FcepsilonRI regulation, function and inhibition. Nat Rev Immunol 2007;7:365–378.

8 Gilfillan AM, Rivera J: The tyrosine kinase network regulating mast cell activation. Immunol Rev 2009; 228:149–169.

9 Shalit M, Levi-Schaffer F: Challenge of mast cells with increasing amounts of antigen induces desensitization. Clin Exp Allergy 1995;25:896–902.

10 Kepley CL: Antigen-induced reduction in mast cell and basophil functional responses due to reduced Syk protein levels. Int Arch Allergy Immunol 2005; 138:29–39.

11 Morales AR, Shah N, Castells M: Antigen-IgE desensitization in signal transducer and activator of transcription 6-deficient mast cells by suboptimal doses of antigen. Ann Allergy Asthma Immunol 2005;94:575–580.
12 Wendel GD Jr, Stark BJ, Jamison RB, Molina RD, Sullivan TJ: Penicillin allergy and desensitization in serious infections during pregnancy. N Engl J Med 1985;312:1229–1232.
13 Gadde J, Spence M, Wheeler B, Adkinson NF Jr: Clinical experience with penicillin skin testing in a large inner-city STD clinic. JAMA 1993;270:2456–2463.
14 Green GR, Rosenblum AH, Sweet LC: Evaluation of penicillin hypersensitivity: value of clinical history and skin testing with penicilloyl-polylysine and penicillin G. A cooperative prospective study of the penicillin study group of the American Academy of Allergy. J Allergy Clin Immunol 1977;60:339–345.
15 Park MA, Li JT: Diagnosis and management of penicillin allergy. Mayo Clin Proc 2005;80:405–410.
16 Salkind AR, Cuddy PG, Foxworth JW: The rational clinical examination. Is this patient allergic to penicillin? An evidence-based analysis of the likelihood of penicillin allergy. JAMA 2001;285:2498–2505.
17 Sogn DD, Evans R 3rd, Shepherd GM, et al: Results of the National Institute of Allergy and Infectious Diseases Collaborative Clinical Trial to test the predictive value of skin testing with major and minor penicillin derivatives in hospitalized adults. Arch Intern Med 1992;152:1025–1032.
18 Park MA, Koch CA, Klemawesch P, Joshi A, Li JT: Increased adverse drug reactions to cephalosporins in penicillin allergy patients with positive penicillin skin test. Int Arch Allergy Immunol 2010;153: 268–273.
19 Kelkar PS, Li JT: Cephalosporin allergy. N Engl J Med 2001;345:804–809.
20 Saxon A, Adelman DC, Patel A, Hajdu R, Calandra GB: Imipenem cross-reactivity with penicillin in humans. J Allergy Clin Immunol 1988;82:213–217.
21 Romano A, Viola M, Guéant-Rodriguez RM: Imipenem in patients with immediate hypersensitivity to penicillins. N Engl J Med 2006;354: 2835–2837.
22 Burrows JA, Toon M, Bell SC: Antibiotic desensitization in adults with cystic fibrosis. Respirology 2003;8:359–364.
23 Legere HJ 3rd, Palis RI, Rodriguez Bouza T, et al: A safe protocol for rapid desensitization in patients with cystic fibrosis and antibiotic hypersensitivity. J Cyst Fibros 2009;8:418–424.
24 Turvey SE, Cronin B, Arnold AD, Dioun AF: Antibiotic desensitization for the allergic patient: 5 years of experience and practice. Ann Allergy Asthma Immunol 2004;92:426–432.
25 Fruman DA, Wood MA, Gjertson CK, et al: FK506 binding protein 12 mediates sensitivity to both FK506 and rapamycin in murine mast cells. Eur J Immunol 1900;25:563–571.
26 Renz CL, Laroche D, Thurn JD, et al: Tryptase levels are not increased during vancomycin-induced anaphylactoid reactions. Anesthesiology 1998;89: 620–625.
27 Anne S, Middleton E Jr, Reisman RE: Vancomycin anaphylaxis and successful desensitization. Ann Allergy 1994;73:402–404.
28 Kitazawa T, et al: Successful vancomycin desensitization with a combination of rapid and slow infusion methods. Intern Med 2006;45:317–321.
29 Lin RY: Desensitization in the management of vancomycin hypersensitivity. Arch Intern Med 1990; 150:2197–2198.
30 Wazny LD, Daghigh B: Desensitization protocols for vancomycin hypersensitivity. Ann Pharmacother 2001;35:1458–1464.
31 Wong JT, Ripple RE, MacLean JA, et al: Vancomycin hypersensitivity: synergism with narcotics and 'desensitization' by a rapid continuous intravenous protocol. J Allergy Clin Immunol 1994;94:189–194.
32 Gea-Banacloche JC, Metcalfe DD: Ciprofloxacin desensitization. J Allergy Clin Immunol 1996;97: 1426–1427.
33 Shear NH, Spielberg SP, Grant DM, Tang BK, Kalow W: Differences in metabolism of sulfonamides predisposing to idiosyncratic toxicity. Ann Intern Med 1986;105:179–184.
34 Earl HS, Sullivan TJ: Acute desensitization of a patient with cystic fibrosis allergic to both beta-lactam and aminoglycoside antibiotics. J Allergy Clin Immunol 1987;79:477–483.
35 Spigarelli MG, Hurwitz ME, Nasr SZ: Hypersensitivity to inhaled TOBI following reaction to gentamicin. Pediatr Pulmonol 2002;33:311–314.
36 Eisenhauer EA, ten Bokkel Huinink WW, Swenerton KD, et al: European-Canadian randomized trial of paclitaxel in relapsed ovarian cancer: high-dose versus low-dose and long versus short infusion. J Clin Oncol 1994;12:2654–2666.
37 Kwon JS, Elit L, Finn M, et al: A comparison of two prophylactic regimens for hypersensitivity reactions to paclitaxel. Gynecol Oncol 2002;84:420–425.
38 Markman M, Kennedy A, Webster K, et al: Paclitaxel-associated hypersensitivity reactions: experience of the gynecologic oncology program of the Cleveland Clinic Cancer Center. J Clin Oncol 2000;18:102–105.
39 Wiernik PH, Schwartz EL, Strauman JJ, et al: Phase I clinical and pharmacokinetic study of taxol. Cancer Res 1987;47:2486–2493.

40 Schrijvers D, Wanders J, Dirix L, et al: Coping with toxicities of docetaxel (Taxotere). Ann Oncol 1993; 4:610–611.

41 Weiss RB, Donehower RC, Wiernik PH, et al: Hypersensitivity reactions from taxol. J Clin Oncol 1990;8:1263–1268.

42 Price KS, Castells MC: Taxol reactions. Allergy Asthma Proc 2002;23:205–208.

43 Decorti G, Bartoli Klugmann F, Candussio L, Baldini L: Effect of paclitaxel and Cremophor EL on mast cell histamine secretion and their interaction with adriamycin. Anticancer Res 1996;16:317–320.

44 Eschalier A, Lavarenne J, Burtin C, et al: Study of histamine release induced by acute administration of antitumor agents in dogs. Cancer Chemother Pharmacol 1988;21:246–250.

45 Essayan DM, Kagey-Sobotka A, Colarusso PJ, et al: Successful parenteral desensitization to paclitaxel. J Allergy Clin Immunol 1996;97:42–46.

46 Szebeni J, Muggia FM, Alving CR: Complement activation by Cremophor EL as a possible contributor to hypersensitivity to paclitaxel: an in vitro study. J Natl Cancer Inst 1998;90:300–306.

47 Feldweg AM, Lee CW, Matulonis UA, Castells M: Rapid desensitization for hypersensitivity reactions to paclitaxel and docetaxel: a new standard protocol used in 77 successful treatments. Gynecol Oncol 2005;96:824–829.

48 Aabo K, Adnitt P, Alberts DS, Athanazziou A, et al: Chemotherapy in advanced ovarian cancer: four systematic meta-analyses of individual patient data from 37 randomized trials. Advanced Ovarian Cancer Trialists' Group. Br J Cancer 1998;78: 1479–1487.

49 Gomez R, Harter P, Lück HJ, et al: Carboplatin hypersensitivity: does introduction of skin test and desensitization reliably predict and avoid the problem? A prospective single-center study. Int J Gynecol Cancer 2009;19:1284–1287.

50 Gadducci A, Tana R, Teti G, et al: Analysis of the pattern of hypersensitivity reactions in patients receiving carboplatin retreatment for recurrent ovarian cancer. Int J Gynecol Cancer 2008;18: 615–620.

51 Makrilia N, Syrigou E, Kaklamanos I, et al: Hypersensitivity reactions associated with platinum antineoplastic agents: a systematic review. Met Based Drugs 2010;ii:207084.

52 Markman M, Kennedy A, Webster K, et al: Clinical features of hypersensitivity reactions to carboplatin. J Clin Oncol 1999;17:1141.

53 Maindrault-Goebel F, André T, Tournigand C, et al: Allergic-type reactions to oxaliplatin: retrospective analysis of 42 patients. Eur J Cancer 2005;41: 2262–2267.

54 Lee C, Gianos M, Klaustermeyer WB: Diagnosis and management of hypersensitivity reactions related to common cancer chemotherapy agents. Ann Allergy Asthma Immunol 2009;102:179–187, quiz 187–189, 222.

55 Schwartz JR, Bandera C, Bradley A, et al: Does the platinum-free interval predict the incidence or severity of hypersensitivity reactions to carboplatin? The experience from Women and Infants' Hospital. Gynecol Oncol 2007;105:81–83.

56 Polyzos A, Tsavaris N, Kosmas C, et al: Hypersensitivity reactions to carboplatin administration are common but not always severe: a 10-year experience. Oncology 2001;61:129–133.

57 Dizon DS, Sabbatini PJ, Aghajanian C, et al: Analysis of Patients with epithelial ovarian cancer or fallopian tube carcinoma retreated with cisplatin after the development of a carboplatin allergy. Gynecol Oncol 2002;84:378–382.

58 Chung CH, O'Neil BH: Infusion reactions to monoclonal antibodies for solid tumors: immunologic mechanisms and risk factors. Oncology (Williston Park) 2009;23:14–17.

59 Brennan PJ, Rodriguez Bouza T, et al: Hypersensitivity reactions to mAbs: 105 desensitizations in 23 patients, from evaluation to treatment. J Allergy Clin Immunol 2009;124:1259–1266.

60 Brown SG: Clinical features and severity grading of anaphylaxis. J Allergy Clin Immunol 2004;114: 371–376.

61 Breslow RG, Caiado J, Castells MC: Acetylsalicylic acid and montelukast block mast cell mediator-related symptoms during rapid desensitization. Ann Allergy Asthma Immunol 2009;102:155–160.

62 Sancho-Serra M, Simarro M, Castells M: Rapid IgE desensitization is antigen specific and impairs early and late mast cell responses targeting FcεRI internalization. Eur J Immunol 2011;41:1004–1013.

Dr. Mariana Castells
Harvard Medical School, Division of Rheumatology, Allergy and Immunology
Department of Medicine, Brigham and Women's Hospital
1 Jimmy Fund Way, Smith Building, Room 626D
Boston, MA 02115 (USA)
Tel. +1 617 278 0300, E-Mail mcastells@partners.org

Author Index

Subject Index